Apheresis in Neurological Disorders

Apheresis in Neurological Disorders

Editor

Johannes Dorst

MDPI • Basel • Beijing • Wuhan • Barcelona • Belgrade • Manchester • Tokyo • Cluj • Tianjin

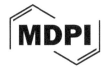

Editor
Johannes Dorst
University of Ulm
Germany

Editorial Office
MDPI
St. Alban-Anlage 66
4052 Basel, Switzerland

This is a reprint of articles from the Special Issue published online in the open access journal *Journal of Clinical Medicine* (ISSN 2077-0383) (available at: https://www.mdpi.com/journal/jcm/special_issues/Apheresis_Neurological_Disorders).

For citation purposes, cite each article independently as indicated on the article page online and as indicated below:

LastName, A.A.; LastName, B.B.; LastName, C.C. Article Title. *Journal Name* **Year**, *Article Number*, Page Range.

ISBN 978-3-03943-585-2 (Hbk)
ISBN 978-3-03943-586-9 (PDF)

Contents

About the Editor

Johannes Dorst studied medicine in Marburg, Germany. He is currently working as a Senior Neurologist at Ulm University, Germany, focusing on neurodegenerative and neuroinflammatory diseases. Since 2013, he has been the head of the Neurological Center of Apheresis and Therapies in Ulm. He has vast experience in the treatment of autoimmune disorders with apheresis, in particular immunoadsorption. Over the years, he has published numerous studies investigating the efficacy of immunoadsorption in various neurological indications, most notably a randomized controlled study comparing immunoadsorption and plasma exchange in steroid-refractory multiple sclerosis.

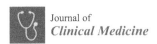

Journal of
Clinical Medicine

Editorial

Apheresis in Neurological Disorders

Johannes Dorst

Department of Neurology, University of Ulm, Oberer Eselsberg 45, 89081 Ulm, Germany;
johannes.dorst@uni-ulm.de; Tel.: +49-731-177-5285

Received: 30 September 2020; Accepted: 2 October 2020; Published: 6 October 2020

1. Introduction

Plasma exchange (PE) and immunoadsorption (IA) constitute important options in the treatment of various autoimmune disorders across different medical disciplines. Their pathophysiological rationale is mainly based on the removal of auto-antibodies and a beneficial modulation of the immune system. From a theoretical point of view, apheresis offers an attractive therapeutical option since its effect relies on eliminating pathogenic components rather than administering drugs which may cause significant side effects. Neurological indications include, amongst others, steroid-refractory relapse of multiple sclerosis (MS), myasthenia gravis, autoimmune encephalitis (AE), Guillain–Barré syndrome (GBS), and chronic inflammatory demyelinating polyneuropathy (CIDP). Although frequently applied in clinical practice, evidence regarding efficacy and safety for the use of PE and IA in the aforementioned indications is generally low, which is directly related to the fact that drugs and medical devices are handled differently with regard to regulatory approvals in most countries, i.e., adequate, indication-specific phase III studies are generally not required in order to introduce medical devices into clinical practice. Therefore, little is known about the efficacy of PE and IA compared to each other and compared to other treatment options. Likewise, knowledge about optimal treatment regimens for conduction of PE and IA is completely lacking.

Therefore, this Special Issue of the Journal of Clinical Medicine focuses on articles which either present novel original data improving the evidence for efficacy and safety of PE and IA in specific neurological indications or review the existing literature in order to understand their significance in various autoimmune neurological diseases and to provide recommendations for their use in clinical practice. Furthermore, various articles highlight potential future areas of application, even beyond classical autoimmune-mediated diseases.

1.1. Methodological Differences between Plasma Exchange and Immunoadsorption

Although both PE and IA primarily focus on removing auto-antibodies from the blood, it is important to understand that both methods imply further immune-modulating mechanisms, including up- and down regulation of anti- and pro-inflammatory proteins [1] and potentially other alterations not yet explored. While, in PE, the plasma including all proteins is removed and substituted by human albumin or fresh frozen plasma, IA is more selective, mainly removing immunoglobulins while largely sparing other plasma constituents. Therefore, theoretically speaking, IA is supposed to offer a low-risk alternative compared to PE, since the preservation of coagulation factors should imply fewer bleeding complications, and since no volume replacement solution is needed, a lower risk of allergic reactions has to be expected. On the other hand, evidence for efficacy for IA is even lower compared to PE for many indications, which does not necessarily imply inferiority compared to PE, but may be simply explained by the fact that IA is the most recent method, and therefore, fewer clinical trials have been performed. Furthermore, preservation of certain pro-inflammatory proteins might compromise the efficacy of IA compared to PE, which may be a concern especially in autoimmune diseases like MS and CIDP, in which distinct disease-related auto-antibodies have not been characterized in the majority of patients. As long as the immunological mechanisms underlying both the diseases and the treatments are not fully understood, therapeutic decisions solely depend on the outcomes of clinical studies comparing different treatment options.

1.2. The Importance of Specific Treatment Regimens

While at least some studies to date have addressed the question of whether to prefer IA or PE in various indications, the question of which specific treatment regimen offers the best ratio between efficacy and safety has so far been completed neglected. Theoretically speaking, a wide array of treatment regimens is possible for both PE and IA with regard to plasma volumes (PVs) processed per treatment, number and frequency of treatments, time intervals between treatments, and peri-procedural medication such as antibiotics, anticoagulants, immunoglobulins, and volume substitution solutions. Due to missing evidence, generally accepted guidelines are lacking, and treatment regimens are therefore chosen based on local expertise and preference. The importance of considering specific treatment regimens is highlighted by our data presented in this Special Issue [2], which show that the advantages of IA compared to PE regarding safety and tolerability, as previously described [3], completely disappear when reducing the PV exchanged during each session in PE. On the other hand, it has, of course, to be questioned if a low-volume PE is equally effective. These questions can only be addressed by future comparative randomised controlled trials (RCTs).

1.3. Evidence for the Use of Plasma Exchange and Immunoadsorption in Specific Indications

In this Special Issue, several articles address the use of PE and/or IA in specific auto-immune mediated neurological diseases by either systematically analysing the existing literature or presenting original data.

1.3.1. Multiple Sclerosis

PE constitutes an established treatment option in MS, mainly based on the RCT published by Weinshenker et al. in 1999 [4] which found a superiority of PE compared to sham treatment in patients with steroid-refractory relapse. Although this study is well done and represents one of the very few examples of an RCT investigating the efficacy of apheresis, the low number of subjects ($n = 22$) must be kept in mind when interpreting the results. In 2019, we finalized an RCT comparing PE and IA in 60 patients with steroid-refractory relapse [5]. In this study, patients in both groups showed significant improvements of clinical outcome parameters. Although PE patients responded faster, IA patients showed significantly larger improvements after 4 weeks, indicating a potential superiority of IA. In this study, we found no difference with regard to safety. In this Special Issue, Mark Lipphardt and colleagues present a systematic meta-analysis [6] including all observational studies and RCTs to date. They found response rates of 76.6% for PE and 80.6% of IA, indicating an about equal and good efficacy for both methods, while safety was also equal.

Steffen Pfeuffer and colleagues investigated a related, equally important question: should another ultra-high-dose methyl-prednisolone (MP) therapy be interpolated after an initial, unsuccessful high-dose MP treatment, or should apheresis be performed directly? In their retrospective database study in 145 patients [7], they found a surprisingly clear result in favour for the direct apheresis (PE) approach, which seriously questions the recommendations of many national and international guidelines and highlights the importance for a sufficiently powered RCT addressing this issue.

Finally, Leoni Rolfes and colleagues provided a comprehensive review about the topic [8] including special situations like treatment of children and pregnant women.

1.3.2. Immune-Mediated Neuropathies

GBS and CIDP constitute the most important autoimmune-mediated neuropathies. GBS represents the acute form and is generally treated with either PE or intravenous immunoglobulins (IVIg) based on several RCTs and a recent Cochrane review [9] which, in summary, suggest equal efficacy. Evidence regarding the efficacy of IA is rather low and mainly relies on retrospective case reports and series. CIDP is often considered as the chronic form of GBS, although it features strong heterogeneity with regard to clinical symptoms and natural courses, which makes treatment and its evaluation difficult. MP, IVIg, and PE are generally considered as the main treatment options of CIDP, and there is no convincing evidence of which approach should be preferred with regard to efficacy and safety. Additionally, immunosuppressive drugs such as azathioprine and rituximab are sometimes used in therapy-refractory cases. Regarding IA, one small RCT suggested superior short-term effects compared to PE [10], while we have demonstrated recently that repeated IA may offer a promising long-term treatment option in therapy-refractory, chronic progressive cases [11].

Although to date distinct disease-related antibodies are not detected in the majority of patients, the discovery of potential pathogenic auto-antibodies against proteins of the node of Ranvier and paranodal regions [12] have corroborated the importance of auto-antibodies in at least a subgroup of patients with immune-mediated neuropathies and therefore supported the rationale to apply treatments which target these antibodies. Alexander Davies and colleagues [13] investigated whether the existence of such antibodies may predict the response to apheresis in patients with GBS and CIDP. Interestingly, they did not find a clear correlation between the presence of known auto-antibodies and treatment response, suggesting that further, undiscovered antibodies may be present.

1.3.3. Autoimmune Encephalitis

The term autoimmune encephalitis (AE) refers to a group of diseases which are characterized by antibodies against neuronal surfaces and synaptic proteins and feature a large spectrum of clinical pictures, including focal neurological, psychiatric, and cognitive symptoms. As opposed to the aforementioned indications, specific auto-antibodies against proteins like N-methyl-D-aspartate (NMDA), gamma-aminobutyric acid (GABA), leucine-rich, glioma inactivated protein 1 (LGI1), and many others have been described and associated with typical clinical presentations. Since high-level evidence is lacking, no universally accepted treatment standards exist. Besides apheresis, current therapeutic strategies include high-dose MP, IVIg, and long-term immunosuppressive drugs such as cyclophosphamide and rituximab. IA is increasingly recognized as a promising therapeutic approach in AE and is even considered as a first-line option in many centers. In their article [14], Rosa Rössling and Harald Prüss review the most relevant studies regarding the use of therapeutic apheresis in AE. Based on their evaluation, they conclude that apheresis constitutes a promising treatment option in AE which should be applied early after disease onset, while they found no evidence that prior treatment with IVIg or steroids yields any additional advantages. Furthermore, they found a clear benefit for patients with antibodies against surface or synaptic antigens, while the effect on patients with onco-neuronal antibodies is less clear.

1.3.4. Chronic Fatigue Syndrome

Myalgic encephalomyelitis / chronic fatigue syndrome (ME/CFS) is a disease characterized by severe fatigue as well as various cognitive, autonomic, and immunological symptoms. The pathophysiological background seems to be complex and has not been fully understood to date. Various auto-antibodies have been described to be associated with the disease, most notably antibodies against the muscarinic acetylcholine receptors (MAR) and β_2-adrenoreceptors (β_2AR). In their previous pilot study [15], Carmen Scheibenbogen and colleagues reported that 7/10 patients with ME/CSF showed rapid clinical improvement and significant reductions of β_2AR antibodies after IA therapy. In this special issue, they present follow-up data from 5 patients who had previously responded to IA treatment and who underwent a subsequent, adjusted IA protocol 2 years later [16]. They found a positive response in 4/5 patients, confirming their previous results that IA may constitute a viable treatment option in ME/CSF, although further controlled studies with higher numbers of patients are certainly needed.

1.3.5. Potential Future Indications and Outlook

This Special Issue also features two articles which focus on potential future areas of application, including diseases which are not generally considered to feature pronounced autoimmune-mediated mechanisms.

Stefan Kayser and colleagues review potential indications for C-reactive protein (CRP) apheresis [17], aiming at removing CRP from the patients' blood by using specific adsorbers. The pathophysiological background of this approach is based on the finding that CRP—most commonly known as an inflammatory biomarker—in fact plays an important role in immunological processes itself by mediating phagocytosis of damaged cells. Under certain conditions including myocardial infarction and ischemic stroke, these mechanisms may have negative impacts as they imply destruction of potentially salvageable tissue. The authors describe preliminary results from a multi-center trial on CRP apheresis in myocardial infarction as well as an upcoming trial in ischemic stroke. They also briefly touch on further potential indications for this interesting approach.

Finally, Sylvia Stracke and colleagues describe the IMAD trial (Efficacy of immunoadsorption for treatment of persons with Alzheimer dementia and agonistic autoantibodies against alpha 1A-adrenoceptor) [18] which tests a novel therapeutic approach for Alzheimer dementia using immunoadsorption. The study is based on the finding that agonistic autoantibodies against α_1- and β_2-adrenoceptors are present in 50% of patients with dementia and expands on a previous small trial in 8 patients [19] which demonstrated that IA was safe and able to significantly reduce α_1-adrenoceptor antibodies. Furthermore, the Mini Mental State Examination (MMSE) scores of these patients remained rather stable over the following 12–18 months. The IMAD trial aims at investigating the effects of IA on brain perfusion and disease progression on 15 patients with Alzheimer dementia and agonistic auto-antibodies.

2. Conclusions

The articles presented in this Special Issue reveal a broad spectrum of present as well as potential future indications for therapeutic apheresis and unanimously support the view that both PE and IA constitute promising, low-risk therapeutic options in the treatment of various autoimmune neurological diseases. However, they also highlight the need to improve indication-specific evidence, which can mainly be achieved by conducting sufficiently-powered RCTs which aim at comparing different treatment options. Along with a better understanding of underlying immunological processes and development of novel prognostic biomarkers, such studies will facilitate adequate therapeutic decision-making and eventually improve clinical outcomes of patients with autoimmune-mediated diseases.

Funding: This research received no external funding.

Conflicts of Interest: The author received honoraria and research grants from Fresenius Medical Care GmbH and Fresenius Medical Care Deutschland GmbH.

Disclosures: J.D. serves as the invited editor for the Special Issue "Apheresis in Neurological Disorders" in the Journal of Clinical Medicine.

References

1. Baggi, F.; Ubiali, F.; Nava, S.; Nessi, V.; Andreetta, F.; Rigamonti, A.; Maggi, L.; Mantegazza, R.; Antozzi, C. Effect of IgG immunoadsorption on serum cytokines in MG and LEMS patients. *J. Neuroimmunol.* **2008**, *201*, 104–110. [CrossRef] [PubMed]
2. Dorst, J.; Fillies, F.; Dreyhaupt, J.; Senel, M.; Tumani, H. Safety and Tolerability of Plasma Exchange and Immunoadsorption in Neuroinflammatory Diseases. *J. Clin. Med.* **2020**, *9*, 2874. [CrossRef] [PubMed]
3. Schneider-Gold, C.; Krenzer, M.; Klinker, E.; Mansouri-Thalegani, B.; Mullges, W.; Toyka, K.V.; Gold, R. Immunoadsorption versus plasma exchange versus combination for treatment of myasthenic deterioration. *Ther. Adv. Neurol. Disord.* **2016**, *9*, 297–303. [CrossRef] [PubMed]

4. Weinshenker, B.G.; O'Brien, P.C.; Petterson, T.M.; Noseworthy, J.H.; Lucchinetti, C.F.; Dodick, D.W.; Pineda, A.A.; Stevens, L.N.; Rodriguez, M. A randomized trial of plasma exchange in acute central nervous system inflammatory demyelinating disease. *Ann. Neurol.* **1999**, *46*, 878–886. [CrossRef]

5. Dorst, J.; Fangerau, T.; Taranu, D.; Eichele, P.; Dreyhaupt, J.; Michels, S.; Schuster, J.; Ludolph, A.C.; Senel, M.; Tumani, H. Safety and efficacy of immunoadsorption versus plasma exchange in steroid-refractory relapse of multiple sclerosis and clinically isolated syndrome: A randomised, parallel-group, controlled trial. *EClinicalMedicine* **2019**, *16*, 98–106. [CrossRef] [PubMed]

6. Lipphardt, M.; Wallbach, M.; Koziolek, M.J. Plasma Exchange or Immunoadsorption in Demyelinating Diseases: A Meta-Analysis. *J. Clin. Med.* **2020**, *9*, 1597. [CrossRef] [PubMed]

7. Pfeuffer, S.; Rolfes, L.; Bormann, E.; Sauerland, C.; Ruck, T.; Schilling, M.; Melzer, N.; Brand, M.; Pul, R.; Kleinschnitz, C.; et al. Comparing Plasma Exchange to Escalated Methyl Prednisolone in Refractory Multiple Sclerosis Relapses. *J. Clin. Med.* **2019**, *9*, 35. [CrossRef] [PubMed]

8. Rolfes, L.; Pfeuffer, S.; Ruck, T.; Melzer, N.; Pawlitzki, M.; Heming, M.; Brand, M.; Wiendl, H.; Meuth, S.G. Therapeutic Apheresis in Acute Relapsing Multiple Sclerosis: Current Evidence and Unmet Needs-A Systematic Review. *J. Clin. Med.* **2019**, *8*, 1623. [CrossRef] [PubMed]

9. Chevret, S.; Hughes, R.A.; Annane, D. Plasma exchange for Guillain-Barré syndrome. *Cochrane Database Syst. Rev.* **2017**, *2*. [CrossRef] [PubMed]

10. Lieker, I.; Slowinski, T.; Harms, L.; Hahn, K.; Klehmet, J. A prospective study comparing tryptophan immunoadsorption with therapeutic plasma exchange for the treatment of chronic inflammatory demyelinating polyneuropathy. *J. Clin. Apher.* **2017**, *32*, 486–493. [CrossRef] [PubMed]

11. Dorst, J.; Ludolph, A.C.; Senel, M.; Tumani, H. Short-term and long-term effects of immunoadsorption in refractory chronic inflammatory demyelinating polyneuropathy: A prospective study in 17 patients. *J. Neurol.* **2018**, *265*, 2906–2915. [CrossRef] [PubMed]

12. Querol, L.; Devaux, J.; Rojas-Garcia, R.; Illa, I. Autoantibodies in chronic inflammatory neuropathies: Diagnostic and therapeutic implications. *Nat. Rev. Neurol.* **2017**, *13*, 533–547. [CrossRef] [PubMed]

13. Davies, A.J.; Fehmi, J.; Senel, M.; Tumani, H.; Dorst, J.; Rinaldi, S. Immunoadsorption and Plasma Exchange in Seropositive and Seronegative Immune-Mediated Neuropathies. *J. Clin. Med.* **2020**, *9*, 2025. [CrossRef] [PubMed]

14. Rössling, R.; Prüss, H. Apheresis in Autoimmune Encephalitis and Autoimmune Dementia. *J. Clin. Med.* **2020**, *9*, 2683. [CrossRef] [PubMed]

15. Scheibenbogen, C.; Loebel, M.; Freitag, H.; Krueger, A.; Bauer, S.; Antelmann, M.; Doehner, W.; Scherbakov, N.; Heidecke, H.; Reinke, P.; et al. Immunoadsorption to remove ß2 adrenergic receptor antibodies in Chronic Fatigue Syndrome CFS/ME. *PLoS ONE* **2018**, *13*, e0193672. [CrossRef] [PubMed]

16. Tölle, M.; Freitag, H.; Antelmann, M.; Hartwig, J.; Schuchardt, M.; van der Giet, M.; Eckardt, K.U.; Grabowski, P.; Scheibenbogen, C. Myalgic Encephalomyelitis/Chronic Fatigue Syndrome: Efficacy of Repeat Immunoadsorption. *J. Clin. Med.* **2020**, *9*, 2443. [CrossRef] [PubMed]

17. Kayser, S.; Brunner, P.; Althaus, K.; Dorst, J.; Sheriff, A. Selective Apheresis of C-Reactive Protein for Treatment of Indications with Elevated CRP Concentrations. *J. Clin. Med.* **2020**, *9*, 2947. [CrossRef] [PubMed]

18. Stracke, S.; Lange, S.; Bornmann, S.; Kock, H.; Schulze, L.; Klinger-König, J.; Böhm, S.; Vogelgesang, A.; von Podewils, F.; Föel, A.; et al. Immunoadsorption for Treatment of Patients with Suspected Alzheimer Dementia and Agonistic Autoantibodies against Alpha1a-Adrenoceptor-Rationale and Design of the IMAD Pilot Study. *J. Clin. Med.* **2020**, *9*, 1919. [CrossRef] [PubMed]

19. Hempel, P.; Heinig, B.; Jerosch, C.; Decius, I.; Karczewski, P.; Kassner, U.; Kunze, R.; Steinhagen-Thiessen, E.; Bimmler, M. Immunoadsorption of Agonistic Autoantibodies Against α1-Adrenergic Receptors in Patients With Mild to Moderate Dementia. *Ther. Apher. Dial.* **2016**, *20*, 523–529. [CrossRef] [PubMed]

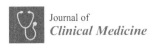

Article

Safety and Tolerability of Plasma Exchange and Immunoadsorption in Neuroinflammatory Diseases

Johannes Dorst [1],*, Frank Fillies [1], Jens Dreyhaupt [2], Makbule Senel [1] and Hayrettin Tumani [1]

[1]   Department of Neurology, University of Ulm, 89081 Ulm, Germany; frank.fillies@uni-ulm.de (F.F.);
      makbule.senel@uni-ulm.de (M.S.); hayrettin.tumani@uni-ulm.de (H.T.)
[2]   Institute for Epidemiology and Medical Biometry, University of Ulm, 89081 Ulm, Germany;
      jens.dreyhaupt@uni-ulm.de
*   Correspondence: Johannes.dorst@uni-ulm.de

Received: 13 August 2020; Accepted: 3 September 2020; Published: 5 September 2020

Abstract: Plasma exchange (PE) and immunoadsorption (IA) are frequently used for treatment of various autoimmune-mediated neurological diseases, including multiple sclerosis (MS), chronic inflammatory demyelinating polyneuropathy (CIDP), and Guillain–Barré syndrome (GBS). Although both methods are generally regarded as well-tolerated treatment options, evidence for safety and tolerability is low for most indications and largely relies on small case series. In this study, we retrospectively analysed adverse events (AEs) and laboratory changes in 284 patients with various neurological indications who received either PE ($n = 65$, 113 cycles) or IA ($n = 219$, 435 cycles) between 2013 and 2020 in our Neurology department. One standard treatment cycle for PE as well as IA consisted of five treatments on five consecutive days. During every treatment, the 2.0–2.5-fold individual plasma volume (PV) was treated in IA, while in PE, the 0.7-fold individual PV was replaced by human albumin solution. Overall, both methods showed an excellent safety profile; no deaths of life-threatening adverse events were recorded. Severe AEs (corresponding to grade 3 on the Common Terminology Criteria for Adverse Events grading scale v5.0) including three patients with sepsis, one pneumonia, and one pneumothorax were present in 5/435 IA cycles (1.1%); in the PE group, no severe AEs were recorded. Furthermore, although advantageous tolerability is generally considered the main advantage of IA over PE, we found that overall frequency of AEs (including grades 1 and 2) was higher in IA (67.1% of all cycles) compared to PE (35.4%; $p < 0.001$). The low incidence of AEs in PE might be caused by the lower PV exchanged during each treatment (0.7-fold) compared to previous studies which predominantly exchanged the 1.0–1.5-fold PV. In order to verify this hypothesis as well as confirming the efficacy of this lower-dosed scheme, prospective studies comparing different treatment regimens are needed.

Keywords: therapeutic plasma exchange; immunoadsorption; neurological diseases; multiple sclerosis; chronic inflammatory demyelinating polyneuropathy

1. Introduction

Plasma exchange (PE) and immunoadsorption (IA) are used in various autoimmune-mediated neurological diseases in order to remove autoimmune antibodies and other pathological constituents from the patients' blood. Currently, indications include multiple sclerosis (MS), myasthenia gravis, autoimmune encephalitis, chronic inflammatory demyelinating polyneuropathy (CIDP), Guillain–Barré syndrome (GBS), and many others. Although PE constitutes the standard technique for most diseases, IA is increasingly recognized as a more specific alternative and generally appreciated for its potentially advantageous safety profile. However, safety and tolerability of both methods have rarely been directly compared under standardized, monocentric conditions.

Originally, both treatment options primarily aimed at removing auto-antibodies from the blood, although various additional immune-modulating mechanisms like up- and downregulation of anti- and pro-inflammatory interleukins have been discussed [1]. Substantial methodological differences have to be considered which may affect efficacy as well as safety. Since in PE the plasma is removed and substituted by a volume replacement solution (human albumin or fresh frozen plasma (FFP)), all circulating proteins are removed, including coagulation factors. In contrast, IA relies on adsorbers which selectively bind human immunoglobulins (Ig) while largely sparing other plasma proteins; the processed plasma is led back to the patient, and no replacement solution is needed. Theoretically speaking, these factors should favor IA in terms of adverse events (AEs), while on the other hand the preservation of pro-inflammatory cytokines and other pathogenetically important proteins may weaken its efficacy dependent on the specific immunology of the respective disease, which is however, not fully understood in many cases. Furthermore, it has been shown that even in IA other plasma proteins are also affected which might explain its efficacy in diseases which are not regarded to be primarily antibody-mediated [2].

Apart from the method itself, specific techniques and treatment regimens have to be taken into account when assessing efficacy and safety of PE and IA. Various regenerable (protein A, recombinant proteins) and non-regenerable (tryptophan, phenylalanine) IA adsorbers are routinely used in clinical practice which feature different binding characteristics with regard to immunoglobulin classes, subclasses, and other plasma proteins [3,4]. For example, protein A adsorbers have a stronger binding affinity to IgG compared to IgA and IgM [3]. Furthermore, various treatment regimens can be applied for PE and IA with regard to number and frequency of treatments as well as the plasma volume (PV) treated during each session. Usually, 5–7 treatments are performed in both PE and IA, while treatment frequencies vary between daily and 2-day applications depending on fibrinogen levels. In IA, processing of the 2.0–2.5-fold individual PV constitutes the standard [5], which allows a daily treatment regimen for regenerable protein A and recombinant protein adsorbers, while a two-day treatment regimen with fixed PV (usually 2 or 2.5 L) is usually applied for non-regenerable tryptophan and phenylalanine adsorbers (due to loss of fibrinogen) [6–8]. In PE, various regimens with different PVs have been used. For example, the original randomized controlled trial (RCT) which built the foundation for the use of PE in MS applied 7 treatments within 14 days, exchanging the 1.1-fold PV during each session [9], while a more recent RCT showed that a daily treatment regime with 5 sessions and replacement of the 0.7-fold PV during each session was also effective [5]. Importantly, across all neurological indications there are no RCTs which directly compare different treatment regimens, and only few regimens have been tried; therefore, it seems very likely that the optimal regimen with regard to efficacy and safety has not yet been found.

Furthermore, specific peri- and intra-procedural measures vary between centers. In order to prevent blood in the extracorporeal circuit from clotting, heparin and/or citrate are most commonly used which carry various potential complications like heparin-induced thrombopenia and hypocalcemia. Some centers replace immunoglobulins after each treatment in order to account for the immunodeficiency induced by the therapy, while others rely on the periprocedural prophylactic administration of antibiotics. For all these measures, no reliable evidence exists.

Previous studies comparing PE and IA with regard to safety and tolerability in neurological diseases predominantly reported either no differences [6,8,10], or advantages for IA [11,12]. Since PE is unspecific, various complications due to loss of coagulation factors and other plasma constituents have been reported such as thrombosis, bleeding, hypotension (due to volume-shift), and sepsis [13,14]. Furthermore, the need of a volume replacement solution carries the risk of severe allergic reactions [13]. Life-threatening complications have been reported in 0.12% of patients [14], and a higher risk of adverse events in patients with neurological diseases compared to non-neurological diseases has been described [13]. On the other hand, IA has repeatedly been described as a safe and well-tolerated procedure [3,4,15]. Two studies in myasthenia gravis found that side effects were reduced in IA compared to PE [11,12]. In MS, the majority of studies did however not report any differences between

IA and PE with regard to safety [5,6,8] which was confirmed by a recent meta-analysis [10]. The only prospective study comparing IA and PE in CIDP [16] reported a good safety profile for both methods and comparable incidences of AEs. One retrospective study reported that both PE and IA were safely applied in 19 patients with GBS [17]. In summary, safety data for PE and IA in neurological diseases largely rely on studies with rather low numbers of subjects, which might explain the large range of reported incidences of AEs as well as the diverging assessments of safety profiles for both methods.

Considering the lack of RCTs regarding the use of PE and IA in neurological diseases, the extensive differences with regard to treatment regimens and peri-procedural measures, and the absence of reliable therapeutic standards for specific disease entities, it is of crucial importance to collect systematic clinical data. In this study, we retrospectively analyzed tolerability and safety data (including adverse events and laboratory abnormalities) in 284 patients (548 treatment cycles, 2470 treatments) with various neurological indications who were treated with either PE ($n = 65$) or IA ($n = 219$) between 2013 and 2020 in our center. We primarily aimed at (1) verifying the advantageous safety and tolerability profile of IA as proposed by previous studies and (2) evaluating our specific PE-regimen which features a comparatively low PV treated per session (0.7-fold) compared to previous publications, allowing daily treatments.

2. Methods

2.1. Patients

All patients who were treated with either PE or IA between 2013 and 2020 in the Department of Neurology, University of Ulm, were analysed. All clinical information including medical history, neurological status, adverse events, laboratory data, and clinical scales were collected by reviewing the complete medical records of each patient, including discharge letters, diagnostic findings, and monitoring documents. We included patients with all neurological diagnoses who received at least one treatment of PE or IA. Overall, 284 patients (65 PE, 219 IA) were identified. Because some patients received more than one cycle, 548 cycles (113 PE, 435 IA) were performed and analysed. Reasons for multiple cycles per patient included chronic diseases like CIDP which necessitate the application of multiple cycles in regular time intervals, or insufficient treatment response. One cycle consisted of 5 treatments, resulting in a total of 2740 treatments (565 PE, 2175 IA) which were separately documented and analysed.

All patients with MS fulfilled the 2017 MacDonald diagnostic criteria for MS [18] or CIS at the time of treatment. Patients with CIDP fulfilled the European Fedaration of Neurological Societies (EFNS) criteria for possible, probable, or definite CIDP. Patients with GBS showed the typical clinical picture including rapidly progressive bilateral limb weakness and sensory deficits, hypo-/areflexia, electrophysiological signs of demyelination, and increased protein levels in cerebrospinal fluid. Patients with other diseases were likewise diagnosed based on the respective internationally accepted guidelines.

2.2. Indication for PE/IA

All patients were treated in the Neurological Department of Ulm University, Neurological Center of Apheresis and Therapies (Neurologisches Apherese- und Therapiezentrum, NATZ). The decision to perform PE or IA was based on individual evaluation, taking into account diagnosis, clinical and diagnostic findings, and response to previous treatments. In patients with MS or clinically isolated syndrome (CIS), prerequisite for apheresis was the unsuccessful application of at least one cycle of high-dose intravenous methyl-prednisolone (MP). In cases of incomplete improvement, a second cycle of high-dose intravenous MP was performed in some patients. In CIDP, apheresis was only applied in therapy-refractory cases, i.e., patients who deteriorated despite MP and/or IVIg therapy (usually both). In case of a positive treatment effect, apheresis was applied in regular time intervals, based on the individual course of disease, i.e., PE/IA was performed when symptoms began to worsen again after the initial improvement. In GBS, apheresis was used as a first-line therapy as an alternative to

IVIg. In some cases, PE/IA was performed after an initial unsuccessful application of IVIg. In all other indications, apheresis was usually performed as an escalation therapy after unsatisfying response to the first-line/standard therapies. The decision for the specific method (PE or IA) was individually made based on current evidence, personal preference/experience, pathophysiological considerations, and comorbidities/contraindications in a process of shared decision-making after in-depth information of each individual patient about all therapeutic options. In 21 patients (8 MS, 2 CIDP, 3 GBS, and 8 other) PE was switched to IA, and in 22 patients (4 MS, 4 CIDP, 3 GBS, and 11 other) IA was switched to PE after one initial unsuccessful cycle.

2.3. Procedures

PE and IA were both applied on 5 consecutive days. The majority of patients received a Shaldon catheter in the right jugular vein. In patients who received several cycles over a prolonged period of time (mainly CIDP), a cubital arteriovenous shunt was used in a few cases. Heparin and citrate were used as anticoagulants, and no prophylactic antibiotics or post-procedural IVIg were given. Before each treatment, a systemic infection was ruled out by blood and urine analysis, and ACE inhibitors were paused at least 3 days before IA. Patients were extensively informed about risks as well as alternative treatment options and gave their written informed consent. During each treatment, a continuous monitoring was performed including blood pressure, heart rate, and oxygen saturation. Laboratory testing including blood count, CRP, electrolytes, liver, and kidney parameters were routinely done on a daily basis during PE/IA.

During PE, a fixed PV of 2 L (corresponding to a mean individual 0.7-fold PV) was exchanged until 07/2018; afterwards, we instead exchanged the 0.7-fold individual PV. Since comparative studies regarding different treatment regimens for PE/IA are completely lacking, these parameters are mainly based on local experience and expertise. A COM.TEC cell separator (Fresenius Kabi Deutschland GmbH, Bad Homburg, Germany) was used during PE.

During IA, the 2.0-fold individual plasma volume was processed on the first day, and the 2.5-fold individual plasma volume was processed on days 2–5. The individual plasma volume was calculated according to the formula published by Sprenger et al. [19]. Three different regenerable double-column adsorbers were used: protein A (Immunosorba, Fresenius Medical Care, Bad Homburg, Germany), Peptid-GAM (Globaffin, Fresenius Medical Care, Bad Homburg, Germany), and recombinant proteins (Miltenyi Biotec, Bergisch Gladbach, Germany). All three adsorbers selectively bind human immunoglobulins while largely sparing other plasma proteins. The choice of adsorber was mainly based on availability. ADAsorb (medicap clinic GmbH, Ulrichstein, Germany) and Life 21 (Miltenyi Biotec, Bergisch Gladbach, Germany) were used as immunoadsorption devices; COM.TEC (Fresenius Kabi Deutschland GmbH, Bad Homburg, Germany) and ART Universal (Fresenius Medical Care, Bad Homburg, Germany) were used for cell separation.

2.4. Outcome Parameters

Adverse events were retrospectively collected by reviewing the medical reports and monitoring curves of each patient and treatment. Laboratory changes were assessed based on daily laboratory reports. Adverse events were classified as Grade 1–5 according to the Common Terminology Criteria for Adverse Events grading scale v5.0.

Efficacy parameters before and after treatment were collected as documented in the medical reports. In patients with MS, these include the Expanded Disability Status Scale (EDSS) and the Multiple Sclerosis Functional Composite (MSFC) as the best validated and frequently used standardized clinical scales. In patients with CIDP, we routinely performed the CIDP score [20], which incorporates the Inflammatory Neuropathy Cause and Treatment (INCAT) score [21], the Oxford muscle strength grading score, and vibration sensitivity testing with a 256-Hz Ryder-Seiffel tuning fork. Since no generally accepted and adequately validated standardized scale exists for GBS, evaluation of efficacy in these patients was based on neurological examination before and after PE/IA and classified as large, partial, equivocal, or no improvement. For other indications, no systematic evaluation of efficacy was done due to low numbers of patients. Efficacy data refer to subgroups of patients with sufficient clinical data and have been published previously [5,20,22].

2.5. Statistical Analysis

Adverse events and laboratory changes were evaluated per cycle. Adverse events were additionally analysed on a per-patient basis in order to exclude bias based on the per-cycle approach (i.e., one patient may present one specific AE during multiple cycles, causing an overestimation of this AE). Statistical analysis was based on absolute/relative frequencies (categorial variables) and median/interquartile range (continuous variables). For evaluation of laboratory changes, we calculated the change between baseline and second day of PE/IA (not shown) as well as fifth day of PE/IA (before last treatment); we also recorded the share of cycles/patients with pathological values for each laboratory parameter.

Changes of patient related continuous data were investigated with the Wilcoxon signed rank test. Group comparisons for patient related continuous data were performed using the Mann–Whitney-U-test. Group comparisons for patient related categorical data were carried out with the chi-square test or Fisher's exact test as appropriate. Group comparisons for cycle related continuous data were investigated using linear mixed effects regression models in order to account for patients receiving multiple cycles. Group comparisons for cycle related binary data were investigated using mixed effects regression models for binary outcomes.

The level of significance was set as $p \leq 0.05$ (two-sided). To estimate treatment effects, we calculated median differences including a two-sided 95% confidence interval. Statistical analyses were done using SAS, version 9.4, and GraphPad Prism, version 7.05. Because of the explorative nature of this study, all results from statistical tests have to be interpreted as hypothesis-generating rather than proof of efficacy. No adjustment for multiple testing was done.

3. Results

3.1. Demographics and Clinical Characteristics

Demographic and clinical characteristics are depicted in Table 1. PE and IA patients were not different with regard to age, sex distribution, and body mass index (BMI). For more detailed clinical information for patients with the most common diagnoses (MS, CIDP, and GBS) see Tables S1–S3. Prognostic factors in patients with MS, CIDP, and GBS were evenly distributed between PE and IA.

Table 1. Baseline Characteristics.

	IA	PE	Total	*p*
Patients (cycles)	219 (435)	65 (113)	284 (548)	
Treatments per cycle	5	5		
Processed PV per treatment	2.0–2.5-fold	0.7-fold		
Age (years)	51.0 (36.0 to 62.0)	45.5 (34.5 to 63.0)	50.0 (36.0 to 62.0)	0.68
Sex				0.89
male	94 (42.9%)	27 (41.5%)	121 (42.6%)	
female	125 (57.1%)	38 (58.5%)	163 (57.4%)	
BMI (kg/m^2)	24.3 (21.8 to 27.8)	25.2 (21.6 to 27.5)	24.6 (21.8 to 27.8)	0.67
Diagnosis				
MS	72 (32.9%)	21 (32.3%)	93 (32.7%)	
CIS	28 (12.8%)	10 (15.4%)	38 (13.4%)	
NMOSD	3 (1.4%)	2 (3.1%)	5 (1.8%)	
AE	15 (6.8%)	2 (3.1%)	17 (6.0%)	
CIDP	30 (13.7%)	4 (6.2%)	34 (12.0%)	

Table 1. *Cont.*

	IA	PE	Total	*p*
GBS	17 (7.8%)	10 (15.4%)	27 (9.5%)	
MG	4 (1.8%)	0	4 (1.4%)	
SPS	3 (1.4%)	1 (1.5%)	4 (1.4%)	
SLE	1 (0.5%)	2 (3.1%)	3 (1.1%)	
Other	46 (21.0%)	12 (18.4%)	58 (20.4%)	

IA—immunoadsorption; PE—plasma exchange; PV—individual plasma volume; BMI—body mass index; MS—multiple sclerosis; CIS—clinically isolated syndrome; NMOSD—neuromyelitis optica spectrum disorder; AE—autoimmune encephalitis; CIDP—chronic inflammatory demyelinating polyneuropathy; GBS—Guillain–Barré syndrome; MG—myasthenia gravis; SPS—stiff person syndrome; SLE—systemic lupus erythematodes.

3.2. Adverse Events

Overall, both methods showed an excellent safety profile; no treatment-associated deaths or life-threatening adverse events were recorded. Severe AEs (corresponding to grade 3 on the Common Terminology Criteria for Adverse Events grading scale) in the IA group included three patients with sepsis, one severe pneumonia, and one pneumothorax, corresponding to 5/435 affected IA cycles (1.1%). In the PE group, no severe AEs were recorded.

Importantly, all three patients with sepsis were diagnosed with CIDP, two-thirds were older than 80 years and multimorbid. One patient had type 2 diabetes mellitus and recurrent urinary infections in medical history. Primary focus was the Shaldon catheter in all three cases. All patients recovered with antibiotic treatment. One severe pneumonia occurred in a 49 year old female with severe myasthenic crisis who was monitored on intensive care unit and dependent on non-invasive ventilation when IA was initiated; she eventually recovered. The pneumothorax (IA group) was a complication of Shaldon catheter placement and necessitated a Bülau drainage as well as a short stay on intensive care unit. The patient recovered completely and received several IA cycles afterwards without any further complications.

Surprisingly, we found that mild and moderate adverse events per cycle (grade 1 and 2; Table 2) were more frequent in the IA group (67.1%) compared to PE (35.4%; *p* < 0.001). With the exception of fatigue, all adverse events were more frequent in the IA group. Most common were intermittent hypotonia (24.0% of all patients), hematoma caused by Shaldon placement (16.4%), and mild infections (6.9%). All adverse events were uncomplicated and did not necessitate any specific therapy. Thrombotic events included deep venous thromboses, most commonly of the Shaldon-affected jugular vein, which were treated with oral anticoagulants and healed without permanent consequences in all cases. Thrombotic events were most frequently seen in patients with GBS.

Table 2. Adverse Events per Cycle.

	MS		CIDP		GBS		Overall		
Adverse Event	PE (*n* = 27)	IA (*n* = 100)	PE (*n* = 18)	IA (*n* = 80)	PE (*n* = 15)	IA (*n* = 22)	PE (*n* = 113)	IA (*n* = 435)	Total (*n* = 550)
Hypotonia	7.4	23.0	5.6	16.3	0.0	31.8	8.8	28.0	24.0
Hematoma (Shaldon)	3.7	18.0	16.7	6.3	13.3	9.1	11.5	17.7	16.4
Mild Infections	0.0	4.0	5.6	7.5	20.0	13.6	5.3	7.4	6.9
Technical Complications	0.0	6.0	0.0	7.5	0.0	13.6	0.8	5.7	4.7
Nausea	3.7	3.0	0.0	1.3	0.0	9.1	3.5	4.8	4.5
Tachycardia	0.0	3.0	0.0	7.5	13.3	4.5	1.8	4.6	4.0
Edema	0.0	3.0	0.0	3.8	0.0	4.5	0.0	4.8	3.8
Allergic Skin Reaction	0.0	10.0	5.6	2.5	0.0	4.5	0.8	4.6	3.8
Thrombosis	3.7	0.0	0.0	3.8	6.7	13.6	2.7	3.4	3.3
Thoracic Pain	0.0	3.0	0.0	1.3	0.0	13.6	0.8	3.9	3.3
Fatigue	0.0	0.0	5.6	1.3	6.7	0.0	3.5	1.1	1.6
Thrombosis	3.7	0.0	0.0	3.8	6.7	13.6	2.7	3.4	3.3

Data are %. Table presents all adverse events that occurred in >3% of patients in at least one of the treatment groups. IA—immunoadsorption; PE—plasma exchange; MS—Multiple Sclerosis; CIDP—Chronic Inflammatory Demyelinating Polyneuropathy; GBS—Guillain–Barré syndrome.

Per-patient analysis yielded similar results as per-cycle analysis (not shown). Albeit CIDP patients were older and had more co-morbidities compared to MS, we did not detect any meaningful disease-specific characteristics with regard to AEs.

3.3. Laboratory Changes

Median laboratory changes between the day of last treatment (before last treatment) compared to baseline of each cycle in both groups are displayed in Table 3. While loss of thrombocytes was more pronounced in IA, loss of erythrocytes was more pronounced in PE. IA patients showed larger decreases of potassium and calcium; sodium was rather stable in PE as well IA. The substitution of proteins masks the assumedly larger loss of plasma proteins in PE compared to IA. Importantly, fibrinogen levels were similar in PE and IA. As described previously, we found that in the IA group IgG was removed more effectively than IgA and IgM; consistently, IgG reduction was more pronounced in IA, while IgA and IgM reduction were more pronounced in PE. Supplementing the absolute changes, Table 4 displays the share of patients above/below the pathological threshold for each laboratory parameter per group which yielded congruent results.

Table 3. Laboratory Changes.

Parameter	PE (n = 113)		IA (n = 435)		P
Leukocytes (G/L)	−0.3	(−1.6 to 0.9)	0.1	(−1.4 to 1.3)	0.98
Erythrocytes (T/L)	−0.55	(−0.72 to −0.21)	−0.35	(−0.59 to −0.14)	**<0.001**
Hemoglobin (g/L)	−15	(−23 to −8)	−10	(−17 to −4)	**<0.001**
Hematocrit (%)	−4	(−2 to −6)	−3	(−1 to −5)	**<0.001**
Thrombocytes (G/L)	−53	(−90 to −26)	−91	(−128 to −55)	**<0.001**
MPV(fL)	0.1	(−0.3 to 0.4)	0.4	(0.1 to 0.8)	**<0.001**
Quick (%)	−24	(−37 to −12)	−10	(−39 to 2)	0.18
INR	0.13	(0.07 to 0.44)	0.06	(−0.01 to 0.37)	0.66
pTT (s)	11.6	(4.6 to 32.3)	6.5	(3.1 to 26.0)	0.52
Fibrinogen (g/L)	−1.7	(−1.9 to −0.1)	−1.6	(−3.4 to −0.8)	0.96
Sodium (mmol/L)	1	(−1 to 3)	2	(1 to 4)	**0.003**
Potassium (mmol/L)	−0.23	(−0.60 to 0.08)	−0.47	(−0.77 to −0.17)	**<0.001**
Calcium (mmol/L)	0.02	(−0.08 to 0.10)	−0.17	(−0.25 to −0.06)	**<0.001**
Urea (mmol/L)	−0.12	(−0.98 to 0.76)	−0.94	(−2.14 to 0.05)	**0.019**
Creatinine (µmol/L)	−1.5	(−8.5 to 1.8)	2	(−5.5 to 8)	**0.002**
GFR (ml/min)	2.0	(−3.5 to 10.5)	−2.5	(−13 to 7.3)	**0.002**
AST (U/L)	9.0	(−6.25 to 13.8)	1.0	(−4.0 to 10.0)	0.98
ALT (U/L)	−6.0	(−13.0 to 7.0)	−3.5	(−9.3 to 9.0)	0.85
GGT (U/L)	−17.0	(−27.5 to −12.0)	−9.0	(−22.0 to −4.0)	0.92
AP (U/L)	−39.0	(−43.0 to −26.0)	−19.0	(−30.3 to −12.0)	**0.03**
Bilirubin (µmol/L)	3.5	(0.5 to 5.3)	0.1	(−2.4 to 11.4)	0.09
Protein (g/L)	−5.9 *	(−9.4 to −1.8)	−19.9	(−23.9 to −15.8)	**<0.001**
CRP (mg/L)	0.08	(−1.02 to 1.40)	0.81	(−0.28 to 3.81)	0.23
IgA (mg/L)[#]	−866	(−572 to −1100)	−1362	(−1197 to −1536)	**<0.001**
IgG (mg/L)[#]	−6639	(−5428 to −7367)	−5770	(−5562 to −6582)	**<0.001**
IgM (mg/L)[#]	−711	(−316 to −924)	−713	(−324 to −1066)	**0.008**

Median laboratory changes (IQR) between the day of last treatment compared to baseline of each cycle in both groups. IA—immunoadsorption; PE—plasma exchange; MPV—mean platelet volume; INR—international normalized ratio; pTT—partial thromboplastin time; GFR—glomerular filtration rate; AST—aspartate aminotransferase; ALT—alanine aminotransferase; GGT—gamma glutamyl transferase; AP—alkaline phosphatase; CRP—C-reactive protein; * after substitution with human albumin solution; # Immunoglobulins A, G, and M were measured in a subset of 61 MS patients who participated in a randomized controlled study [5]. Bold *p*-values mark significant values.

Table 4. Pathological Laboratory Parameters at Last Day of Apheresis (Before Last Treatment).

Parameter	PE (n = 113)	IA (n = 435)	p
Leukocytes (G/L)	18.3%	19.0%	0.64
Erythrocytes (T/L)	53.9%	38.5%	**0.05**
Hemoglobin (g/L)	58.7%	46.0%	0.08
Hematocrit (%)	54.8%	45.8%	0.09
Thrombocytes (G/L)	12.6%	41.5%	**<0.001**
MPV(fL)	4.9%	6.1%	0.46
Quick (%)	44.8%	37.5%	0.15
INR	90.0%	91.0%	0.82
pTT (s)	78.6%	79.9%	0.85
Fibrinogen (g/L)	80.0%	66.7%	0.82
Sodium (mmol/L)	5.8%	0.3%	0.13
Potassium (mmol/L)	9.7%	27.0%	**0.001**
Calcium (mmol/L)	5.2%	17.8%	0.11
Urea (mmol/L)	8.3%	7.1%	0.90
Creatinine (μmol/L)	23.4%	28.1%	0.80
GFR (ml/min)	85.3%	82.6%	0.42
AST (U/L)	33.3%	23.8%	0.07
ALT (U/L)	18.2%	20.6%	0.49
GGT (U/L)	0.0%	15.7%	0.15
AP (U/L)	100.0%	88.5%	0.64
Bilirubin (μmol/L)	16.7%	11.4%	0.52
Protein (g/L)	92.0%*	99.1%	**0.004**
CRP (mg/L)	24.5%	40.3%	0.23

Share of patients with values below or above the pathological threshold for each parameter at last day of apheresis in each group. IA—immunoadsorption; PE—plasma exchange; MPV—mean platelet volume; INR—international normalized ratio; pTT—partial thromboplastin time; GFR—glomerular filtration rate; AST—aspartate aminotransferase; ALT—alanine aminotransferase; GGT—gamma glutamyl transferase; AP—alkaline phosphatase; CRP—C-reactive protein; * after substitution with human albumin solution. Bold p-values mark significant values.

3.4. Efficacy

Efficacy data for patients with sufficient standardized data have previously been published. These data refer to subsets of the study population investigated in the current study and were treated with the same IA and PE protocols.

In steroid-refractory MS, we conducted a randomized controlled trial in 61 patients (31 IA vs. 30 PE, 5 treatments on 5 consecutive days as outlined above) [5]. We found a significant improvement of symptoms after four weeks compared to pre-treatment in both groups as measured by MSFC and EDSS. In the PE group, median MSFC improved from 0.22 (–0.27 to 0.55) to 0.57 (0.15 to 0.82; $p < 0.001$), and median EDSS improved from 3.0 (2.0 to 3.5) to 2.0 (1.0 to 3.5; $p < 0.001$). In the IA group, median MSFC improved from 0.09 (–0.19 to 0.39) to 0.63 (0.21 to 0.90; $p < 0.001$), and median EDSS improved from 3.0 (2.0 to 4.0) to 2.0 (1.0 to 3.1; $p < 0.001$). Although improvement started earlier in the PE group, MSFC improvement (0.385 vs. 0.265; $p = 0.03$) and response rates (86.7% vs. 76.7%) after four weeks were larger in the IA group.

In CIDP, we performed a prospective observational study in 17 patients with therapy-refractory courses (insufficient response to steroids and/or IVIg) who underwent IA [20]. Overall, median CIDP scores improved from 308.0 (266.0 to 374.5) pre-treatment to 330.0 (290.0 to 393.5; $p = 0.02$) after two weeks. Furthermore, we were able to stabilize disease progression in 6/7 patients who received long-term IA treatments in regular intervals. Before IA, these patients lost 6.7 (3.0 to 13.1) points of CIDP score per month, while during IA, they lost 0.1 (0.0 to 0.8) points. Due to the insufficient number of patients treated with PE, we cannot provide any comparative results.

A retrospective analysis of 20 patients with GBS [22] yielded response rates of 61.5% for IA and 71.4% for PE after the last treatment based on the documented neurological examinations.

4. Discussion

This study aimed at evaluating safety and tolerability of PE and IA as main options of apheresis in autoimmune-mediated neurological diseases. Pre-existing evidence suggested that IA may be superior to PE in this regard, although comparative studies with high numbers of patients are missing. For this purpose, we analysed data from 284 patients (548 cycles, 2740 treatments) who were treated with either PE or IA between 2013 and 2020 in our center under standardized conditions. Importantly, we used an adjusted protocol for PE, aiming for a comparatively small volume of exchanged plasma volume per day (0.7-fold individual PV per day) compared to other commonly used regimens which imply higher volumes (1.0–1.5-fold individual PV per day). This protocol is based on our own clinical experience, including a randomized controlled trial in MS [5] which suggested an excellent safety and good efficacy profile for this specific regimen. The retrospective nature of this study has to be mentioned as a limitation, since we cannot exclude that AEs occurred or diagnoses changed after discharge. We regard the high number of treatments under standardized, monocentric conditions and the continuous, systematic recording of safety data as strengths of this study.

Overall, we found that both methods were very safe across all neurological indications, since we did not record any life-threatening complications or deaths, and grade 3 AEs were recorded in only 1.1% of IA cycles while in PE, we did not record any grade 3 AEs. Therefore, the incidence of serious AEs was even rarer in PE compared to IA. Surprisingly, we found that the share of mild and moderate AEs, including thrombosis, hypotonia, allergic reactions, nausea, and vegetative symptoms were also lower in PE which contradicts the common conception of IA as a better tolerated method of apheresis. However, a closer look at current literature reveals that this question has not been conclusively answered as highlighted by several studies in MS [6,8] as well as a recent meta-analysis [10] which found similar incidences of adverse events. The generally favourable safety profile of both PE and IA should also be considered when weighing against alternative treatment options, for example whether a second high-dose MP cycle should be performed in steroid-refractory MS relapse before apheresis. As highlighted by a recent publication [23], sparing a second MP cycle and applying apheresis directly may be superior in terms of efficacy and safety.

Data about complication rates of PE are heterogenous, varying between 4.2% and 25.6% [13,24–26], most likely due to heterogenous treatment regimens with regard to PV treated per session, type and dosage of applied anticoagulants, type of venous access (peripheral or central), and type of volume substitution (human albumin or FFP). Basic-Jukic et al. found moderate allergic reactions in 1.6% of 509 patients treated with PE as well as severe anaphylactic reactions in five cases; accordingly, Schneider-Gold et al. found a higher incidence of allergic reactions in patients with myasthenia gravis treated with PE compared to IA [11]. However, the incidence of allergic reactions in PE may presumably be lowered by using human albumin solution instead of FFP, since allergic reactions are commonly associated with FFP [27], but very rarely with human albumin solution [28]. Accordingly, the incidence of allergic reactions was extremely low in our PE study population (0.8%), and lower compared to IA (4.6%). Since no volume substitution is needed in IA, the higher incidence of allergic reactions in IA may be associated with the higher amounts of anticoagulants needed for IA, especially heparin. Furthermore, it cannot be ruled out completely that adsorber substances may be reinfused.

Importantly, in order to utilize the advantageous safety profile of human albumin solution compared to FFP in PE, it is essential to limit fibrinogen loss by either reducing the frequency of treatments (i.e., performing treatments on a two-day instead of a daily basis) or reducing the PV processed during each treatment. Based on our data, it was possible to perform daily PE treatments with 0.7-fold PV without any treatment interruptions while maintaining acceptable fibrinogen plasma levels, i.e., fibrinogen levels remained above 0.8 g/L before each treatment. Applying this scheme, we found comparable fibrinogen levels in PE and IA, suggesting that (1) fibrinogen loss in PE can be sufficiently controlled by attenuating PV per treatment, and (2) significant loss of fibrinogen is also present in IA. In line with our finding of similar and acceptable fibrinogen levels in both PE and IA, we did not record any bleeding complications with both measures, while the incidence of thrombotic events was similar (2.7% in PE, 3.4% in IA). Therefore, we can conclude that maintaining higher fibrinogen levels during PE may contribute to improve safety, since bleeding complications have previously been described to occur more frequently in PE (3.1% of treatments) compared to IA (1.3%) [15].

In addition to allergic reactions and bleeding complications, infections induced by the immune-modulating effects of PE/IA are a major concern. Based on our data, both measures were very safe in this regard. We found severe infections with consecutive sepsis in three patients who were all diagnosed with CIDP; two of them were >80 years old. Therefore, we conclude that these clinical characteristics constitute risk factors which have to be considered. Mild infections occurred in only 5.3% (PE) and 7.4% (IA), respectively. These data corroborate the conception that peri-procedural prophylactic application of antibiotics or immunoglobulins is not needed. We could not confirm the finding of Schneider-Gold et al. who found a higher frequency of respiratory infections in PE compared to IA [11]. Again, different treatment regimens (0.7-fold vs. up to 1.5-fold PV treated in PE patients) do most likely account for this discrepancy, since treating lower PVs per session implies a higher preservation of antibodies and other anti-infective plasma proteins. Accordingly, we found that overall reduction rates of immunoglobulins were about similar in PE and IA; regarding subclasses, we found that reduction rates of IgA and IgM were higher in PE, while reduction rate of IgG was higher in IA. This was expected since the applied IA adsorbers feature a higher IgG affinity [29].

Regarding mild adverse events such as hypotonia, nausea, and palpitations, we generally found higher incidences in the IA group. This finding is not necessarily caused by technical differences of PE and IA, but may simply be explained by the significantly prolonged treatment times in IA. Applying the treatment regimens outlined above and dependent on the patient's individual PV, one IA treatment requires about the double amount of time compared to PE due to the excessive amount of blood treated during each session. Apart from the higher incidence of adverse events which are associated with longer treatment times, this also implies a larger burden for the patient.

Subclinical laboratory changes were unproblematic in all cases and did not necessitate specific treatment, with the exception of potassium and protein substitution which are routinely done in PE as well as IA. Interestingly, we found a higher incidence of anemia in PE, but a higher incidence of thrombopenia in IA, confirming previous findings [5]. The latter may possibly be explained by the higher demand for heparin during IA, since the external blood circuit has to be maintained for a longer timeframe and heparin may cause heparin-induced thrombopenia (HIT). While cell count abnormalities can be contributed to the procedures themselves, changes of plasma constituents like liver transaminases or urea do not necessarily imply organic disturbances, but rather signify that these substances are removed by the procedures. Regarding electrolytes, hypokalemia and hypocalcemia (due to citrate binding) are both known phenomena in PE and IA. In our study electrolyte disturbances were more frequent in the IA group.

Despite the lower incidence of AEs and laboratory abnormalities found for the low-PV PE treatment regimen compared to IA, this finding has to be interpreted carefully because of the following limitations of this study: First, the safety profile was compared with IA, which is quite a novel therapeutic approach itself, especially with regard to neurological diseases. A superiority of our PE regimen compared to other commonly applied regimens can however only be proven by conducting a direct comparative prospective study. Secondly, lowering the PV treated each day may compromise the efficacy of the procedure, which cannot be adequately analysed by means of a retrospective study design. We investigated the efficacy of this approach in a randomized controlled study in patients with steroid-refractory MS relapse versus IA [5]. Indeed, we found that after four weeks, IA patients showed a significantly larger improvement of the MSFC; however, the difference between PE and IA was rather small.

In summary, we conclude that:

1. PE and IA constitute safe and generally well-tolerated therapeutic options in autoimmune-mediated neurological diseases.

2. Contrary to previous publications, we found a lower incidence of adverse events in the PE group—possibly due to the low-volume per treatment regimen (0.7-fold PV per day), which allows to use human albumin solution while maintaining sufficient fibrinogen levels.

3. Safety and efficacy of this specific PE treatment regimen have to be further evaluated by means of a directly comparative, prospective study.

4. This study highlights the importance to consider specific treatment regimens with regard to safety and efficacy in general when assessing apheresis studies.

Supplementary Materials: The following are available online at http://www.mdpi.com/2077-0383/9/9/2874/s1, Supplementary Table S1: Baseline Characteristics of patients with MS/CIS; Supplementary Table S2: Baseline Characteristics of patients with CIDP; Supplementary Table S3: Baseline Characteristics of patients with GBS.

Author Contributions: Conceptualization, J.D. (Johannes Dorst); data curation, J.D. (Johannes Dorst) and F.F.; formal analysis, J.D. (Johannes Dorst), F.F., and J.D. (Jens Dreyhaupt); investigation, J.D. (Johannes Dorst) and F.F.; methodology, J.D. (Johannes Dorst), F.F., and J.D. (Jens Dreyhaupt); project administration, J.D. (Johannes Dorst); resources, J.D. (Johannes Dorst), M.S., and H.T.; supervision, J.D. (Johannes Dorst); validation, J.D. (Johannes Dorst), F.F., J.D. (Jens Dreyhaupt), M.S., and H.T.; visualization, J.D. (Johannes Dorst); writing—original draft, J.D. (Johannes Dorst); writing—review and editing, J.D. (Johannes Dorst), F.F., J.D. (Jens Dreyhaupt), M.S., and H.T.; and funding acquisition, N/A. All authors have read and agreed to the published version of the manuscript.

Funding: This research received no external funding.

Acknowledgments: The authors would like to thank Helmut Lehner and his team for their excellent care for the patients in our Neurological Center of Apheresis and Therapies (NATZ).

Conflicts of Interest: J.D. (Johannes Dorst) received honoraria and research grants from Fresenius Medical Care GmbH and Fresenius Medical Care Deutschland GmbH. MS has received consulting and/or speaker honoraria from Alexion, Bayer, Biogen, Merck, Roche, and Sanofi Genzyme. She has received travel funding from Celgene, and TEVA. She has received research funding from the Hertha-Nathorff-Program. H.T. reports funding for research projects, lectures, and travel from Bayer, Biogen, Genzyme, Merck, Novartis, Roche, Teva, and received research support from DMSG and BMBF. F.F. and J.D. (Jens Dreyhaupt) report no conflicts of interest.

References

1. Baggi, F.; Ubiali, F.; Nava, S.; Nessi, V.; Andreetta, F.; Rigamonti, A.; Maggi, L.; Mantegazza, R.; Antozzi, C. Effect of IgG immunoadsorption on serum cytokines in MG and LEMS patients. *J. Neuroimmunol.* **2008**, *201–202*, 104–110. [CrossRef] [PubMed]

2. Trebst, C.; Bronzlik, P.; Kielstein, J.T.; Schmidt, B.M.; Stangel, M. Immunoadsorption therapy for steroid-unresponsive relapses in patients with multiple sclerosis. *Blood Purificat.* **2012**, *33*, 1–6. [CrossRef] [PubMed]

3. Belak, M.; Borberg, H.; Jimenez, C.; Oette, K. Technical and clinical experience with protein A immunoadsorption columns. *Transfus. Sci.* **1994**, *15*, 419–422. [CrossRef]

4. Hohenstein, B.; Passauer, J.; Ziemssen, T.; Julius, U. Immunoadsorption with regenerating systems in neurological disorders –A single center experience. *Atheroscler. Suppl.* **2015**, *18*, 119–123. [CrossRef] [PubMed]

5. Dorst, J.; Fangerau, T.; Taranu, D.; Eichele, P.; Dreyhaupt, J.; Michels, S.; Schuster, J.; Ludolph, A.C.; Senel, M.; Tumani, H. Safety and efficacy of immunoadsorption versus plasma exchange in steroid-refractory relapse of multiple sclerosis and clinically isolated syndrome: A randomised, parallel-group, controlled trial. *EClinicalMedicine* **2019**, *16*, 98–106. [CrossRef]

6. Muhlhausen, J.; Kitze, B.; Huppke, P.; Muller, G.A.; Koziolek, M.J. Apheresis in treatment of acute inflammatory demyelinating disorders. *Atheroscler. Suppl.* **2015**, *18*, 251–256. [CrossRef]

7. Schimrigk, S.; Faiss, J.; Köhler, W.; Günther, A.; Harms, L.; Kraft, A.; Ehrlich, S.; Eberl, A.; Fassbender, C.; Klingel, R.; et al. Escalation therapy of steroid refractory multiple sclerosis relapse with tryptophan immunoadsorption - Observational multicenter study with 147 patients. *Eur. Neurol.* **2016**, *75*, 300–306. [CrossRef]

8. Lipphardt, M.; Muhlhausen, J.; Kitze, B.; Heigl, F.; Mauch, E.; Helms, H.-J.; Müller, G.A.; Koziolek, M.J. Immunoadsorption or plasma exchange in steroid-refractory multiple sclerosis and neuromyelitis optica. *J. Clin. Apher.* **2019**, *30*, 381–391. [CrossRef]

9. Weinshenker, B.G.; O'Brien, P.C.; Petterson, T.M.; Noseworthy, J.H.; Lucchinetti, C.F.; Dodick, D.W.; Pineda, A.A.; Stevens, L.N.; Rodriguez, M. A randomized trial of plasma exchange in acute central nervous system inflammatory demyelinating disease. *Ann. Neurol.* **1999**, *46*, 878–886. [CrossRef]

10. Lipphardt, M.; Wallbach, M.; Koziolek, M.J. Plasma exchange or immunoadsorption in demyelinating diseases: A meta-analysis. *J. Clin. Med.* **2020**, *9*, 1597. [CrossRef]

11. Schneider-Gold, C.; Krenzer, M.; Klinker, E.; Mansouri-Thalegani, B.; Müllges, W.; Toyka, K.V.; Gold, R. Immunoadsorption versus plasma exchange versus combination for treatment of myasthenic deterioration. *Ther. Adv. Neurol. Disord.* **2016**, *9*, 297–303. [CrossRef] [PubMed]

12. Kohler, W.; Bucka, C.; Klingel, R. A randomized and controlled study comparing immunoadsorption and plasma exchange in myasthenic crisis. *J. Clin. Apher.* **2011**, *26*, 347–355. [CrossRef] [PubMed]

13. Bramlage, C.P.; Schröder, K.; Bramlage, P.; Ahrens, K.; Zapf, A.; Müller, G.A.; Koziolek, M.J. Predictors of complications in therapeutic plasma exchange. *J. Clin. Apher.* **2009**, *24*, 225–231. [CrossRef] [PubMed]

14. Basic-Jukic, N.; Kes, P.; Glavas-Boras, S.; Brunetta, B.; Bubic-Filipi, L.; Puretic, Z. Complications of therapeutic plasma exchange: Experience with 4857 treatments. *Ther. Apher. Dial.* **2005**, *9*, 391–395. [CrossRef]

15. Zöllner, S.; Pablik, E.; Druml, W.; Derfler, K.; Rees, A.; Biesenbach, P. Fibrinogen reduction and bleeding complications in plasma exchange, immunoadsorption and a combination of the two. *Blood Purif.* **2014**, *38*, 160–166. [CrossRef]

16. Lieker, I.; Slowinski, T.; Harms, L.; Hahn, K.; Klehmet, J. A prospective study comparing tryptophan immunoadsorption with therapeutic plasma exchange for the treatment of chronic inflammatory demyelinating polyneuropathy. *J. Clin. Apher.* **2017**, *32*, 486–493. [CrossRef]

17. Marn Pernat, A.; Buturovic-Ponikvar, J.; Svigelj, V.; Ponikvar, R. Guillain-Barre syndrome treated by membrane plasma exchange and/or immunoadsorption. *Ther. Apher. Dial.* **2009**, *13*, 310–313. [CrossRef]

18. Thompson, A.J.; Banwell, B.L.; Barkhof, F.; Carroll, W.M.; Coetzee, T.; Comi, G.; Correale, J.; Fazekas, F.; Filippi, M.; Freedman, M.S.; et al. Diagnosis of multiple sclerosis: 2017 revisions of the McDonald criteria. *Lancet Neurol.* **2018**, *17*, 162–173. [CrossRef]

19. Sprenger, K.B.; Huber, K.; Kratz, W.; Henze, E. Nomograms for the prediction of patient's plasma volume in plasma exchange therapy from height, weight, and hematocrit. *J. Clin. Apher.* **1987**, *3*, 185–190. [CrossRef]

20. Dorst, J.; Ludolph, A.C.; Senel, M.; Tumani, H. Short-term and long-term effects of immunoadsorption in refractory chronic inflammatory demyelinating polyneuropathy: A prospective study in 17 patients. *J. Neurol.* **2018**, *265*, 2906–2915. [CrossRef]

21. Merkies, I.S.; Schmitz, P.I.; van der Meche, F.G.; Samijn, J.P.; van Doorn, P.A. Clinimetric evaluation of a new overall disability scale in immune mediated polyneuropathies. *J. Neurol. Neurosurg. Psychiatry* **2002**, *72*, 596–601. [CrossRef] [PubMed]

22. Davies, A.J.; Fehmi, J.; Senel, M.; Tumani, H.; Dorst, J.; Rinaldi, S. Immunoadsorption and plasma exchange in seropositive and seronegative immune-mediated neuropathies. *J. Clin. Med.* **2020**, *9*, 2025. [CrossRef] [PubMed]

23. Pfeuffer, S.; Rolfes, L.; Bormann, E.; Sauerland, C.; Ruck, T.; Schilling, M.; Melzer, N.; Brand, M.; Pul, R.; Kleinschnitz, C.; et al. Comparing plasma exchange to escalated methyl prednisolone in refractory multiple sclerosis relapses. *J. Clin. Med.* **2020**, *9*, 35. [CrossRef] [PubMed]

24. Mokrzycki, M.H.; Kaplan, A.A. Therapeutic plasma exchange: Complications and management. *Am. J. Kidney Dis.* **1994**, *23*, 817–827. [CrossRef]

25. Samtleben, W.; Blumenstein, M.; Liebl, L.; Gurland, H.J. Membrane plasma separation for treatment of immunologically mediated diseases. *Trans. Am. Soc. Artif. Intern. Organs* **1980**, *26*, 12–16.

26. Sprenger, K.B.; Rasche, H.; Franz, H.E. Membrane plasma separation: Complications and monitoring. *Artif. Organs* **1984**, *8*, 360–363.

27. Pandey, S.; Vyas, G.N. Adverse effects of plasma transfusion. *Transfusion* **2012**, *52* (Suppl. 1), 65S–79S. [CrossRef]

28. Vincent, J.L.; Wilkes, M.M.; Navickis, R.J. Safety of human albumin—serious adverse events reported worldwide in 1998-2000. *Br. J. Anaesth.* **2003**, *91*, 625–630. [CrossRef]

29. Gjörstrup, P.; Watt, R.M. Therapeutic protein A immunoadsorption. A review. *Transfus. sci.* **1990**, *11*, 281–302. [CrossRef]

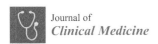

Journal of
Clinical Medicine

MDPI

Article

Myalgic Encephalomyelitis/Chronic Fatigue Syndrome: Efficacy of Repeat Immunoadsorption

Markus Tölle [1], Helma Freitag [2], Michaela Antelmann [2], Jelka Hartwig [2], Mirjam Schuchardt [1], Markus van der Giet [1], Kai-Uwe Eckardt [1], Patricia Grabowski [2,†] and Carmen Scheibenbogen [2,3,*,†]

1   Department of Nephrology and Medical Intensive Care, Charité—Universitätsmedizin Berlin, Corporate Member of Freie Universität Berlin, Humboldt Universität zu Berlin, and Berlin Institute of Health, 12203 Berlin, Germany; Markus.Toelle@charite.de (M.T.); Mirjam.Schuchardt@charite.de (M.S.); Markus.vanderGiet@charite.de (M.v.d.G.); Kai-Uwe.Eckardt@charite.de (K.-U.E.)
2   Institute of Medical Immunology, Charité—Universitätsmedizin Berlin, Corporate Member of Freie Universität Berlin, Humboldt Universität zu Berlin, and Berlin Institute of Health, 13353 Berlin, Germany; Helma.Freitag@charite.de (H.F.); Michaela.Antelmann@charite.de (M.A.); Jelka.Hartwig@charite.de (J.H.); Patricia.Grabowski@charite.de (P.G.)
3   Berlin-Brandenburg Center for Regenerative Therapies (BCRT), 13353 Berlin, Germany
*   Correspondence: Carmen.Scheibenbogen@charite.de
†   Shared senior.

Received: 13 July 2020; Accepted: 28 July 2020; Published: 30 July 2020

Abstract: (1) Myalgic Encephalomyelitis/Chronic Fatigue Syndrome (ME/CFS) is a complex neuroimmunological disease. There is evidence for an autoimmune mechanism for ME/CFS with an infection-triggered onset and dysfunction of ß$_2$-adrenoreceptor antibodies (ß$_2$AR-AB). In a first proof-of-concept study, we could show that IA was effective to reduce ß$_2$AR-AB and led to improvement of various symptoms. (2) Five of the ME/CFS patients who had clinical improvement following treatment with a five-day IA were retreated in the current study about two years later with a modified IA protocol. The severity of symptoms was assessed by disease specific scores during a follow-up period of 12 months. The antibodies were determined by ELISA. (3) The modified IA treatment protocol resulted in a remarkable similar clinical response. The treatment was well tolerated and 80–90% decline of total IgG and ß$_2$AR-AB was achieved. Four patients showed a rapid improvement in several clinical symptoms during IA therapy, lasting for six to 12 months. One patient had no improvement. (4) We could provide further evidence that IA has clinical efficacy in patients with ME/CFS. Data from our pilot trial warrant further controlled studies in ME/CFS.

Keywords: Myalgic Encephalomyelitis/Chronic Fatigue Syndrome; immunoadsorption; ß$_2$ adrenoreceptor autoantibody

1. Introduction

Myalgic encephalomyelitis/chronic fatigue syndrome (ME/CFS) is a debilitating disease that is characterized by persistent fatigue and exertional intolerance with disproportionate worsening after physical or cognitive exertion. Furthermore, it is accompanied by a variety of other symptoms that are related to immunological and autonomous dysfunction [1]. With an estimated prevalence of 0.1–0.5%, ME/CFS is a frequent and chronic disease that is often triggered by an acute infection [2]. Around 2.5 million Americans suffer from ME/CFS causing an annual financial cost up to 24 billion dollars per year [3]. ME/CFS affects all races, ages, and socioeconomic groups, with women affected 2–3 times more frequently than men [4,5]. Currently, the exact pathophysiology of ME/CFS is not well understood. There is increasing evidence for an autoimmune pathomechanism in ME/CFS [6].

Autoimmunity-related risk variants in PTPN22 and CTLA4 were found to be associated with ME/CFS with infectious onset in a recent study [7]. Several studies described autoantibodies in ME/CFS, including antibodies against nuclear and membrane structures, cardiolipin, neurotransmitter receptors, and against autoantigens formed by oxidative or nitrosative damage [6,8–10]. Elevated autoantibodies against the muscarinic acetylcholine receptors (MAR-AB) and ß$_2$-adrenoreceptor antibodies (ß$_2$AR-AB) could be detected in a subgroup of patients [11–13]. There is first evidence for a dysfunction of adrenergic receptor antibodies in ME/CFS [14,15]. A recent study showed a correlation between ß$_2$AR-AB and brain network alterations that was associated with pain [16]. Results from two clinical studies in which rituximab was used for depleting CD20+ B lymphocytes provided first evidence that B cells are involved in the pathogenesis of ME/CFS [17,18]. Approximately 60% of patients in the treatment group showed a partial or complete remission of clinical symptoms, lasting for more than six months in several patients. Interestingly, the clinical improvement was only seen after a time delay of three to four months. This indicates that the immediate depletion of CD20+ B cells has no direct effect, because CD20− antibody-producing plasma cells remain unaffected by rituximab treatment. There was a sustained reduction in ß$_2$AR-AB in patients who had a clinical response to rituximab [11].

An effective treatment option for autoantibody-mediated diseases is immunoadsorption (IA). By using specific adsorbers, the plasma concentration of immunoglobulin G (IgG) can be quickly and efficiently reduced [19]. Clinical symptoms of various autoimmune diseases that are associated with autoantibodies, including dilative cardiomyopathy, therapy refractive lupus erythematosus, and various neurological diseases, could be improved quickly by IA [20–22]. Recently, we described a proof-of-concept prospective observational IA study in ten patients with ME/CFS, in whom ß$_2$AR-AB were elevated [23]. Five cycles of IA were conducted on days one–three and six–seven. In nine patients, the ß$_2$AR-AB decreased rapidly during IA treatment and it was still significantly lower than the pretreatment level after six months. The frequency of memory B cells significantly decreased, whereas the frequency of plasma cells increased after a five-day IA cycle. A rapid improvement of symptoms was reported by 70% of patients already during IA. Three of these patients had long lasting improvement for more than 12 months and four patients had short improvement. However, two patients had a marked worsening of symptoms during IA and could not receive the fifth IA.

Here, we present data of a conformational trial. Patients who had responded to the first IA (IA1) were retreated with a modified IA protocol (IA2) about two years later. Here, IA cycles were given with longer intervals.

2. Materials and Methods

2.1. Patients

For the conformational trial, we adjusted the treatment protocol (IA2, see Figure 1). Five of the ten participants of our first study in 2016 were included in the current study. These patients had a transient or long-lasting improvement of clinical symptoms after the first IA therapy. Detailed inclusion criteria were described before [23]. In short, all of the patients fulfilled the Canadian Consensus Criteria [1], had increased ß$_2$AR-AB levels, and an infection-triggered disease onset.

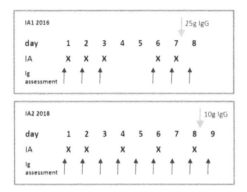

Figure 1. Treatment protocols of both studies. X indicates the point of time when immunoadsorption (IA) was conducted, black arrows when blood samples were collected, and blue arrow for immunoglobulin G (IgG) supplementation.

2.2. Study Protocol

During the IA1 study, we learned that repeated IA can worsen fatigue. Four patients had worsening of fatigue towards the end of treatment despite improvement of other symptoms. To improve the tolerability of the treatment, we extended the treatment period and reduced the dose of IgG replacement. IA was performed at day one, two, four, six, and eight (Figure 1) using Globaffin® columns (Fresenius, Bad Homburg, Germany), a broadband-immunoadsorber containing synthetic peptide-GAM® as ligand capable of binding IgG and immune complexes independent from their antigen specificity and, thus, useful for the removal of autoantibodies. Patients received 10 g polyclonal immunoglobulin substitution intravenously (Octagam, Octapharma, Langenfeld, Germany or Gammunex, Grifols, Frankfurt/M., Germany) to restore IgG plasma levels after the final IA session. The study was approved by the Ethics Committee of Charité - Universitätsmedizin Berlin (project code: EA2/063/15 from 10 September, 2018) in accordance with the 1964 Declaration of Helsinki and its later amendments. All of the patients gave written informed consent.

2.3. Assessment of Autoantibodies, Ig, Albumin and Fibrinogen

$ß_1AR$-/$ß_2AR$-AB and M3AR-/M4AR-AB were determined using ELISA technology by CellTrend GmbH (Luckenwalde, Germany), as in our previous study [23]. Total serum IgG, IgA, IgM, albumin, and fibrinogen were determined at the Charité diagnostics laboratory (Labor Berlin GmbH, Berlin, Germany).

2.4. Symptom Assessment by Scores

We assessed the presence and severity of symptoms, as described in our previous study [23]. In short, the patients quantified the severity of symptoms of the Canadian consensus criteria using a questionnaire that was developed by Fluge et al. [17,18]. After the determination of a baseline value, patients stated the improvement or worsening of symptoms (0–3: worsening; 3: no change from baseline; 3–6: improvement). The patients filled this questionnaire daily during treatment and monthly during follow-up. Furthermore, patients evaluated fatigue and cognitive impairment monthly using FACT-F questionnaire [24].

2.5. Statistical Analysis

We conducted statistical data analyses using GraphPad Prism version 6.0 software similarly to the first proof-of-concept study [23]. In short, we used nonparametric statistical methods, median and interquartile range (IQR) for continuous variables. For univariate comparisons, we used Wilcoxon matched-pairs signed-rank test and Mann–Whitney-U test or Fisher's exact test for independent groups. A two-tailed *p*-value of <0.05 was considered to be statistically significant.

3. Results

3.1. Patient Characteristics and IA Treatment

All of the patients had an infection-triggered onset of ME/CFS and all showed elevated levels of ß$_1$/ß$_2$-AR-AB and M3/M4-AR-AB (except patient 8 only ß$_2$). Bell disability scale indicating the severity of disease ranged from 30–75 (median of 45) and the median was significantly higher than before the first IA study in 2016 (median of 30, range 10–50, *p* = 0.01, Figure S1) corresponding to an increase of the ability to perform desk work from 2–3 h to 4 h daily [25]. Table 1 shows patient characteristics. The intervals between the cycles were extended in the present protocol in order to improve the tolerability of the treatment. Five cycles of IA were conducted within eight days (day 1, 2, 4, 6, and 8). A citrate-based anticoagulation was used. We observed a drop of fibrinogen and albumin levels in a similar extent compared to the first study (Figure S2). No albumin substitution was necessary and there was no bleeding episode. Immediately after the fifth IA, all apatients received 10 g IgG intravenously, as compared to 25 g in the first proof-of-concept study.

Table 1. Patients' characteristics.

Patient No. from 2016 Study	Gender	Age	ME/CFS Onset	Disease Severity Bell Score before IA1	Disease Severity Bell Score before IA2
2	f	60	2011	30	45
4	m	50	2000	20	35
5	f	37	2012	40	75
6	f	32	2002	50	60
8	f	32	2005	10	30

3.2. Course of IgG and Autoantibodies

Before IA treatment, the total IgG levels were within the normal range in all patients (median 9.85 g/L, range 8.99 to 13.26 g/L). As expected, the absolute IgG levels were strongly reduced already after the first IA with a minimum IgG level after the fourth IA (median 0.95, range 0.64 to 1.68 g/L). The absolute level of autoantibodies decreased in a comparable way, as shown in Figure 2. Figure 3 shows the relative decrease in IgG and autoantibody concentrations in each individual patient. The IgA and IgM levels did not change significantly (Figure S3).

3.3. Clinical Course

Before IA1, all of the patients suffered from severe exhaustion and post-exertional malaise grade 6–10 (0 none, 10 most severe symptoms) and from concentration impairment grade 4–10, muscle pain (*n* = 4), and immune-associated symptoms of sore throat, flu-like symptoms, and painful lymph nodes (Figure 4). Two years later, before the IA2, the total score of symptoms had improved in three of the five patients (patient 2, 4, and 5), was similar in patient 6, and slightly worse in patient 8 (shown in Figure 4). However, the Bell score was improved in patient 8 from 10 to 30 as she could not walk before the first IA due to marked muscle fatigue, which had considerably improved following the IA1.

The assessment of symptoms was performed daily during the IA2 (Figure 5) and afterwards monthly until month 12 (Figure 6). Interestingly, the course of symptoms was similar in IA2 as compared to IA1. Patients 2 and 8 (Figure 5) showed rapid improvement of all symptoms during IA2. In patient 4, muscle pain and immune symptoms improved. In patient 5, muscle pain disappeared during IA and cognitive and immune symptoms slightly improved, but fatigue worsened. Patient 6, who had a short-term improvement of cognition during IA1, had no improvement during the IA2. Patients 5, 6, and 8 had a transient worsening of symptoms after IgG infusion at day eight.

The course of symptoms during the 12 months after IA2 was again similar to the IA1 in all patients (Figure 6). Patient 2, 4, and 5 again showed a sustained improvement in symptoms for ten to 12 months, although with some fluctuations. Patient 8 had marked improvement for six months. When patient 8 worsened at month six a further IA treatment was offered, but she preferred to receive plasmapheresis on month 9 in her local hospital, which again almost completely resolved the symptoms. Patient 6, who had a two months improvement during IA1 with consecutive worsening, experienced an immediate worsening under IA2.

Further patients filled in FACT-F questionnaire monthly, assessing the severity of fatigue showing a similar course to IA1. A strong improvement of fatigue was reported by patients 5 and 8, while patient 2 and 4 only had a slight improvement of fatigue in accordance to the fatigue that was reported in the symptom score (Figures 6 and 7).

Regarding tolerability, three of the five patients had a worsening of fatigue from day 6 on during IA1, but two patients had marked worsening of fatigue also during IA2.

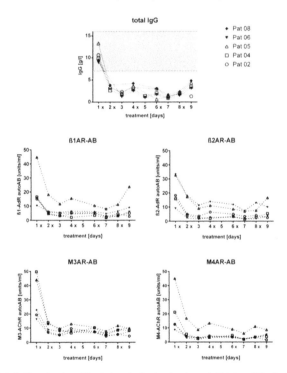

Figure 2. Absolute IgG and autoantibody levels during treatment. Total and β_1, β_2, M3, and M4 IgG in the serum before and during IA. X indicates the point of time when IA was conducted. Gray area indicates reference range of serum levels.

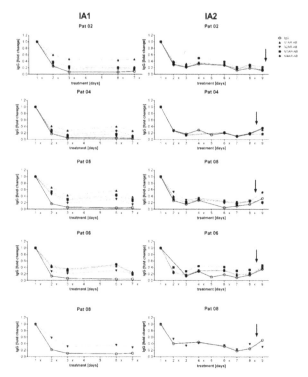

Figure 3. Relative IgG and autoantibody levels during treatment. Relative changes of total IgG and ß₁, ß₂, M3, and M4 autoantibody concentration in the serum before and during first IA 2016 (left) and second IA (right). The daily levels are depicted as x-fold change to day 1 level for each single patient. X indicates the single IA, arrow when patients received 10 g IgG i.v.

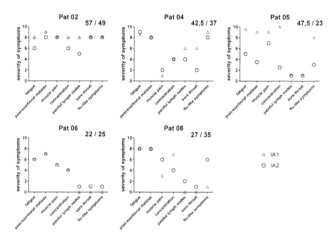

Figure 4. Patients condition before first and second treatment. Symptom scores before first IA (triangle) and second IA (circle). Symptoms are indicated as 0 (absent) to 10 (most severe). Sum of each patient is displayed in the upper right corner (left: IA1, right: IA2).

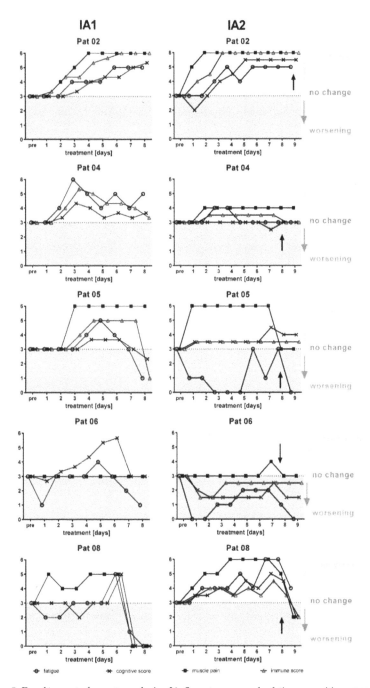

Figure 5. Development of symptoms during IA. Symptom scores for fatigue, cognitive score, muscle pain and immune score during IA1 (left) and IA2 (right) are shown for each patient (3 unchanged, 4 slight, 5 marked improvement, 6 complete disappearance, 2 slight increase, 1 marked increase). The line indicates level 3 for unchanged symptoms.

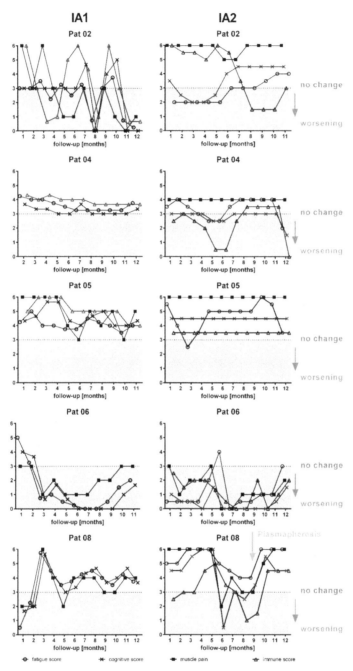

Figure 6. Development of symptoms during 12 months follow-up. Symptom scores for fatigue, cognitive score, muscle pain and immune score during first IA (left) and second IA (right) are shown for each patient (3 unchanged, 4 slight, 5 marked improvement, 6 complete disappearance, 2 slight increase, 1 marked increase). The line indicates level 3 for unchanged symptoms.

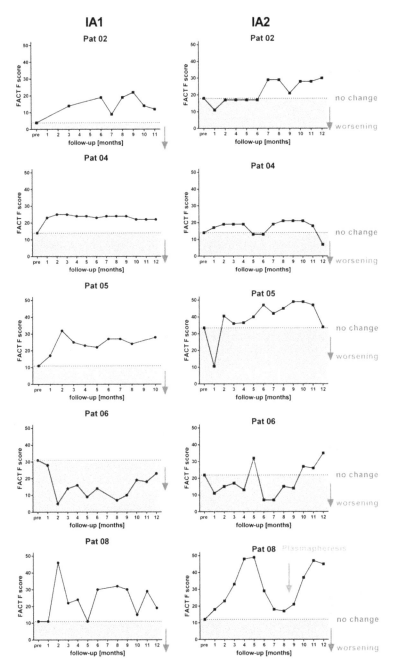

Figure 7. FACT-F score follow-up. Score of FACT-F questionnaire assessing severity of fatigue before and up to 12 months after first IA (left) in comparison to second IA (right) for each patient. Scoring of FACT-F fatigue questionnaire ranges from 0 (strongly fatigued) to a maximum of 52 (without fatigue). Dotted line indicates the individual pretreatment score before IA.

4. Discussion

In our first proof-of-concept study in ten patients with infection-triggered ME/CFS, we observed that IA caused a rapid decrease in ß$_2$AR-AB levels in nine of ten patients. Moreover, an improvement in clinical symptoms could be achieved in seven of the patients, which lasted, in three patients, for more than 12 months [23]. Furthermore, the ME/CFS patients frequently suffer from endothelial dysfunction, which was also improved following IA [26]. These results provided first evidence that IA may be a therapeutic option in ME/CFS patients and the rapid relief from clinical symptoms may be explained by the removal of autoantibodies. We also found a decrease of memory B cells following IA1 and significantly lower ß$_2$AR-AB after six months, suggesting that IA may have an effect on autoreactive memory B cells as well. Repeated IA were shown in other autoimmune diseases to enhance efficacy or induce a second remission [19–21].

Therefore, we conducted a conformational study in five patients with a clinical response in the first study and retreated them with second IA. Remarkably, disease severity was still improved before IA2 when compared to before IA1 two years earlier, with a higher Bell score in all five patients. During IA1, two patients had considerable worsening of all ME/CFS symptoms, which may be attributed to their enhanced susceptibility to stress and changes in the water and electrolyte balance. In addition, four patients had worsening of fatigue during IA1. Despite longer intervals between the cycles during IA2, two patients, however, had again marked worsening of fatigue. When compared to the IA1 protocol, the IA2 protocol resulted in a comparable decrease in IgG and autoantibody concentrations.

As in the IA1 study, the clinical symptoms that were associated with ME/CFS were assessed with a questionnaire quantifying the most important symptoms of the CCC [1,17] The descriptions of subjective self-reported symptom correlated well with the objective activity tracking of steps per day in IA1 [23]. Similar to IA1, we could observe an improvement of several clinical symptoms during IA in four of five patients lasting with some fluctuations for 6–12 months. The patient who experienced marked worsening also only had a moderate and transient improvement in symptoms after IA1.

Of interest is that one patient received a plasmapheresis nine months after IA2, which again almost completely resolved the symptoms. Plasmapheresis constitutes another possibility to eliminate pathogenic antibodies by exchange of patient with donor plasma, but its efficacy has not been assessed in ME/CFS to our knowledge. In other diseases, it was shown that IA and plasmapheresis both resulted in comparable clinical efficacy [27].

Our observations are in line with the clinical results of IA in neuro-immunological diseases or dilative cardiomyopathy [27,28]. Dilative cardiomyopathy is often associated with ß$_1$AR-AB, which could be effectively reduced by IA leading to a long-term improvement in the clinical outcome [28]. Clinical features of a refractory lupus erythematosus, like proteinuria, SLEDAI (activity index for systemic lupus erythematosus disease) and autoantibody concentrations, could be successfully improved and stabilized at levels that meet the criteria of remission in the long term by the regular use of an IA for up to ten years [20].

In our first study, a sustained decrease of ß$_2$ IgG was observed at month six, which could also be shown in responder to the rituximab therapy [11]. The long-term decline of autoantibody concentrations may be explained due to enhanced B cell differentiation with a higher apoptosis rate of autoreactive B cells and consecutive loss of short living autoreactive plasma cells [11]. This hypothesis would correspond to the observed decrease in ß$_2$AR-AB six months after IA1, when the levels of total IgG and tetanus and pneumococcal IgG corresponded to the pretreatment ones [11]. However, the effect of adrenergic stimulation on immune cells is complex and does not directly correlate with levels of ß$_2$AR-AB [14]. ß$_2$AR-AB belong to a network of natural antibodies against G-protein coupled receptors, which has been described to be dysregulated in various autoimmune diseases [29]. In our recent study, we found that ß$_2$AR-AB activate the ß$_2$AR. The ß$_2$AR activation by IgG was attenuated in ME/CFS patients, which could explain many symptoms of ME/CFS [14]. As IA removes total IgG, we have, however, no direct evidence from our study that the removal of ß$_2$AR itself leads to improvement. Several other autoantibodies were reported in ME/CFS [6].

J. Clin. Med. **2020**, *9*, 2443

In this study, the patients received a single IgG infusion at the end of IA protocol in order to partially restore the strong IgG depletion. IgG treatment is also effective in autoantibody-mediated autoimmune diseases [30]. Doses applied for treatment of autoimmune disease are usually above 1.0 g/kg body weight. In the current study, an approximately 10-fold lower and single dose of IgG was applied, so that the treatment effect due to the IgG administration seems unlikely.

Limitations of the current trial are the small number of patients and the lack of a placebo control group. One aspect of this study was to investigate the reproducibility of the effect of IA on clinical symptoms in a subset of patients from the first study. In all patients, the effect of IA treatment could be reproduced. Although some placebo-treated patients showed an improvement in randomized placebo-controlled trials (RCT) in ME/CFS [18,31], the reproducibility and the long lasting symptom improvement associated with a significantly decreased frequency of memory B cells, increased frequency of plasma cells, and lower autoantibody concentration six month after IA1 rather speaks against an unspecific effect. Further, although being considered unlikely, IgG replacement at the end of IA may have an immunomodulatory effect. Therefore, we have intentionally kept the IgG dose in the current study lower to minimize this potential effect.

Our study was designed to get further evidence for efficacy and tolerability prior to performing a consecutive RCT. We have evidence for similar clinical and immunological efficacy of this schedule.

5. Conclusions

In summary, the current study provides further evidence that IA is effective in ME/CFS. This result warrants further studies of repeat IA therapy to maintain clinical remission, as shown for other autoimmune diseases [20]. Another option is to include IA in a therapy algorithm as initial therapy for autoantibody-positive ME/CFS patients in order to achieve rapid symptom relief and, therefore, shorten the known time latency of four months or longer until the onset of efficacy of B cell-targeting therapies.

Supplementary Materials: The following are available online at http://www.mdpi.com/2077-0383/9/8/2443/s1, Figure S1: Initial Bell score., Figure S2: Albumin and fibrinogen serum concentrations., Figure S3: IgA and IgM serum concentrations.

Author Contributions: Conceptualization, M.T., P.G. and C.S.; methodology, M.T., H.F. and C.S.; validation, M.T., H.F., M.S., M.v.d.G. and K.-U.E.; formal analysis, M.T., H.F., J.H., P.G. and C.S.; investigation, M.T., H.F., M.A., J.H., P.G. and C.S.; data curation, H.F.; writing—original draft preparation, M.T., H.F. and C.S.; writing—review and editing, M.T., H.F., M.S., M.v.d.G., K.-U.E., P.G. and C.S.; visualization, H.F.; supervision, M.T. and C.S.; project administration, M.T. and C.S.; funding acquisition, M.T. and C.S. All authors have read and agreed to the published version of the manuscript.

Funding: This investigator-initiated trial was funded Fresenius Medical Care Germany GmbH and the Weidenhammer Zöbele foundation.

Acknowledgments: We thank Rene Stipp, Fresenius, for his technical support.

Conflicts of Interest: M.T. received research grants from Fresenius Medical Care, speaker's honoraria from Baxter International, and Diamed Medizintechnik. C.S. received research grants and speakers' honoraria from Fresenius Medical Care. All other authors declare no conflict of interest.

References

1. Carruthers, B.M.; van de Sande, M.I.; De Meirleir, K.L.; Klimas, N.G.; Broderick, G.; Mitchell, T.; Staines, D.; Powles, A.C.; Speight, N.; Vallings, R.; et al. Myalgic Encephalomyelitis: International Consensus Criteria. *J. Intern. Med.* **2011**, *270*, 327–338. [CrossRef]
2. Chu, L.; Valencia, I.J.; Garvert, D.W.; Montoya, J.G. Onset Patterns and Course of Myalgic Encephalomyelitis/Chronic Fatigue Syndrome. *Front. Pediatr.* **2019**, *7*, 12. [CrossRef]
3. Clayton, E.W.; Biaggionni, I.; Cockshell, S.; Vermeculen, R.; Snell, C.; Rove, K. *Beyond Myalgic Encephalomyelitis/Chronic Fatigue Syndrome: Redefining an Illness*; The National Academies Press: Washington, DC, USA, 2015.

4. Rowe, P.C.; Underhill, R.; Friedman, K.J.; Gurwitt, A.; Medow, M.S.; Schwartz, M.S.; Speight, N.; Stewart, J.M.; Vallings, R.; Rowe, K.S. Myalgic Encephalomyelitis/Chronic Fatigue Syndrome Diagnosis and Management in Young People: A Primer. *Front. Pediatr.* **2017**, *5*. [CrossRef]

5. Valdez, A.R.; Hancock, E.E.; Adebayo, S.; Kiernicki, D.J.; Proskauer, D.; Attewell, J.R.; Bateman, L.; DeMaria, A.J.; Lapp, C.W.; Rowe, P.C.; et al. Estimating Prevalence, Demographics, and Costs of ME/CFS Using Large Scale Medical Claims Data and Machine Learning. *Front. Pediatr.* **2019**, *6*, 412. [CrossRef]

6. Sotzny, F.; Blanco, J.; Capelli, E.; Castro-Marrero, J.; Steiner, S.; Murovska, M.; Scheibenbogen, C. Myalgic Encephalomyelitis/Chronic Fatigue Syndrome—Evidence for an autoimmune disease. *Autoimmun. Rev.* **2018**, *17*, 601–609. [CrossRef]

7. Steiner, S.; Becker, S.C.; Hartwig, J.; Sotzny, F.; Lorenz, S.; Bauer, S.; Löbel, M.; Stittrich, A.B.; Grabowski, P.; Scheibenbogen, C. Autoimmunity-Related Risk Variants in PTPN22 and CTLA4 Are Associated With ME/CFS With Infectious Onset. *Front. Immunol.* **2020**, *11*. [CrossRef]

8. Klein, R.; A Berg, P. High incidence of antibodies to 5-hydroxytryptamine, gangliosides and phospholipids in patients with chronic fatigue and fibromyalgia syndrome and their relatives: Evidence for a clinical entity of both disorders. *Eur. J. Med. Res.* **1995**, *1*, 21–26.

9. Maes, M.; Mihaylova, I.; Kubera, M.; Leunis, J.C.; Twisk, F.N.; Geffard, M. Igm-Mediated Autoimmune Responses Directed against Anchorage Epitopes Are Greater in Myalgic Encephalomyelitis/Chronic Fatigue Syndrome (Me/Cfs) Than in Major Depression. *Metab. Brain Dis.* **2012**, *27*, 415–423. [CrossRef] [PubMed]

10. Ortega-Hernandez, O.-D.; Cuccia, M.; Bozzini, S.; Bassi, N.; Moscavitch, S.; Diaz-Gallo, L.M.; Blank, M.; Agmon-Levin, N.; Shoenfeld, Y. Autoantibodies, Polymorphisms in the Serotonin Pathway, and Human Leukocyte Antigen Class II Alleles in Chronic Fatigue Syndrome. *Ann. N. Y. Acad. Sci.* **2009**, *1173*, 589–599. [CrossRef] [PubMed]

11. Löbel, M.; Grabowski, P.; Heidecke, H.; Bauer, S.; Hanitsch, L.; Wittke, K.; Meisel, C.; Reinke, P.; Volk, H.-D.; Fluge, Ø.; et al. Antibodies to β adrenergic and muscarinic cholinergic receptors in patients with Chronic Fatigue Syndrome. *Brain Behav. Immun.* **2016**, *52*, 32–39. [CrossRef] [PubMed]

12. Tanaka, S.; Kuratsune, H.; Hidaka, Y.; Hakariya, Y.; Tatsumi, K.-I.; Takano, T.; Kanakura, Y.; Amino, N. Autoantibodies against muscarinic cholinergic receptor in chronic fatigue syndrome. *Int. J. Mol. Med.* **2003**, *12*, 225–230. [CrossRef] [PubMed]

13. Yamamoto, S.; Ouchi, Y.; Nakatsuka, D.; Tahara, T.; Mizuno, K.; Tajima, S.; Onoe, H.; Yoshikawa, E.; Tsukada, H.; Iwase, M.; et al. Reduction of [11C](+)3-MPB Binding in Brain of Chronic Fatigue Syndrome with Serum Autoantibody against Muscarinic Cholinergic Receptor. *PLoS ONE* **2012**, *7*, e51515. [CrossRef] [PubMed]

14. Hartwig, J.; Sotzny, F.; Bauer, S.; Heidecke, H.; Riemekasten, G.; Dragun, D.; Meisel, C.; Dames, C.; Grabowski, P.; Scheibenbogen, C. IgG stimulated β2 adrenergic receptor activation is attenuated in patients with ME/CFS. *Brain Behav. Immun. Health* **2020**, *3*. [CrossRef]

15. Wirth, K.; Scheibenbogen, C. A Unifying Hypothesis of the Pathophysiology of Myalgic Encephalomyelitis/Chronic Fatigue Syndrome (ME/CFS): Recognitions from the finding of autoantibodies against ß2-adrenergic receptors. *Autoimmun. Rev.* **2020**, *19*, 102527. [CrossRef]

16. Fujii, H.; Sato, W.; Kimura, Y.; Matsuda, H.; Ota, M.; Maikusa, N.; Suzuki, F.; Amano, K.; Shin, I.; Yamamura, T.; et al. Altered Structural Brain Networks Related to Adrenergic/Muscarinic Receptor Autoantibodies in Chronic Fatigue Syndrome. *J. Neuroimaging* **2020**. [CrossRef]

17. Fluge, Ø.; Bruland, O.; Risa, K.; Storstein, A.; Kristoffersen, E.K.; Sapkota, D.; Næss, H.; Dahl, O.; Nyland, H.; Mella, O. Benefit from B-Lymphocyte Depletion Using the Anti-CD20 Antibody Rituximab in Chronic Fatigue Syndrome. A Double-Blind and Placebo-Controlled Study. *PLoS ONE* **2011**, *6*, e26358. [CrossRef]

18. Fluge, Ø.; Risa, K.; Lunde, S.; Alme, K.; Rekeland, I.G.; Sapkota, D.; Kristoffersen, E.K.; Sørland, K.; Bruland, O.; Dahl, O.; et al. B-Lymphocyte Depletion in Myalgic Encephalopathy/Chronic Fatigue Syndrome. An Open-Label Phase II Study with Rituximab Maintenance Treatment. *PLoS ONE* **2015**, *10*, e0129898. [CrossRef]

19. Padmanabhan, A.; Connelly-Smith, L.; Aqui, N.; Balogun, R.A.; Klingel, R.; Meyer, E.; Pham, H.P.; Schneiderman, J.; Witt, V.; Wu, Y.; et al. Guidelines on the Use of Therapeutic Apheresis in Clinical Practice—Evidence-Based Approach from the Writing Committee of the American Society for Apheresis: The Eighth Special Issue. *J. Clin. Apher.* **2019**, *34*, 171–354. [CrossRef]

20. Stummvoll, G.; Schmaldienst, S.; Smolen, J.S.; Derfler, K.; Biesenbach, P. Lupus nephritis: Prolonged immunoadsorption (IAS) reduces proteinuria and stabilizes global disease activity. *Nephrol. Dial. Transplant.* **2011**, *27*, 618–626. [CrossRef]

21. Dandel, M.; Wallukat, G.; Englert, A.; Hetzer, R. Immunoadsorption therapy for dilated cardiomyopathy and pulmonary arterial hypertension. *Atheroscler. Suppl.* **2013**, *14*, 203–211. [CrossRef]

22. Wallukat, G.; Müller, J.; Hetzer, R. Specific Removal of β1-Adrenergic Autoantibodies from Patients with Idiopathic Dilated Cardiomyopathy. *N. Engl. J. Med.* **2002**, *347*, 1806. [CrossRef] [PubMed]

23. Scheibenbogen, C.; Loebel, M.; Freitag, H.; Krueger, A.; Bauer, S.; Antelmann, M.; Doehner, W.; Scherbakov, N.; Heidecke, H.; Reinke, P.; et al. Immunoadsorption to remove ß2 adrenergic receptor antibodies in Chronic Fatigue Syndrome CFS/ME. *PLoS ONE* **2018**, *13*, e0193672. [CrossRef] [PubMed]

24. Cella, D. The Functional Assessment of Cancer Therapy-Anemia (FACT-An) Scale: A new tool for the assessment of outcomes in cancer anemia and fatigue. *Semin. Hematol.* **1997**, *34*, 13–19. [PubMed]

25. Bell, D.S. *The Doctor's Guide to Chronic Fatigue Syndrome: Understanding, Treating, and Living with Cfids*; Reprint, Reprint edition (18 January 1995); Da Capo Press: Boston, MA, USA, 1995.

26. Scherbakov, N.; Szklarski, M.; Hartwig, J.; Sotzny, F.; Lorenz, S.; Meyer, A.; Grabowski, P.; Doehner, W.; Scheibenbogen, C. Peripheral endothelial dysfunction in myalgic encephalomyelitis/chronic fatigue syndrome. *ESC Heart Fail.* **2020**, *7*, 1064–1071. [CrossRef]

27. Heine, J.; Ly, L.-T.; Lieker, I.; Slowinski, T.; Finke, C.; Prüss, H.; Harms, L. Immunoadsorption or plasma exchange in the treatment of autoimmune encephalitis: A pilot study. *J. Neurol.* **2016**, *263*, 2395–2402. [CrossRef]

28. Dandel, M.; Wallukat, G.; Englert, A.; Lehmkuhl, H.; Knosalla, C.; Hetzer, R. Long-Term Benefits of Immunoadsorption in B1-Adrenoceptor Autoantibody-Positive Transplant Candidates with Dilated Cardiomyopathy. *Eur. J. Heart. Fail.* **2012**, *14*, 1374–1388. [CrossRef]

29. Cabral-Marques, O.; Marques, A.; Giil, L.M.; De Vito, R.; Rademacher, J.; Günther, J.; Lange, T.; Humrich, J.Y.; Klapa, S.; Schinke, S.; et al. GPCR-specific autoantibody signatures are associated with physiological and pathological immune homeostasis. *Nat. Commun.* **2018**, *9*, 5224. [CrossRef]

30. Perez, E.E.; Orange, J.S.; Bonilla, F.; Chinen, J.; Chinn, I.K.; Dorsey, M.; El-Gamal, Y.; Harville, T.O.; Hossny, E.; Mazer, B.; et al. Update on the use of immunoglobulin in human disease: A review of evidence. *J. Allergy Clin. Immunol.* **2017**, *139*, S1–S46. [CrossRef]

31. Whiting, P.F.; Bagnall, A.-M.; Sowden, A.J.; Cornell, J.E.; Mulrow, C.D.; Ramirez, G. Interventions for the Treatment and Management of Chronic Fatigue Syndrome. *JAMA* **2001**, *286*, 1360–1368. [CrossRef]

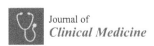

Journal of
Clinical Medicine

Article

Immunoadsorption and Plasma Exchange in Seropositive and Seronegative Immune-Mediated Neuropathies

Alexander J. Davies [1], Janev Fehmi [1], Makbule Senel [2], Hayrettin Tumani [2], Johannes Dorst [2,†] and Simon Rinaldi [1,*,†]

[1] Nuffield Department of Clinical Neurosciences, University of Oxford, Oxford OX3 9DU, UK; alexander.davies@ndcn.ox.ac.uk (A.J.D.); janev.fehmi@sjc.ox.ac.uk (J.F.)
[2] Department of Neurology, University of Ulm, 89081 Ulm, Germany; makbule.senel@uni-ulm.de (M.S.); hayrettin.tumani@uni-ulm.de (H.T.); johannes.dorst@uni-ulm.de (J.D.)
* Correspondence: simon.rinaldi@ndcn.ox.ac.uk
† These authors contributed equally to this work.

Received: 19 May 2020; Accepted: 24 June 2020; Published: 27 June 2020

Abstract: The inflammatory neuropathies are disabling conditions with diverse immunological mechanisms. In some, a pathogenic role for immunoglobulin G (IgG)-class autoantibodies is increasingly appreciated, and immunoadsorption (IA) may therefore be a useful therapeutic option. We reviewed the use of and response to IA or plasma exchange (PLEx) in a cohort of 41 patients with nodal/paranodal antibodies identified from a total of 573 individuals with suspected inflammatory neuropathies during the course of routine diagnostic testing (PNAb cohort). 20 patients had been treated with PLEx and 4 with IA. Following a global but subjective evaluation by their treating clinicians, none of these patients were judged to have had a good response to either of these treatment modalities. Sequential serology of one PNAb+ case suggests prolonged suppression of antibody levels with frequent apheresis cycles or adjuvant therapies, may be required for effective treatment. We further retrospectively evaluated the serological status of 40 patients with either Guillain-Barré syndrome (GBS) or chronic inflammatory demyelinating polyneuropathy (CIDP), and a control group of 20 patients with clinically-isolated syndrome/multiple sclerosis (CIS/MS), who had all been treated with IgG-depleting IA (IA cohort). 32 of these patients (8/20 with CIDP, 13/20 with GBS, 11/20 with MS) were judged responsive to apheresis despite none of the serum samples from this cohort testing positive for IgG antibodies against glycolipids or nodal/paranodal cell-adhesion molecules. Although negative on antigen specific assays, three patients' pre-treatment sera and eluates were reactive against different components of myelinating co-cultures. In summary, preliminary evidence suggests that GBS/CIDP patients without detectable IgG antibodies on routine diagnostic tests may nevertheless benefit from IA, and that an unbiased screening approach using myelinating co-cultures may assist in the detection of further autoantibodies which remain to be identified in such patients.

Keywords: Inflammatory neuropathy; chronic inflammatory demyelinating polyneuropathy; Guillain-Barré syndrome; multiple sclerosis; paranodal antibodies; plasmapheresis; plasma exchange; immunoadsorption

---

1. Introduction

The inflammatory neuropathies are a heterogeneous group of disorders in which peripheral nerve function and structure are disturbed by largely ill-defined immunological mechanisms [1]. They can broadly be divided into acute and chronic forms, typified by the umbrella terms Guillain-Barré syndrome (GBS) and chronic inflammatory demyelinating polyneuropathy (CIDP), respectively.

Humoral and cellular immunity are likely to play a role in the pathogenesis of both syndromes. For some clinically defined subtypes, a role for the humoral immune system and pathogenic autoantibodies appears to be more prominent [2,3], but particularly at the level of the individual patient, a direct and consistent link between the clinical syndrome, serological profile, and underlying immunopathological mechanism remains difficult to establish.

Randomised controlled trials have demonstrated that therapeutic plasma exchange (PLEx) speeds up recovery from GBS [4], and provides at least a short-term improvement in disability in CIDP [5]. In both conditions there is evidence that intravenous immunoglobulin (IVIg) has similar efficacy [6,7]. Two small, randomised studies have compared immunoadsorption (IA) with PLEx or IVIg in CIDP. Response rates to IA (6/9 using tryptophan-based columns [8] and 4/5 using protein A [9]) were not significantly different to their respective comparators. The trial comparing IA (using protein A) with IVIg had a high drop-out rate and was excluded from the relevant Cochrane review due to a high risk of bias [9]. Two further reports described the crossover from PLEx to IA in CIDP, in a single patient each, reaching opposite conclusions about which was more efficacious [10,11]. A number of retrospective case series and case reports have favourably evaluated immunoadsorption in both GBS and CIDP [12–21]. A retrospective Japanese report of IA in GBS found that patients who received IA within 6 days of onset of their neuropathy had a more rapid improvement in disability compared to those who received supportive care alone, whereas patients who received IA later than this in their disease course did not [22]. However, high-quality evidence demonstrating the efficacy of IA in the inflammatory neuropathies is lacking [23]. There is also some evidence that apheresis can improve recovery from multiple sclerosis relapses, and these approaches are often used after inadequate responses to corticosteroids [24,25].

Certain subtypes of GBS are associated with immunoglobulin (Ig) G ganglioside antibodies [26], with a handful of small studies showing an effective reduction of antibody titres using IA [19,27]. More recently a subset of CIDP-like neuropathies have been linked to predominantly IgG4-subclass antibodies directed against nodal or paranodal cell-adhesion molecules [28–32]. It has been speculated that patients with such antibodies may respond particularly well to selective IgG immunoadsorption [33]. A recent case series of four patients with CIDP and neurofascin-155 (NF155) antibodies reported that PLEx was effective in 3, and partially effective in 1, whilst tryptophan-based IA was ineffective in one such patient [34].

There are of course substantial differences between PLEx and IA. The former removes a broad range of circulating molecules and requires the use of replacement fluid, typically fresh frozen plasma, or albumin. Replacement fluid is not required in IA, and the range of circulating factors removed is more limited. This is advantageous in reducing complications, such as those due to the unwanted removal of coagulation factors [35], but may also lead to a loss of therapeutic effect if this depends on the removal of pro-inflammatory cytokines, or other pathogenically-relevant molecules, rather than immunoglobulins. It is also important to appreciate that there are variations in the biological effects between the different types of IA, which may also influence their clinical efficacy. For example, Yuki and colleagues have previously demonstrated that tryptophan-based columns are more effective than phenylalanine for adsorbing anti-ganglioside antibodies [36]. IA using protein A or synthetic ligands has been proposed as a method to remove a larger fraction of circulating IgG more selectively and quickly, whilst more modestly affecting IgM and IgA levels, and leaving complement, albumin and fibrinogen largely unaffected [37].

Intuitively, it may be assumed that patients who respond to "Ig-selective" IA do so because pathogenic Ig is being removed from the circulation. However, previous assessments of IA efficacy rarely report serological status. It is therefore currently unclear as to whether the presence of known serum autoantibodies in GBS and CIDP prospectively identifies a subpopulation of patients who are likely to respond more favourably to IA. It is also unclear as to whether any particular IA system or treatment programme is more likely to produce a positive outcome.

In this study we provide a retrospective evaluation of apheresis in two serologically-defined patient cohorts. We first reviewed the subjective clinician-reported overall impression of response to IA or PLEx in a cohort of neuropathy patients identified during routine diagnostic testing (PNAb cohort), and compared patients in which nodal/paranodal antibodies were or were not detected. We present the detailed case history and parallel serological analysis of a patient with NF155 antibodies who was treated with IA. Finally, we perform a retrospective analysis of the serological status of a sample of 60 patients who had been treated with IgG-depleting IA (IA cohort) and compare this with clinician-reported outcomes.

2. Experimental Section

2.1. Paranodal Antibody (PNAb) Patient Cohort

Since 2015, 88 patients with confirmed or suspected inflammatory neuropathies presenting to the neuropathy clinic in Oxford have been recruited to an observational study. This study was approved by the National Health Service (NHS) National Research Ethics Service Committee (South Central–Oxford A, 14/SC/0280). Patients recruited prior to 2017 were tested retrospectively, and those recruited from 2017 prospectively, for nodal/paranodal antibodies by the methods described in Appendix A. Since August 2017, serum samples from a further 537 external patients with confirmed or suspected inflammatory neuropathies have been received for diagnostic nodal/paranodal antibody testing by the Oxford laboratory. Clinical information was requested for all patients, including details of treatments used, and a clinician-led, subjective, overall impression of their efficacy.

2.2. IA Patient Cohort

The IA cohort consisted of 60 subjects (20 with CIDP, 20 with GBS, and a control group of 20 with multiple sclerosis/clinically-isolated syndrome, MS/CIS) who were selected from patients treated with IA between June 2013 and January 2018 in the University of Ulm, Department of Neurology based on the inclusion criteria outlined below. The study was reviewed by the appropriate ethics committee of the University of Ulm (approval number 20/10) and was performed in accordance with the ethical standards of the Declaration of Helsinki from 1964. Written informed consent for the sample collection was obtained from all patients participating in this study.

2.2.1. CIDP

All patients with CIDP fulfilled the EFNS criteria for possible, probable, or definite CIDP, had a continuously progressive course of disease, and had previously received several cycles of steroids ($n = 5$), IVIg ($n = 2$) or both ($n = 13$), with insufficient response. Fifteen patients who had previously received IVIg showed further disease progression under IVIg therapy, therefore we opted for a new therapeutic approach with IA. In 5 patients who had never received IVIg we chose IA instead of IVIg based on our favourable clinical experience with IA in CIDP. Two patients had never been treated with prednisolone because of severe diabetes mellitus. Further treatments included azathioprine ($n = 5$), cyclophosphamide ($n = 1$), mycophenolate mofetil ($n = 2$), and methotrexate ($n = 1$). Assessment of the clinical outcome directly and 2 weeks after IA was based on the Inflammatory Neuropathy Cause and Treatment (INCAT) score [38] and the Ulmer CIDP score, which includes the INCAT, the Oxford muscle strength grading scale (Medical Research Council, MRC), and vibration sensitivity testing [33].

2.2.2. GBS

All patients with GBS showed the typical clinical picture including rapidly progressive bilateral limb weakness and sensory deficits, hypo-/areflexia, electrophysiological signs of demyelination, and increased protein levels in cerebrospinal fluid. Anti-ganglioside antibodies were not tested prospectively. In contrast to CIDP and MS, IA was a first-line therapy in 4 GBS patients, and used as an escalation therapy in 9 more. In order to establish equally sized subgroups, the GBS group included

7 patients who received PLEx rather than IA. Classification of the clinical outcome (no improvement, equivocal improvement, partial improvement, large improvement) directly after the last treatment was retrospectively based on the neurological examination as documented in the medical records (discharge letter) of each patient.

2.2.3. MS/CIS

All patients fulfilled the 2017 MacDonald diagnostic criteria for MS [39] or CIS. All patients treated with IA suffered from a steroid-refractory relapse, i.e., an acute relapse without complete remission after one or more cycles of high dose intravenous methylprednisolone (IVMP) therapy (at least 3×1000 mg). Assessment of the clinical outcome directly after the last treatment was based on the Expanded Disability Status Scale (EDSS).

2.3. IA Treatment

One cycle of IA consisted of five treatments on 5 consecutive days. The total plasma volume of each patient was calculated using body weight, height, and haematocrit. Two plasma volumes were processed during the first treatment, and 2.5 plasma volumes were processed during all the subsequent treatments. The Adsorber system (ADAsorb, medicap clinic GmbH, Ulrichstein, Germany) contained two regenerating protein A columns (Immunosorba, Fresenius Medical Care, Bad Homburg, Germany).

2.4. Sample Collection and Storage

Eluate samples were obtained during each IA treatment and buffered with bicarbonate (pH 7.0). Serum samples were obtained before and after each IA treatment. A standardized protocol for serum and eluate collection was applied as previously recommended [40]. All biosamples were stored according to the predefined standard operating procedure (SOPs) at the local biobank in Ulm at minus 80 °C within two hours. Later they were transferred for measurement on dry ice to Oxford for further analysis.

2.5. Serological Analysis

Sera and eluates from the 3 patient cohorts and from control subjects were analysed using a nodal/paranodal antibody cell-based assay, paranodal, ganglioside and sulfatide ELISA, and against myelinating co-cultures. Methodological details for these experiments are given in Appendix A.

3. Results

3.1. Nodal/Paranodal Antibody (PNAb) Diagnostic Cohort

3.1.1. Demographics, Clinical and Serological Characteristics

Since August 2018, serum samples from 537 different patients with confirmed or suspected inflammatory neuropathies have been received for diagnostic nodal/paranodal antibody testing by the Oxford laboratory, and we have tested a further 88 patients from our own research cohort. Overall, 42/625 patients (6.7%) were positive for nodal/paranodal antibodies (PNAb+), comprising 16 (2.6%) with NF155 specific antibodies, 1 (0.2%) with NF186 specific antibodies, 6 (1%) with pan-neurofascin antibodies, 12 (1.9%) with contactin-1 (CNTN1) antibodies and 7 (1.1%) with contactin-associated protein (Caspr1) or CNTN1/Caspr1-complex antibodies. The median age of the PNAb+ patients was 58 (range 15 to 79) and 30/42 (71.4%) were male. The initial clinical diagnosis was CIDP in 28 (66.6%), GBS in 13 (31.0%) and atypical multifocal motor neuropathy in 1 (2.4%). In one patient, the diagnosis of CIDP was subsequently revised to motor neuron disease; the diagnosis of an inflammatory neuropathy was retained at follow up in all other antibody positive cases. The remaining 583 patients were paranodal antibody negative (PNAb-negative), with clinical data available for 185 patients. The median age of the PNAb-negative patients was 62 (range 4 to 90) and 120/185 (64.9%) were male. The initial clinical diagnosis was CIDP in 100 (53.8%), combined central and peripheral demyelination in 3 (1.6%), GBS in 38 (20.4%), and multifocal motor neuropathy in 16 (8.6%). In 9/131 (6.9%) patients for whom follow up data was available, the diagnosis was subsequently revised away from that of an inflammatory neuropathy. Summary demographic and clinical details of the subgroups of apheresis treated PNAb-positive and PNAb-negative patients are given in Table 1. There was no significant difference in the median age, sex distribution, clinical diagnosis, or other serological results between the 2 subgroups. There was a non-significant trend towards more severe disease and more frequent IgG and less frequent IgM paraprotein detection in PNAb-positive patients. The frequencies of prior IVIg, steroid, PLEx and immunosuppressant use was also similar between the groups, while rituximab and IA were significantly more likely to have been used in the PNAb-positive group. PLEX aside, there was, however, no statistically significant difference in the clinician reported responses to these therapies between the 2 groups, although there was a trend to rituximab being more often judged effective in the PNAb-positive compared to PNAb-negative group.

Table 1. Summary characteristics of apheresis treated patients from the PNAb cohort.

	PNAb Positive (*n* = 21)	PNAb Negative (*n* = 33)	Significance (PNAb+ v PNAb-neg)		
Age: median, (range)	58 (35–79)	62 (5–90)	ns	$p = 0.94$	Mann-Whitney
Male sex: *n*, (%)	16 (76.2%)	23 (69.7%)	ns	$p = 0.76$	Fisher's exact
Initial clinical diagnosis:					
• GBS: *n* (%)	6 (28.6%)	10 (30.3%)	ns	$p > 0.99$	Fisher's exact (GBS or not)
• CIDP: *n* (%)	14 (66.7%)	18 (54.5%)	ns	$p = 0.41$	Fisher's exact (CIDP or not)
• Other: *n* (%)	1 (4.7%)	5 (15.1%)	ns	$p = 0.39$	Fisher's exact (Other or not)
Peak severity/nadir mRs (median, range)	5 (2–6)	4 (2–5)	ns	$p = 0.10$	Mann-Whitney
Other serology: *n/n* (%)					
Any ganglioside Ab	1/16 (6.3%)	3/18 (16.7%)	ns	$p = 0.60$	Fisher's exact
• GM1	1/16 (6.3%)	2/18 (11.1%)	ns	$p > 0.99$	Fisher's exact
• GQ1b	0/16	1/18 (5.6%)	ns	$p > 0.99$	Fisher's exact
MAG	0/4	1/8 (12.5%)	ns	$p > 0.99$	Fisher's exact
Paraprotein	2/17 (11.8%)	6/26 (23.1%)	ns	$p = 0.45$	Fisher's exact
• IgM	0/17	5/26 (19.2%)	ns	$p = 0.14$	Fisher's exact
• IgG	2/17 (11.8%)	1/26 (3.8%)	ns	$p = 0.55$	Fisher's exact

Treatment % treated (% of those judged to have good response)			Difference in proportion treated/proportion with good response		
IVIg	90.5 (5.3%)	87.9% (3.4%)	ns/ns	$p > 0.99/p > 0.99$	Fisher's exact
Steroids	85.7% (0)	75.8% (8%)	ns/ns	$p = 0.50/p = 0.50$	Fisher's exact
PLEx	95.2% (0)	100% (24.2%)	ns/*	$p = 0.39/*p = 0.01$	Fisher's exact
IA	19% (0)	0 (0)	***/ns	***$p < 0.001/ p > 0.99$	Fisher's exact
Rituximab	66.7% (64.3%)	18.2% (16.7%)	***/ns	***$p < 0.002/p = 0.14$	Fisher's exact
Other immuno-suppression	33.3% (28.6%)	24.2% (12.5%)	ns/ns	$p = 0.54/p = 0.47$	Fisher's exact

GBS, Guillain-Barré syndrome; CIDP, chronic inflammatory demyelinating polyneuropathy; GM1, monosialoganglioside GM1; GQ1b, tetrasialoganglioside GQ1b; MAG, myelin associated glycoprotein; IVIg, intravenous immunoglobulin; PLEx, plasma exchange; IA, immunoadsorption, * and ***, indicate statistical significance.

3.1.2. Physician-Reported Subjective Evaluation of Responses to Plasma Exchange or Immunoadsorption

Of the PNAb+ patients, 17 were treated with PLEx alone, 1 with IA alone, and 3 with both modalities. Protein A columns were used for three of the IA treated patients, the other (described in detail below) was treated with a GAM-peptide-ligand-based column (Globaffin, Fresenius Medical Care (UK) Ltd, Sutton-in-Ashfield, UK). Serial disability measures are available for only one other PNAb+ patient: a 68-year-old lady with a clinical diagnosis of GBS. Neither her overall neuropathy limitations score (ONLS, 12/12) nor inflammatory neuropathy Rasch-built overall disability score (iRODS, 0/48) improved following 2 cycles 5 treatments of PLEx starting on days 40 and 69 of her illness, prior to her death on day 110 from infectious complications. For all other PNab+ patients, only clinician-reported, retrospective, and subjective evaluations of response were available. None of the treating clinicians judged that either PLEx or IA had produced a subjectively "good" response in any of the PNAb+ patients. With PLEx, 5 patients (25.0%) were reported as having had a partial response, 2 (10.0%) an equivocal response, 12 (60.0%) no response, and one to have deteriorated (5.0%). With IA, 1 (25%) partial response, and 1 (25%) equivocal response were reported, with 2 patients (50%) reported as showing no response (Figure 1A,B). The proportion of PNAb+ patients subjectively judged as showing a partial or better response to PLEx (25.0%) versus IA (25.0%) was identical.

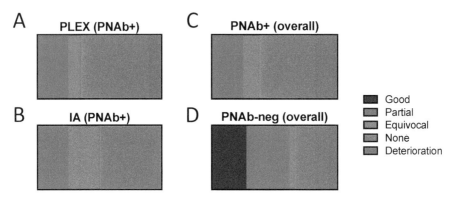

Figure 1. Physician-reported subjective evaluation of response to plasma exchange or immunoadsorption in paranodal antibody positive and negative patients. Paranodal antibody positive patients treated with (**A**) plasma exchange (*n* = 17), (**B**) immunoadsorption (*n* = 4), or (**C**) either modality (*n* = 21), compared to (**D**) paranodal antibody negative patients (*n* = 33) (all treated with plasma exchange).

Of the PNAb-negative patients, 33 were treated with PLEx: 8 patients (24.2%) were subjectively reported as having a good response, 10 (30.3%) a partial response, 1 (3.0%) an equivocal response, 8 (24.2%) no response, and 2 (6.1%) as deteriorating. For 4 patients, the response to PLEx was not reported. Amongst the 3 ganglioside antibody positive patients, 2 were reported as having a partial response, and 1 no response, to PLEx. Apheresis, with or without IA, was significantly more likely to have been reported by treating clinicians to have produced partial or better response in the PNAb-negative patients (62.1%) compared to the PNAb+ patients (25.0%) (*p* = 0.01, Fisher's exact test, OR 4.9 (95% CI 1.52 to 14.88) (Figure 1C,D). It should be emphasised that this is a comparison of the physicians' subjective overall impression of response, rather than an evaluation of the true efficacy, or otherwise, of these treatments.

3.2. Detailed Profile of an NF155 Antibody Positive Patient Treated with Immunoadsorption

This 46-year-old male first presented to neurology in July 2019 with a 6-week history of ascending numbness and paraesthesia in his feet, then hands. He had lost the ability to run and found walking to be unsteady. On examination, power was full, but there was global areflexia with distal sensory loss to temperature, pin-prick, vibration and proprioception. His gait was broad-based and unsteady and Rhomberg's test was positive after 20 s of eye closure. There was a postural tremor of both hands without cerebellar or extrapyramidal signs. The presentation was felt to be consistent with sensory ataxic CIDP. Neurofascin-155 antibody mediated disease was high in the differential. A positive result on the NF155 CBA and ELISA was duly returned 2 days later, at an initial titre of 1:6400. IgG4 was the dominant subclass, with IgG1 and IgG2 also represented (Figure 2A,B). CSF was acellular with an elevated protein (1.8 g/L). Nerve conduction studies showed absent median but preserved sural sensory nerve action potentials. Distal motor latencies and F-wave latencies were significantly prolonged, with slowing of intermediate motor conduction velocities. There was conduction block without temporal dispersion in the sampled peroneal nerve between the ankle and fibular head. Pulsed dexamethasone was commenced 4 days later (40mg per day for 4 days every 4 weeks for 3 cycles). There was no change in the examination findings. A progressive deterioration in symptoms and disability measures prompted a trial of IVIg (2 g/kg over 5 days) which resulted in a pompholyx-type skin rash, and no neurological benefit over the next 6 weeks. Approval was then sought for rituximab, and IA was arranged as a potential temporising measure.

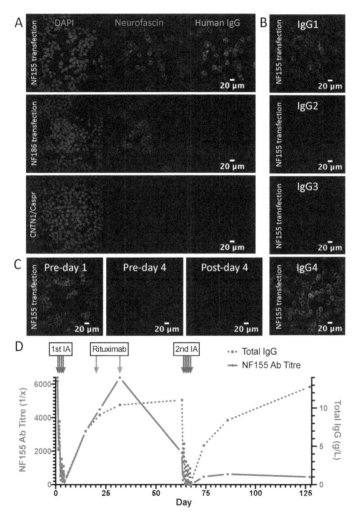

Figure 2. Serological results of NF155 antibody positive patient at baseline and during IA treatment. (**A**) Serum contains IgG (green) which binds to the cell membrane of NF155-transfected HEK293T cells, and co-localises with a commercial pan-neurofascin antibody (red). No signal is seen with NF186 or CNTN1/Caspr1-transfected cells. (**B**) The predominant IgG subclass of the NF155 antibodies is IgG4, with IgG1>IgG2 also represented. (**C**) The antibody signal intensity at 1:100 before, during and immediately after the first cycle of IA shows a progressive decline. (**D**) NF155 antibody titre (red) and total IgG levels (blue) over 2 cycles of IA, before and after rituximab.

Four treatment sessions of 2–2.5 plasma volumes were given on 4 consecutive days using a multiple pass, GAM-peptide-ligand-based column (Globaffin, Fresenius Medical Care Ltd, Sutton-in-Ashfield, UK). IA was effective in rapidly and substantially reducing the NF155 antibody titre (Figure 2C), but this had returned to baseline by 1 month (Figure 2D) and there was no observed clinical benefit. Rituximab was then given (1g on 2 occasions 2 weeks apart) followed by a second cycle of 5 treatments sessions of IA 1 month later. This was again associated with a rapid and substantial reduction in NF155 antibody titre, which on this occasion recovered more slowly and incompletely (Figure 2D). This more persistent suppression of antibody titres was associated with a progressive improvement in symptoms and disability, which is currently ongoing (Figure 3).

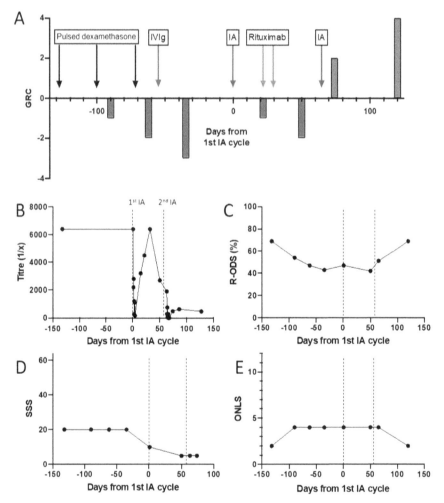

Figure 3. Antibody titres and outcome/disability measures during treatment of a patient with an NF155-antibody-mediated neuropathy. (**A**) Patient global rating of change after treatment with dexamethasone, IVIg, IA and rituximab. (**B**) NF155 antibody titre. (**C**) Inflammatory neuropathy Rasch-built Overall Disability Score. (**D**) Sensory sum score. (**E**) Overall neuropathy limitations score.

3.3. Demographics and Clinical Characteristics of the IA Treated Cohort

3.3.1. CIDP

Details of this cohort are given in Appendix B (Table A1). Sixteen of these 20 CIDP patients have been described in a previous publication [33]. 16/20 (80%) were male. At the start of IA treatment, the cohort had a median age of 66 (range 27 to 80), and a median disease duration of 95.5 months (range 63 to 139). All had progressive disease and met the European Federation of Neurological Societies (EFNS) criteria for definite, probable, or possible CIDP [41]. 18/20 had been previously treated with corticosteroids and 14/20 with IVIg, with sub-optimal responses. Six patients were treated with at least one of azathioprine, cyclophosphamide, mycophenolate mofetil or methotrexate. Nine patients received multiple (range 2–9) cycles of IA. Five patients showed improvements in their Inflammatory Neuropathy Cause and Treatment (INCAT) disability score when assessed 2 weeks after initial IA treatment, and 8 patients showed substantial improvements (at least 10 points) in the CIDP score.

3.3.2. GBS

Details of this cohort are given in Appendix B (Table A2). 10/20 patients (50%) were male. At the start of IA or PLEx treatment, the cohort had a median age of 66 (range 31 to 89). IA was applied to 13/20 patients. IA was used as a first-line therapy in 3, as a second-line therapy (after unsuccessful treatment with IVIg) in 9, and as a third-line therapy (after both IVIg and PLEx) in 1 patient. This subgroup was supplemented with 7 patients who received PLEx, instead of IA. In these patients, PLEx was used as a first-line therapy in 6, and as a second-line therapy (after IVIg) in 1 patient. 18/20 patients received 1 cycle of IA or PLEx, and only 2 patients received 2 cycles. 4/20 (3/13 IA, 1/7 PLEx) patients showed no clinical improvement after the last treatment, 3 patients (2/13 IA, 1/7 PLEx) showed equivocal improvement, 8 patients (4/13 IA, 4/7 PLEx) showed partial improvement, and 5 patients (4/13 IA, 1/ PLEx) showed large improvement.

3.3.3. MS/CIS

Details of this cohort are given in Appendix B (Table A3). 15/20 patients (75%) were female. At the start of IA treatment, the cohort had a median age of 29 (range 15 to 57). Patients were diagnosed with MS (16/20) or CIS (4/20), and had all been treated unsuccessfully with at least one cycle of high-dose intravenous methyl prednisolone (MP). 8 patients had received 2 or more cycles of high-dose IVMP. 11/20 patients showed an improvement of EDSS after the last IA treatment, while 9/20 patients did not improve.

3.4. Glycolipid and Nodal/Paranodal Antibodies in the IA Cohort

Pre-treatment serum samples from the IA cohort were tested for sulfatide and GM1- and GQ1b-ganglioside IgG antibodies by ELISA. None of these sera were positive on these assays. Serum samples taken pre and post-treatment, as well as first treatment session eluates from the IA cohort (20 CIDP, 20 GBS and 20 MS/CIS patients), were tested by both cell-based assay (CBA) and ELISA for antibodies to nodal (neurofascin-186) and paranodal (neurofascin-155, contactin-1 and Caspr) cell adhesion molecules. None of the sera were positive on either assay. One eluate from the MS/CIS cohort (patient 09) was positive on the neurofascin-155 CBA (blind scored as '2+' at 1:100, end-point titre 1:200, Figure 4A) (For scoring method see Appendix A.1). The sole detected subclass was IgG1. The corresponding pre-treatment serum was negative for NF155 antibodies at 1:100, the standard screening titre for this assay, but scored 3+ when repeated at 1:20. Two further eluates, one from the MS/CIS cohort and one from the CIP cohort, also produced faint membrane binding (1+) on the neurofascin-155 CBA that was not sufficient to be called positive at 1:100. Repeat testing of these eluates at 1:20 increased the signal to 2+ and 3+ respectively. However, this titre is below the usual positivity cut-off for this assay, and no signal was produced with any of the IgG subclass-specific secondary antibodies. All of these eluates were negative on the neurofascin-155 ELISA and negative for all other antigens by both CBA (including neurofascin-186, Figure 4B) and ELISA (results not shown).

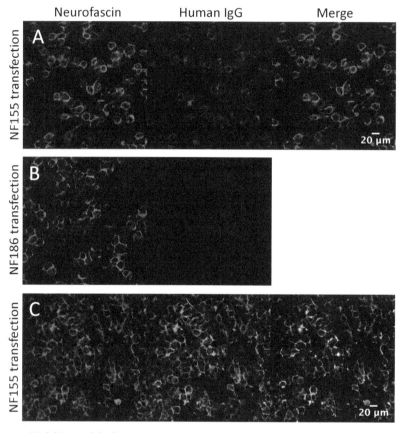

Figure 4. Nodal/paranodal cell-based assays. (**A**) MS/CIS eluate weakly positive on the neurofascin-155 CBA at 1:100 (Score 2+, end-point titre 1:200) and (**B**) negative on the neurofascin-186 CBA. (**C**) Strong positive at 1:100 (Score 4+, end-point titre 1:3200) from the antibody positive CIDP cohort shown for comparison.

3.5. Screening the IA Eluates for Novel Antibodies Using Myelinating Co-Cultures

In this experiment, eluates from the first treatment session of each IA cohort were compared with purified IgG from the serum of 22 healthy control volunteers (gratefully received from A/Prof Sarosh Irani, University of Oxford) isolated by Protein G purification. Serum was not available in sufficient quantities from PNAb cohort to purify IgG and these samples were therefore not tested in this experiment. IgG from IA eluates (1:50 dilution) and protein G purification (1:12.5 dilution) were applied to myelinated human sensory neuron cultures in a 96 well, flat-bottom imaging plate format enabling high-throughput staining and imaging. The mean IgG concentration after dilution was not significantly different between the groups (One-Way ANOVA: $F(3,78) = 1.500$, $p = 0.2211$) (Figure 5A). Out of 82 samples tested, 1 CIDP (patient 11), 1 GBS (patient 07, who was also concurrently identified as HIV positive, see Appendix B.2 for further detail) and 1 MS/CIS (patient 13) sample were scored as 'positive' for either axonal, glial or nodal IgG deposition by an observer blinded to the patient group; a further 1 MS/CIS patient sample with weak IgG labelling was marked 'equivocal'. All 4 of these sera and IA eluates were negative on the glycolipid and paranodal antibody assays, as above. Pre-treatment serum from MS patient 13 was also negative on our in-house live CBAs for aquapaorin-4 and MOG antibodies. Neither of the MS/CIS eluates which produced a weak signal on the neurofascin-155 CBA were positive on the co-culture assay.

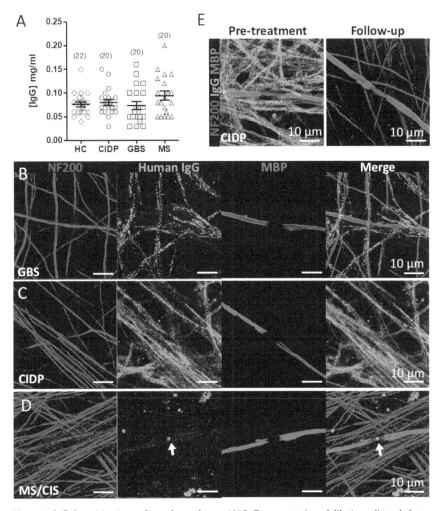

Figure 5. IgG deposition in myelinated co-cultures. (**A**) IgG concentration of dilution-adjusted eluates used for screening on myelinated cultures. (**B–D**) Immunofluorescence images of IgG binding patterns in myelinating co-cultures of IA eluates (1:50) from three patients with neurological disease identified in the screening assay: B) GBS (patient 07), C) CIDP (patient 11), and D) MS/CIS (patient 13) (arrow indicates IgG deposition at the node of Ranvier). (**E**) IgG labelling in myelinated co-cultures of serum (1:50) sampled from the CIDP (patient 11) before (Pre-treatment) and after IA (Follow-up). Note all IgG immunoreactivity is lost at follow-up. NF200, neurofilament 200; MBP, myelin basic protein.

Serum samples taken pre- and post-IA from the four candidate patients (1:50 dilution) were further validated on myelinated cultures plated on 13 mm coverslips with careful attention paid to media changes and washing steps. Strong IgG deposition aligned with neurofilament positive axons was observed in the serum and IA eluate of the GBS (patient 07) (Figure 5B) and CIDP (patient 11) (Figure 5C) patients. We confirmed nodal reactive IgG in the serum and IA eluate of one MS patient

(Figure 5D and Video S1), which was absent from post-IA serum. The post-treatment follow-up serum from the CIDP (patient 11) patient was negative for any IgG reactivity (Figure 5E). No IgG reactivity was observed in the serum or eluate of the MS/CIS patient 13 previously marked as equivocal, confirming this as a false positive. Clinical vignettes describing the patients with IgG deposition on co-cultures are given in Appendix B.

4. Discussion

In the PNAb cohort, we found that PLEx or IA were more often subjectively judged to have been effective in seronegative cases, and that in contrast, detection of at least one of the known nodal/paranodal antibodies in patients with inflammatory neuropathies was not associated with clinicians perceiving a positive response to either treatment. The proportion of PNAb-negative patients judged to have had a partial or better response (62.1%) was similar to the proportion of patients judged to have had a partial or better response in the IA cohort (52.5% overall), all of whom were also negative for known nodal/paranodal antibodies. We emphasise that the evaluation of the PNAb cohort is limited by the retrospective and subjective nature of the patient assessment. In addition, the small number of cases precludes us from reaching any conclusions regarding the objective benefits of one treatment modality compared to the other in this setting. In addition, improvement in neurological symptoms following IA/PLEX may occur after a delay, which may not be reflected in the immediate judgement of the treating physician. Blinding, randomisation, standardised follow up, as well as a control group to judge the natural history of these heterogeneous diseases, are required for a definitive evaluation of apheresis treatment efficacy in these patient groups. However, it is notable that treating physicians were less likely to think that apheresis had been effective in PNAb-positive patients.

Why seropositive patients were rarely assessed to have responded positively to either IA or PLEx is unclear. Our close monitoring of a prospectively-identified neurofascin-155 positive individual showed that while IA given as a mono-therapy was able to effectively reduce antibody titres, levels quickly rebounded and reached pre-treatment levels inside 4 weeks. This transient serological effect was not sufficient to reduce disability. More prolonged suppression of antibody titres, with frequent apheresis cycles or adjuvant therapies, may therefore be required for effective treatment in such cases.

Rituximab has previously been suggested as an effective treatment for paranodal antibody positive patients [42,43], but may take several weeks (or even months) to produce benefit. In this case, a second cycle of IA, 4 weeks after a course of rituximab, produced a more persistent suppression of antibody titres, which was associated with clinical improvement. The extent to which IA contributed to this effect is unclear. Theoretically, the more rapid action of IA might be complementary to the delayed but more sustained effects of rituximab. Whether this combination of treatment offers significant benefit over rituximab alone requires further investigation.

Retrospective analysis of serum samples from 60 IA-treated patients failed to identify any individuals who would have been classified as positive on routine diagnostic testing for previously described nodal/paranodal and glycolipid antibodies. A small number of first-treatment IA eluates did produce a low-level signal on the neurofascin-155 CBA. Whilst the diagnostic importance of low-titre, non-IgG4 results has been doubted [44], a pathogenic role for these antibodies cannot be ruled out.

The apparently better response of seronegative patients to apheresis, particularly IA, has several possible explanations. One is that these differences simply reflect variation in the disease characteristics and natural progression of seropositive versus seronegative inflammatory neuropathies: Overall, seropositive patients tend to have more severe, aggressive disease that is refractory to treatment [30–32]. Conversely, less severely affected, seronegative, patients may be more likely to have a monophasic disease course and stabilise or improve, independent of any particular therapy. Indeed, the median peak disability, measured by nadir modified Rankin score (mRs), of apheresis-treated PNAb+ patients in our series was higher, albeit non-significantly, than that of the apheresis-treated seronegative group (median nadir mRs 5 v 4, $p = 0.1$, Mann-Witney test, Table 1), although there was no significant difference in the use of, or clinician evaluated response to, other treatment modalities. There was also no significant difference in the proportion of patients initially diagnosed as GBS (28.6% and 30.3%, $p > 0.99$) compared to CIDP (66.7% and 54.5%, $p = 0.41$) in the PNAb+ and PNAb-negative groups, respectively (Fisher's exact test, Table 1). However, this does not exclude the possibility that patients in the seronegative group may often have a shorter disease course, with less irreversible axonal degeneration.

Another explanation for perceived apheresis efficacy in seronegative patients is the presence of antibodies below the threshold for positive detection on diagnostic testing, leading to a correspondingly slower rebound in titres following PLEx/IA and a more sustained suppression of antibody levels. A further possibility is that the response to IA in diagnostically seronegative patients is due to the therapeutic removal of as-yet uncharacterised, pathologically relevant antibodies in these patient groups. We therefore tested for further nerve-related antigens by screening eluates from the IA cohort against myelinating co-cultures. Three positive IA eluate samples were identified in the original 96-well co-culture screen and were further validated in a larger 24-well format, confirming similar binding patterns. IgG from one GBS patient co-localised with NF200 suggesting an axonal antigen. One CIDP patient serum and IA eluate showed IgG binding that aligned with NF200-positive axons but may also reflect deposition on non-myelinating Schwann cells.

One patient's serum and IA eluate from the MS/CIS group revealed nodal specific IgG binding. The presence of antibodies against nodal antigens such as neurofascin, has precedence in MS, and although uncommon, is more predominant in chronic progressive forms of the disease [45]. However, this sample was negative for antibodies against both the glial/paranodal and nodal/axonal isoforms of neurofascin (NF155 and NF186, respectively). The original focus on peripheral neuropathies led us to use a sensory neuron system for the myelinating cultures. Nevertheless, multiple peripheral nerve antigens are also found in the CNS (and vice versa), including NF155, CNTN1 and the ganglioside GM1. Therefore, it is quite feasible for the unknown antigen targeted by IgG in this CIS/MS patient to be mutually expressed in the peripheral and central nervous systems (CNS). Other autoantibodies against nerve and glial structures in the CNS including myelin basic protein, myelin-associated lipids, contactin-2, and KIR4.1 are among those proposed in MS patients [46]; however, their presence may not be specific to the disease [47]. For this reason, the inclusion of MS/CIS patients as a control group is potentially problematic. However, as patients with non-autoimmune neurological disease essentially never receive apheresis treatment, the inclusion of this group was a pragmatic way to obtain non-neuropathy IA eluates for use in our unbiased screening assays. With some similarity to the discovery of nodal/paranodal antibodies in chronic neuropathies, MS has recently been separated from other distinct, serologically-defined disorders, characterised by the presence of aquaporin-4 or myelin oligodendrocyte glycoprotein (MOG) directed autoantibodies. Whether the nodal antigen targeted by antibodies in this MS patient has a pathogenic role and might similarly define a non-MS disease entity is currently unknown. Further investigation using brain tissue may help elucidate the antigen target, pathological potential, and clinical relevance. Unfortunately, purified Ig/eluate was not available from the PNAb-negative apheresis cohort, and it is possible that novel autoantibodies are also present in some of these patients.

The two patients for whom follow-up samples were available (CIDP and MS/CIS) had no detectable IgG labelling in their serum after IA compared to pre-treatment. Thus, IA is effective at removing both established and potentially novel pathogenic autoreactive IgG from the circulation. Follow-up serum samples at later time points will help correlate any changes in disease progress with antibody titres.

Development of myelinated hiPSC-derived neuronal cultures in a 96-well format allowed for efficient simultaneous screening of >80 IgG eluates from patients and controls. The benefits of using live cultures for screening are the presence of complex structures including nodes of Ranvier, paranodal and juxtaparanodal regions, and compact myelin internodes, that provide an unbiased substrate for antibody screening against nerve-related antigens in their native conformation. IgG binding patterns ranged from broad axonal coverage to focal nodal localisation, reflecting morphologically distinct antigens. Images were acquired by an experienced observer who was blind to the sample identity.

J. Clin. Med. **2020**, *9*, 2025

Although time-consuming, acquisition in such a supervised manner aids the detection of localised signals, such as the node-specific labelling identified in one MS/CIS patient.

A single sample that was marked as 'equivocal' on the 96-well assay was subsequently confirmed as negative. The minimal occurrence of non-specific IgG labelling in the 96 well format may reflect a lower washing efficiency in the smaller volume of the 96-well plate. Nevertheless, no healthy control samples were identified as positive in the screen, suggesting the cultures are useful as a selective substrate for nerve-targeted autoantibodies.

IA is rarely performed on healthy subjects; therefore control IgG were prepared from the sera of healthy volunteers by protein G purification. IgG concentrations in the healthy samples were normalised to the patient IA eluates such that the mean IgG concentrations were not significantly different, however the variation within each group was maintained in order to reflect the original sample. The detection of specific signals in both the serum and IA eluate of each of the three positive patients suggests that a uniform dilution of 1:50 is sufficient for antibody screening within IA eluates. We cannot, however, exclude the possibility of further antibodies below the level of detection. In summary, our findings of nerve antigen reactive antibodies in three 'seronegative' neurological patients suggest the utility of an unbiased screening system such as we have described here for the myelinating co-cultures. The development of equivalent cultures containing CNS antigens and cell-types may be of further benefit to relevant MS cases.

5. Conclusions

Currently available serological tests do not unambiguously identify patients who are likely to respond to IA or PLEx. In patients with nodal/paranodal antibody associated neuropathies, frequent plasmapheresis and/or additional therapies may be required to produce an acceptable level and duration of clinical improvement. Prospective longitudinal studies involving standardized and validated outcome measures, with serial monitoring of auto-antibodies, are needed to optimise apheresis treatment regimens and accurately assess efficacy.

Supplementary Materials: The following are available online at http://www.mdpi.com/2077-0383/9/7/2025/s1, Video S1: 3D reconstruction of IgG deposition (green) at the node of Ranvier after incubation with MS serum.

Author Contributions: Conceptualization, S.R. and J.D.; methodology, A.J.D., J.F., H.T., J.D., S.R., M.S.; validation, A.J.D., J.F., H.T., M.S., J.D., S.R.; formal analysis, A.J.D., J.D., S.R.; investigation, A.J.D., J.F., H.T., M.S., J.D., S.R.; resources, J.D., S.R.; data curation, A.J.D., J.F., J.D., S.R.; writing—original draft preparation, A.J.D., S.R.; writing—review and editing, A.J.D., J.F., H.T., J.D., S.R., M.S.; visualization, A.J.D., S.R.; supervision, S.R.; project administration, S.R.; funding acquisition, S.R. All authors have read and agreed to the published version of the manuscript.

Funding: This research was funded by Medical Research Council, grant number MR/P008399/1 (awarded to S.R.) and the GBS/CIDP Foundation International Benson Fellowship (awarded to J.F.). A.D. is also supported by a Human Immune Discovery Initiative grant (BRCRCF19-04) from the National Institute for Health Research. Support for assay development was received from the John Fell Fund, University of Oxford.

Acknowledgments: The authors would like to thank Sarosh Irani, University of Oxford, for providing serum samples from control subjects used to prepare the control IgG, and all clinicians who sent samples and completed request forms for nodal/paranodal antibody testing.

Conflicts of Interest: S.R. runs a not-for-profit diagnostic testing service for nodal/paranodal antibodies. He has received a speaker's honorarium and travel expenses from Fresenius Medical Care. A.D. is named inventor on a patent for immune cell therapy in nerve injury and has received travel grants from IASP and Biolegend. M.S. has received consulting and/or speaker honoraria from Bayer, Biogen, Merck, Roche, and Sanofi Genzyme. She has received research funding from the Hertha-Nathorff-Program. J.D. reports research funds and speaker's honoraria from Fresenius Medical Care GmbH and Fresenius Medical Care Deutschland GmbH. The Globaffin IA column used to treat the NF155 PNAb+ patient was provided free of charge by Fresenius on a trial basis. The funders had no role in the design of the study; in the collection, analyses, or interpretation of data; in the writing of the manuscript, or in the decision to publish the results.

Appendix A. Detailed Experimental Methods

Appendix A.1. Nodal/Parnodal Cell-Based Assays

All sera and IA eluates were screened for IgG antibodies to neurofascin-155, neurofascin-186, contatctin-1 and Caspr1 using a live, cell-based assay (CBA), following previously described methods with slight modification [32]. In brief, HEK293T cells on poly-L-lysine coated 13mm coverslips at 80–90% confluence were transiently transfected with human neurofascin-155 (RC228652, Origene) or human neurofascin-186 (courtesy of Jerome Devaux, University of Marseille) mammalian-expression vectors, or co-transfected with both human contactin-1 (CNTN1, EXA1153-MO29 Genecopoeia, Maryland, US) and human Caspr1 (EXMO417-MO2 Genecopoeia, Maryland, US) at equimolar concentrations, using Jet-PEI transfection reagent (101-10; Polyplus). After 16 h, the cells were washed and replaced with Dulbecco's Modified Eagle Medium (DMEM) (Gibco) containing 10% fetal bovine serum (FBS). 24 hours later, sera and eluates diluted 1:100 in DMEM + BSA (1%) were incubated with the cells for 1 h at room temperature. Co-incubation with commercial chicken anti-neurofascin primary antibody, (1:1000) (Cat no. AF3235; R&D Systems, Bio-Techne) was used to confirm successful transfection and to assess for co-localisation with any bound human IgG. Following serum/eluate incubation, cells were washed 3 times with DMEM + HEPES (20 mM), and fixed for 5 minutes in 4% PFA. Secondary antibody incubation was with goat anti-human IgG-Fc specific-Alexa Fluor 488 (1:750) (Cat no. H10120; Life Tech) and goat anti-Chicken Alexa Fluor 546 1:1000 (Cat no. A11040; Life Tech). To determine antibody subclass unconjugated mouse anti-human IgG subclass 1-4 antibodies were used at 1:100 (Cat nos. I2513, I25635, I7260 I7385; Sigma-Aldrich, Merck) followed by a fluorescently tagged tertiary antibody goat anti-mouse Alexa Fluor 488 (1:750) (Cat no. A11029; Life Tech). Positivity was assessed by an observer blinded to the clinical data using fluorescence microscopy. Taking into account the intensity of the membrane signal and co-localisation of the human IgG signal with the commercial antibody, the assay was scored on a 5 point scale as follows: 4+ very strong positive, 3+ strong positive, 2+ positive, 1+ negative (non-specific background or faint/poorly co-localised human IgG signal only), 0 no human IgG binding seen.

Appendix A.2. Nodal/Paranodal ELISA

Individual wells of Nunc Maxisorp ELISA plates (Fisher Scientific) were coated overnight at 4 C with either human recombinant neurofascin-155 (NF155) (8208-NF; R&D systems), NF186 (TP329070; OriGene Technologies) or CNTN1 (10383-H08H; Sino Biological Inc) diluted to 1 g/ml in PBS. The coating solution was then removed and the plate blocked with 5% milk in PBS for 1 h at room temperature. Serum or eluates diluted 1:100 in 5% milk were then applied for 1h at room temperature then washed by 5 cycles of immersion in PBS. Anti-human IgG (Fc specific) peroxidase-conjugated anti-human IgG (A0170; Sigma) was used as the secondary antibody at 1:3000. The detection reaction was performed using 50 l o-Phenylenediamine dihydrochloride solution (OPD fast, Sigma), stopped after 20 minutes by the application of 25 l 4M sulphuric acid, and optical densities measured at 492 nm using a FLUOstar Omega plate reader (BMG Labtech). Wells with ODs greater than 0.1 above uncoated (PBS only) control wells were considered positive.

Appendix A.3. Ganglioside and Sulfatide ELISA

Ganglioside and sulfatide ELISAs were performed using Immunolon 2HB 96 well plates [48]. Wells were coated with 100 ul of GM1 or GQ1b bovine gangliosides diluted to 2 g/ml, or sulfatide to 5 g/ml, in methanol. Negative control wells contained methanol only. Plates were then air-dried overnight in the fume hood, placed at 4 C, and blocked with 2% BSA/PBS. Sera/eluates were diluted 1:100 in 1% BSA/PBS and incubated for 2 h at 4 C. Secondary antibodies and detection were the same as the nodal/paranodal ELISA, except that secondary antibody incubation was performed at 4 C.

Appendix A.4. Protein G IgG Purification

Healthy control sera (100 μl) were diluted 1:1 in sterile PBS, added to protein G columns (Cat. 28-4083-47, Ab SpinTrap, GE Healthcare) prepared according to the manufacturer's instructions. Briefly, samples were incubated 15 min at 4 °C on rollers to bind IgG. Serum was then removed by centrifugation (100 g, 30 s) and columns washed twice with binding buffer (20 mM Na_2PO_4, pH 7.0). IgG were eluted with 320 μl 0.1M glycine (pH 2.6) and neutralised with 80 μl Tris-HCl (pH 8.0). Elution was repeated once more and samples taken forward for IgG quantification.

Appendix A.5. IgG ELISA

IgG in serum and eluates was quantified by enzyme-linked immunosorbent assay (ELISA) using a human IgG ELISA quantification kit (Cat. E80-104, Bethyl Laboratories Inc. TX, US) according to the manufacturer's instructions. Briefly, 96 well plates (Maxisorp, Nunc) were coated with goat anti-human IgG-Fc capture antibody (10 μg/ml) in coating buffer (0.05M carbonate-bicarbonate, pH 9.6) (100 μl/well) for 1h at room temperature (RT). Plates were washed 5 times by immersion in wash buffer (50mM Tris, 0.14M NaCl, 0.05% Tween 20, pH 8.0), blocked for 1h at RT in blocking buffer (50mM Tris, 0.14M NaCl, 1% BSA, pH 8.0), followed again by immersion 5 times in washing buffer. Serum samples and IgG eluates were prepared at 1:10,000 dilution in sample diluent, as well as a dilution series of human reference serum standards (50mM Tris, 0.14M NaCl, 1% BSA, 0.05% Tween 20, pH 8.0). All samples and standards were prepared in duplicate (100 μL/well) and incubated 1h at RT. After 5x immersion washes 100 μL of HRP-conjugated goat anti-human IgG-Fc Detection Antibody (1:200,000) was incubated 1h at RT followed by 5 immersion washes. Plates were developed by the addition of 100 μL of TMB substrate solution (20 min, RT) and reaction stopped by adding equal volume of 0.18M H_2SO_4. Absorbance values were read immediately on a plate reader (FLUO Star Omega, BMG Labtech) at 450nm (signal) and 630nm (background). A standard curve was constructed from the background subtracted absorbance (OD) values obtained from the human serum standards using a 4-parameter function (https://mycurvefit.com/). IgG concentrations of each sample were calculated from averages of the duplicate, background-subtracted OD values, multiplied by the original dilution. All values for diluted samples fell within the standard curve (1–1000 ng/mL).

Appendix A.6. Myelinating Co-Cultures

Myelinating co-cultures were prepared using human induced pluripotent stem cells (hiPSC)-derived sensory neurons and primary rat Schwann cells with some modifications to previously described methods [49]. hiPSCs from control subjects were obtained via the StemBANCC consortium at the University of Oxford (https://www.ndcn.ox.ac.uk/research/stembancc). In brief, hiPSCs were differentiated to sensory neurons using a combination of small-molecule mediated dual-SMAD inhibition and wnt activation. On day 11 of differentiation, sensory neuron precursors were seeded onto 13 mm diameter glass coverslips (approximately 20,000 cells per coverslip) or 96-well flat, glass-bottom imaging plates (Sensoplate Microplate, Greiner-Bio) (approximately 5000 neurons per well) previously coated with poly-D-lysine (PDL) (10 μg/mL) overnight and reduced growth-factor matrigel (Corning). Neurons were maintained in neurobasal media supplemented with N2, B27, Glutamax and anti-anti (all Gibco, Life Technologies) ('complete' neurobasal) plus recombinant human β-NGF (rhNGF) (Cat. 450-01, Peprotech), NT3 (Cat. 450-03, Peprotech), GDNF (Cat. 450-10, Peprotech), and BDNF (Cat. PHC7074, Life Technologies) (all growth factors 25 ng/ml), supplemented with Rho-associated, coiled-coil containing protein kinase (ROCK) inhibitor (10 μM) (Tocris, Bio-Techne) on days 11–12, CHIR99021 (3 μM) (Sigma) on days 11–14 and cytosine arabinoside (Ara-C) (1 μM) (Sigma) on days 12–14. Neurons were incubated at 37 °C in 5% CO_2 for 4 weeks with twice-weekly medium changes prior to addition of Schwann cells for myelination.

Primary Schwann cells were isolated from the sciatic nerves of rat pups (P2-3). Mother and pups were killed by rising concentration of CO_2 in accordance with Schedule 1 of the UK Home Office

Animals (Scientific Procedures) Act 1986. Sciatic nerves were rapidly dissected and digested in a mixture of collagenase (3mg/ml) (Worthington, Lorne Labs) and dispase II (3.5mg/mL) (Roche) for 1 h at 37 °C with frequent gentle agitation. Nerves were washed in DMEM + FBS (10%) and gently triturated using a fire-polished glass Pasteur pipette. Dissociated cells were seeded into tissue culture flasks overnight and expanded in Schwann cell expansion medium containing charcoal-stripped FBS (10%) (Sigma), Forskolin (4 μM), recombinant human NRG1-β1 EGF domain (80 ng/mL) (Cat. 396-HB, R&D Systems) and recombinant murine NGF (10 ng/ml) (Cat. 450-34, Peprotech) in DMEM/F12 (Gibco). Cells were serially treated with 5–10 μM Ara-C to eliminate fibroblasts. Expanded Schwann cells were added to the neuronal cultures (25,000 cells per coverslip or 5000 cell per 96-well) and allowed to proliferate and align with the axons for 1 week in basal media containing: (CS-FBS) (10%), insulin (5 mg/ml) (Sigma), holo-transferrin (100 mg/mL) (Sigma), rhNGF (25 ng/mL) (Peprotech) (Sigma), Selenium (25 ng/mL) (Sigma), 25 ng/ml thyroxine (Sigma), progesterone (30 ng/ml) (Sigma), triiodothyronine (25 ng/mL) (Sigma) and putrescine 8 mg/mL (Sigma) in DMEM/F12 media (Gibco, Life Technologies). From this point on, cultures were maintained in 'myelination medium' containing: 5% CS-FBS, ascorbic acid (25 μg/mL), phenol-free matrigel (1:300) (Corning) and hrNGF (25 ng/mL) in 'complete' neurobasal medium. Myelinating cultures were matured for at least 4 weeks before use in subsequent experiments.

Appendix A.7. Myelinated Co-Culture Immunreactivity Screening

Sera or IgG eluates were diluted in neurobasal 'complete' media (including 1% BSA and human NGF, 50 ng/mL), added to myelinated co-cultures either in a 96 well plate (100 μL/well) or coverslips in a 24 well plate (300 μL/well) format and incubated for 1h at 37 °C. Serum containing antibodies to known antigens, as well as normal human serum, were run as positive and negative controls, respectively. For 96-well plate screening, serum samples were blinded by an independent investigator. Cultures were then washed 4x with pre-warmed PBS and fixed with 2% PFA in PBS for 30 min at RT. Wells were washed with PBS followed by DMEM plus HEPES (20 mM). Cultures were then labelled with Alex488-conjugated goat anti-human IgG (H+L) (A11013, Life Technologies) secondary antibody (1:750) in DMEM/HEPES plus 1% BSA, 1h at RT followed by washing 2x with DMEM/HEPES and 3x PBS. Cultures were then permeabilised with ice cold methanol (45 min on ice), blocked with 5% normal goat serum and incubated with chicken anti-neurofilament (NF)200 (1:10,000) (ab4680, Abcam) and rat anti-myelin basic protein (MBP) (1:500) (ab7349, Abcam) primary antibodies overnight at 4 °C. After washing in PBS antibodies were labelled with goat anti-chicken biotin (1:500) (BA-9010, Vector Laboratories) and goat anti-rat Alexa 546 (1:1000) (A11081, Life Technologies) secondary antibodies for 1h at RT, followed by streptavidin pacific blue (1:500) (S11222, Life Technologies) 45–60 min at RT. After washing in PBS coverslips were mounted onto glass slides (SuperFrost, ThermoScientific) with Vectorshield (H1000, Vector Laboratories) and stored at −20 °C prior to imaging. 96-well plates were flooded with PBS containing 0.02% NaN₃ and sealed with plate-sealing film. Plates were stored at 4 °C until imaging. Confocal images were acquired with a x63 oil-immersion lens (1024 × 1024 resolution) and exported as maximum intensity projection of 4–5 × 1 μm interval z-section images. Plates were allowed to reach room temperature before imaging.

J. Clin. Med. **2020**, 9, 2025

Appendix B. Baseline Clinical Features of IA Cohorts and Clinical Vignettes of Patients with IgG Deposition in Co-Cultures

Table A1. Baseline characteristics and response to IA treatment of the CIDP cohort.

ID	Age	Sex	Disease Duration (mo)	Steroids Yes/No	IVIg Yes/No	Other Immunosuppression Used [1]	IA Cycles	CIDP-Score Baseline	CIDP Score at 2 Weeks	Progression before IA	Progression after IA
01 *	59	M	83	Y	Y		1	296	298		
02 *	61	M	114	Y	Y	AZA	3	376	416	2.9	0
03 *	58	M	158	Y	N	AZA, CPM, MPM	9	102	118	4.1	0.1
04 *	65	M	114	Y	N		1	434	438		
05 *	67	F	112	Y	Y		1	435	435		
06 *	60	M	104	Y	Y		1	268	313		
07 *	80	M	66	Y	N	AZA	3	306	342	19.3	0.8
08 *	62	M	73	N	Y		5	231	361	13.1	0.7
09 *	68	M	67	Y	Y		4	373	364	6.7	0
10 *	75	M	134	Y	Y		1	326	326		
11 *	66	M	166	Y	Y	AZA, MTX	1	308	316		
12 *	72	M	65	N	Y		3	314	330	8.7	2.0
13 *	66	F	64	Y	N		1	314	282		
14 *	60	M	102	Y	N		2	297	382	3.0	0
15 *	66	F	86	Y	Y		1	393	405		
16 *	68	M	62	Y	N	MPM	1	264	264		
17	67	M	65	Y	N		3	N/A	N/A	N/A	N/A
18	53	M	97	Y	Y		1	N/A	N/A	N/A	N/A
19	67	F	94	Y	Y	AZA	2	N/A	N/A	N/A	N/A
20	67	M	201	Y	Y		1	N/A	N/A	N/A	N/A

* These patients were included in a previous publication [33]. [1] AZA=azathioprine, CPM=cyclophosphamide, MPM=mycophenolate-mofetil, MTX=methotrexate.

Table A2. Baseline characteristics and response to IA treatment of the GBS cohort.

ID	Age	Sex	1st/2nd/3rd-Line	PLEx Yes/No	IVIg Yes/No	PLEx / IA Cycles	Clinical Outcome
01	76	F	2	N	Y	1	0
02	73	M	3	Y	Y	2	(+)
03	36	F	2	N	Y	1	(+)
04	76	M	2	N	Y	2	++
05	64	M	2	N	Y	1	0
06	31	F	1	Y	N	1	++
07	52	M	1	N	N	1	+
08	33	F	1	N	N	1	0
09	53	F	2	N	Y	1	+
10	38	F	2	N	Y	1	++
11	89	M	2	N	Y	1	+
12	75	M	PLEx (1)	Y	N	1	0
13	66	F	PLEx (1)	Y	Y	1	++
14	66	F	PLEx (1)	Y	N	1	+
15	42	M	PLEx (1)	Y	N	1	+
16	77	F	PLEx (1)	Y	N	1	++
17	67	M	2	N	Y	1	++
18	77	M	PLEx (2)	Y	Y	1	(+)
19	62	M	PLEx (1)	Y	N	1	+
20	66	F	2	N	Y	1	+

Outcome: 0 no response; (+) equivocal response; + partial response; ++ good response.

Table A3. Baseline characteristics and response to IA treatment of the MS cohort.

ID	Age	Sex	Diagnosis	DMT	Symptoms	MP	IA Cycles	EDSS before IA	EDSS after IA
01	44	F	CIS	none	ON	5×1g iv	1	2.0	0.0
02	21	M	MS	none	Sensory deficits UE+LE	5×2g iv	1	4.0	3.0
03	48	M	MS	none	Sensory deficits UE+LE	5×1g iv	1	4.0	3.0
04	18	F	CIS	none	ON	7×1g iv	1	1.0	1.0
05	30	F	MS	dimethyl fumarate	Sensory deficits UE	2×5×1g iv / 2×5×1g it	1	1.0	1.0
06	46	F	MS	none	Sensory deficits UE+LE, gait ataxia	5×1g iv	1	6.5	6.5
07	28	F	MS	dimethyl fumarate	Sensomotoric deficits UE+LE	5×1g iv	1	6.5	6.5
08	26	F	MS	dimethyl fumarate	Sensory deficits UE	4×1g iv	1	3.0	3.0
09	19	M	MS	none	Organic psycho syndrome	5×1g iv	2	5.5	3.0
10	20	F	MS	none	ON	5×1g iv	1	2.0	1.0
11	47	F	MS	fingolimod	Motor deficits UE+LE	5×1g iv	1	7.0	6.0
12	19	F	MS	none	ON (bilateral), hemihypesthesia	5×1g iv / 5×2g iv	1	2.5	2.5
13	49	F	MS	fingolimod	ON, paraparesis	5×1g iv	1	4.5	4.5
14	23	F	CIS	none	ON	5×1g iv / 5×1g iv	1	2.0	1.0
15	50	F	MS	none	ON (bilateral), gait ataxia	5×1g iv / 5×2g iv	1	5.0	4.0
16	15	M	MS	none	Dysarthria, dysphagia	12×1g iv	1	4.0	3.0
17	17	F	CIS	none	ON	5×1g iv / 5×1g iv	1	1.0	1.0
18	46	F	MS	interferon beta 1a	Sensory deficits UE+LE, gait ataxia	5×1g iv	1	3.5	3.0
19	57	F	MS	none	Paraparesis, hemihypesthesia	5×1g iv	1	4.0	4.0
20	37	M	MS	none	Paresis LE	5×1g iv / 5×2g iv	1	6.0	5.5

MS—Multiple Sclerosis; CIS—Clinically Isolated Syndrome; ON—optic neuritis; UE—upper extremities; LE—lower extremities; MP—methyl prednisolone; DMT—actual disease-modifying treatment; EDSS—Expanded Disability Status Scale.

Appendix B.1. CIDP (Patient 11)

This 66-year-old male first developed sensory deficits, myalgia, and gait disturbance in 2007, followed in 2009 by asymmetric distal weakness in the legs then arms, and after 3 years, worsening neuropathic pain and trigeminal nerve dysfunction. Routine bloods, serum protein electrophoresis with immunofixation, and an extensive autoantibody screen revealed no abnormalities. Neve conduction studies showed a demyelinating, sensory-motor neuropathy (reduced nerve conduction velocities, prolonged motor distal latencies, prolonged F-wave latencies, and temporal dispersion in multiple nerves), meeting the EFNS criteria for definite CIDP. EMG showed no evidence of myopathy. First line treatment with high dose then tapering corticosteroids was initiated in 2007. This produced some improvement in myalgia but no other benefit and was stopped after a few weeks due to unacceptable side effects (multiple infections). Further progression in 2009 led to the use of IVIg and the introduction of azathioprine, which was again stopped after a few weeks due to adverse reactions. High-dose, pulsed, corticosteroids were again used in 2011, and methotrexate was also introduced. The clinical picture stabilised but these therapies could not be continued due to recurrent urosepsis. The patient then received 1 cycle (5 treatment sessions and 12 plasma volumes in total) of IA in 2015 without further improvement in his clinical picture after 2 weeks.

Appendix B.2. GBS (Patient 07)

This 52-year-old male presented in 2017 with neuropathic pain, limb-weakness, and facio-bulbar cranial nerve dysfunction. There was a rapid worsening over the next few days to complete tetraplegia, with autonomic involvement (bradycardia) and respiratory insufficiency, necessitating transfer to intensive care for ventilatory support. Nerve conduction studies showed a demyelinating, sensory-motor neuropathy. The CSF protein was elevated at 1.2 g/L, as was the CSF white cell count at 19 per mm^3. The white cells were classified as activated lymphocytes and monocytes. No infectious organisms were identified in the CSF despite extensive testing. A subsequent serological HIV test was positive, initially showing 376000 HIV RNA copies per ml. This confirmed a new diagnosis of HIV infection, and raises the possibility that this gentleman's GBS was associated with HIV seroconversion. However, in the absence of serial serological testing, we cannot confirm this unequivocally. The CD4/CD8 ratio was 0.34 (reduced). Standard IVIg treatment did not produce any immediate improvement. Antiretroviral therapy was commenced with an associated decline in viral load over the next few weeks, reducing HIV RNA copies to 100/ml. IA therapy had to be delayed multiple times due to recurrent infections and other complications. It was finally started about 6 weeks after onset of symptoms. Following 5 days of IA, there was a slow improvement in strength over the next 14 days, with a limited return of movement in the arms and legs. After a subsequent cycle of plasma exchange, this slow improvement continued. The patient was transferred to an early rehabilitation clinic about 3 months after onset of symptoms.

Appendix B.3. MS (Patient 13)

This 37-year-old male was diagnosed with highly active multiple sclerosis in 1998. This followed a relapsing-remitting course, with an accumulation of residual deficits producing a persistent spastic tetraparesis. Brain and spinal MRI were performed, showing multiple supra- and infratentorial, as well as spinal T2-hyperintense lesions with Gadolinum-enhancement in the cervical cord. Aquaporin-4- and MOG- antibodies were negative. The patient had previously received multiple disease modifying therapies, including beta-interferon, natalizumab, and currently fingolimod, but continued to experience relapses in the last year. A 2015 relapse with left sided optic neuritis was treated with high-dose prednisolone. This was associated with partial improvement and was followed with 5 days of IA. Further outcome data is not available.

References

1. Rinaldi, S.; Bennett, D.L. Pathogenic mechanisms in inflammatory and paraproteinaemic peripheral neuropathies. *Curr. Opin. Neurol.* **2014**, *27*, 541–551. [CrossRef] [PubMed]
2. Willison, H.J. The immunobiology of Guillain-Barre syndromes. *J. Peripher. Nerv. Syst.* **2005**, *10*, 94–112. [CrossRef] [PubMed]
3. Fehmi, J.; Scherer, S.S.; Willison, H.J.; Rinaldi, S. Nodes, paranodes and neuropathies. *J. Neurol. Neurosurg. Psychiatry* **2017**, *89*, 61–71. [CrossRef] [PubMed]
4. Chevret, S.; Hughes, R.A.; Annane, D. Plasma exchange for Guillain-Barré syndrome. *Cochrane Database Syst. Rev.* **2017**, *2017*, CD001798. [CrossRef]
5. Mehndiratta, M.M.; Hughes, R.A.C.; Pritchard, J. Plasma exchange for chronic inflammatory demyelinating polyradiculoneuropathy. *Cochrane Database Syst. Rev.* **2015**, *2015*, CD003906. [CrossRef]
6. Eftimov, F.; Winer, J.B.; Vermeulen, M.; De Haan, R.; Van Schaik, I.N. Intravenous immunoglobulin for chronic inflammatory demyelinating polyradiculoneuropathy. *Cochrane Database Syst. Rev.* **2013**, CD001797. [CrossRef]
7. Hughes, R.A.C.; Raphaël, J.C.; Swan, A.V.; A Doorn, P. Intravenous immunoglobulin for Guillain-Barré syndrome. *Cochrane Database Syst. Rev.* **2004**, CD002063. [CrossRef]
8. Lieker, I.; Slowinski, T.; Harms, L.; Hahn, K.; Klehmet, J. A prospective study comparing tryptophan immunoadsorption with therapeutic plasma exchange for the treatment of chronic inflammatory demyelinating polyneuropathy. *J. Clin. Apher.* **2017**, *32*, 486–493. [CrossRef]
9. Zinman, L.; Sutton, D.; Ng, E.; Nwe, P.; Ngo, M.; Bril, V. A pilot study to compare the use of the Excorim staphylococcal protein immunoadsorption system and IVIG in chronic inflammatory demyelinating polyneuropathy. *Transfus. Apher. Sci.* **2005**, *33*, 317–324. [CrossRef]
10. Hadden, R.D.M.; Bensa, S.; Lunn, M.; Hughes, R. Immunoadsorption inferior to plasma exchange in a patient with chronic inflammatory demyelinating polyradiculoneuropathy. *J. Neurol. Neurosurg. Psychiatry* **2002**, *72*, 644–646. [CrossRef]
11. Ullrich, H.; Mansouri-Taleghani, B.; Lackner, K.J.; Schalke, B.; Bogdahn, U.; Schmitz, G. Chronic inflammatory demyelinating polyradiculoneuropathy: Superiority of protein A immunoadsorption over plasma exchange treatment. *Transfus. Sci.* **1998**, *19*, 33–38. [CrossRef]
12. Galldiks, N.; Burghaus, L.; Dohmen, C.; Teschner, S.; Pollok, M.; Leebmann, J.; Frischmuth, N.; Höllinger, P.; Nazli, N.; Fassbender, C.; et al. Immunoadsorption in Patients with Chronic Inflammatory Demyelinating Polyradiculoneuropathy with Unsatisfactory Response to First-Line Treatment. *Eur. Neurol.* **2011**, *66*, 183–189. [CrossRef] [PubMed]
13. Yamawaki, T.; Suzuki, N. Can immunoadsorption plasmapheresis be used as the first choice therapy for neuroimmunological disorders? *Ther. Apher.* **1997**, *1*, 348–352. [CrossRef] [PubMed]
14. Pernat, A.M.; Svigelj, V.; Ponikvar, R.; Buturović-Ponikvar, J. Guillain-Barré Syndrome Treated by Membrane Plasma Exchange and/or Immunoadsorption. *Ther. Apher. Dial.* **2009**, *13*, 310–313. [CrossRef]
15. Arakawa, H.; Yuhara, Y.; Todokoro, M.; Kato, M.; Mochizuki, H.; Tokuyama, K.; Kunimoto, F.; Morikawa, A. Immunoadsorption therapy for a child with Guillain-Barre syndrome subsequent to Mycoplasma infection: A case study. *Brain Dev.* **2005**, *27*, 431–433. [CrossRef]
16. Okamiya, S.; Ogino, M.; Ogino, Y.; Irie, S.; Kanazawa, N.; Saito, T.; Sakai, F. Tryptophan-immobilized Column-based Immunoadsorption as the Choice Method for Plasmapheresis in Guillain-Barre Syndrome. *Ther. Apher. Dial.* **2004**, *8*, 248–253. [CrossRef]
17. Haupt, W.; Rosenow, F.; Van Der Ven, C.; Birkmann, C. Immunoadsorption in Guillain-Barré syndrome and myasthenia gravis. *Ther. Apher.* **2000**, *4*, 195–197. [CrossRef]
18. Uetakagaito, M.; Horikawa, H.; Yoshinaka, H.; Tagawa, Y.; Yuki, N. Two Patients with Acute Guillain-Barré Syndrome Treated with Different Apheresis Methods. *Ther. Apher.* **1997**, *1*, 340–342. [CrossRef]
19. Hirai, K.; Kihara, M.; Nakajima, F.; Miyanomae, Y.; Yoshioka, H. Immunoadsorption Therapy in Guillain-Barré Syndrome. *Pediatric Neurol.* **1998**, *19*, 55–57. [CrossRef]
20. Chida, K.; Takase, S.; Itoyama, Y. Development of facial palsy during immunoadsorption plasmapheresis in Miller Fisher syndrome: A clinical report of two cases. *J. Neurol. Neurosurg. Psychiatry* **1998**, *64*, 399–401. [CrossRef]

21. Ruiz, J.C.; Berciano, J.; Polo, J.M.; De Francisco, A.L.M.; Arias, M. Treatment of Guillain-Barré syndrome with protein-A immunoadsorption: Report of two cases. *Ann. Neurol.* **1992**, *31*, 574–575. [CrossRef] [PubMed]
22. Takei, H.; Komaba, Y.; Araki, T.; Iino, Y.; Katayama, Y. Plasma Immunoadsorption Therapy for Guillain-Barré Syndrome: Critical Day for Initiation. *J. Nippon. Med. Sch.* **2002**, *69*, 557–563. [CrossRef] [PubMed]
23. Mahdi-Rogers, M.; Brassington, R.; A Gunn, A.; A Van Doorn, P.; Hughes, R.A. Immunomodulatory treatment other than corticosteroids, immunoglobulin and plasma exchange for chronic inflammatory demyelinating polyradiculoneuropathy. *Cochrane Database Syst. Rev.* **2017**, *2017*, CD003280. [CrossRef] [PubMed]
24. Rolfes, L.; Pfeuffer, S.; Ruck, T.; Melzer, N.; Pawlitzki, M.; Heming, M.; Brand, M.; Wiendl, H.; Meuth, S. Ruck Therapeutic Apheresis in Acute Relapsing Multiple Sclerosis: Current Evidence and Unmet Needs—A Systematic Review. *J. Clin. Med.* **2019**, *8*, 1623. [CrossRef] [PubMed]
25. Lipphardt, M.; Wallbach, M.; Koziolek, M.J. Plasma Exchange or Immunoadsorption in Demyelinating Diseases: A Meta-Analysis. *J. Clin. Med.* **2020**, *9*, 1597. [CrossRef]
26. Willison, H.J.; Yuki, N. Peripheral neuropathies and anti-glycolipid antibodies. *Brain* **2002**, *125*, 2591–2625. [CrossRef]
27. Tagawa, Y.; Yuki, N.; Hirata, K. Ability to remove immunoglobulins and anti-ganglioside antibodies by plasma exchange, double-filtration plasmapheresis and immunoadsorption. *J. Neurol. Sci.* **1998**, *157*, 90–95. [CrossRef]
28. Ng, J.K.M.; Malotka, J.; Kawakami, N.; Derfuss, T.; Khademi, M.; Olsson, T.; Linington, C.; Odaka, M.; Tackenberg, B.; Prüss, H.; et al. Neurofascin as a target for autoantibodies in peripheral neuropathies. *Neurology* **2012**, *79*, 2241–2248. [CrossRef]
29. Querol, L.; Nogales-Gadea, G.; Rojas-García, R.; Martinez-Hernandez, E.; Diaz-Manera, J.; Suárez-Calvet, X.; Navas, M.; Araque, J.; Gallardo, E.; Illa, I. Antibodies to contactin-1 in chronic inflammatory demyelinating polyneuropathy. *Ann. Neurol.* **2012**, *73*, 370–380. [CrossRef]
30. Querol, L.; Nogales-Gadea, G.; Rojas-Garcia, R.; Diaz-Manera, J.; Pardo, J.; Ortega-Moreno, A.; Sedano, M.J.; Gallardo, E.; Berciano, J.; Blesa, R.; et al. Neurofascin IgG4 antibodies in CIDP associate with disabling tremor and poor response to IVIg. *Neurology* **2014**, *82*, 879–886. [CrossRef]
31. Doppler, K.; Appeltshauser, L.; Villmann, C.; Martin, C.; Peles, E.; Krämer, H.H.; Haarmann, A.; Buttmann, M.; Sommer, C. Auto-antibodies to contactin-associated protein 1 (Caspr) in two patients with painful inflammatory neuropathy. *Brain* **2016**, *139*, 2617–2630. [CrossRef]
32. Delmont, E.; Manso, C.; Querol, L.; Cortese, A.; Berardinelli, A.; Lozza, A.; Belghazi, M.; Malissart, P.; Labauge, P.; Taieb, G.; et al. Autoantibodies to nodal isoforms of neurofascin in chronic inflammatory demyelinating polyneuropathy. *Brain* **2017**, *140*, 1851–1858. [CrossRef] [PubMed]
33. Dorst, J.; Ludolph, A.C.; Senel, M.; Tumani, H. Short-term and long-term effects of immunoadsorption in refractory chronic inflammatory demyelinating polyneuropathy: A prospective study in 17 patients. *J. Neurol.* **2018**, *265*, 2906–2915. [CrossRef] [PubMed]
34. Kuwahara, M.; Suzuki, H.; Oka, N.; Ogata, H.; Yanagimoto, S.; Sadakane, S.; Fukumoto, Y.; Yamana, M.; Yuhara, Y.; Yoshikawa, K.; et al. ELectron microscopic abnormality and therapeutic efficacy in chronic inflammatory demyelinating polyneuropathy with anti-neurofascin155 immunoglobulin G4 antibody. *Muscle Nerve* **2017**, *57*, 498–502. [CrossRef] [PubMed]
35. Süfke, S.; Lehnert, H.; Gebauer, F.; Uhlenbusch-Körwer, I. Safety Aspects of Immunoadsorption in IgG Removal Using a Single-Use, Multiple-pass Protein A Immunoadsorber (LIGASORB): Clinical Investigation in Healthy Volunteers. *Ther. Apher. Dial.* **2017**, *21*, 405–413. [CrossRef] [PubMed]
36. Chida, K.; Watanabe, S.; Okita, N.; Takase, S.; Tagawa, Y.; Yuki, N. Immunoadsorption therapy for Fisher's syndrome: Analysis of the recovery process of external ophthalmoplegia and the removal ability of anti-GQ1b antibodies. *Rinsho Shinkeigaku* **1996**, *36*, 551–556.
37. Belak, M.; Borberg, H.; Jimenez, C.; Oette, K. Technical and clinical experience with Protein A Immunoadsorption columns. *Transfus. Sci.* **1994**, *15*, 419–422. [CrossRef]
38. Merkies, I.S.; Schmitz, P.I.M.; A Van Der Meché, F.G.; Samijn, J.; A Van Doorn, P. Clinimetric evaluation of a new overall disability scale in immune mediated polyneuropathies. *J. Neurol. Neurosurg. Psychiatry* **2002**, *72*, 596–601. [CrossRef]
39. Thompson, A.J.; Banwell, B.L.; Barkhof, F.; Carroll, W.M.; Coetzee, T.; Comi, G.; Correale, J.; Fazekas, F.; Filippi, M.; Freedman, M.S.; et al. Diagnosis of multiple sclerosis: 2017 revisions of the McDonald criteria. *Lancet Neurol.* **2017**, *17*, 162–173. [CrossRef]

40. Teunissen, C.E.; Petzold, A.; Bennett, J.L.; Berven, F.S.; Brundin, L.; Comabella, M.; Franciotta, D.; Frederiksen, J.L.; Fleming, J.O.; Furlan, R.; et al. A consensus protocol for the standardization of cerebrospinal fluid collection and biobanking. *Neurology* **2009**, *73*, 1914–1922. [CrossRef]

41. Pns, J.T.F.O.T.E.A.T.; Efns, J.T.F.O.T.; Pns, T. European Federation of Neurological Societies/Peripheral Nerve Society Guideline on management of chronic inflammatory demyelinating polyradiculoneuropathy: Report of a joint task force of the European Federation of Neurological Societies and the Peripheral Nerve Society-First Revision. *J. Peripher. Nerv. Syst.* **2010**, *15*, 1–9. [CrossRef]

42. Querol, L.; Rojas-García, R.; Diaz-Manera, J.; Barcena, J.; Pardo, J.; Ortega-Moreno, A.; Sedano, M.J.; Seró-Ballesteros, L.; Carvajal, A.; Ortiz-Castellon, N.; et al. Rituximab in treatment-resistant CIDP with antibodies against paranodal proteins. *Neurol. Neuroimmunol. Neuroinflammation* **2015**, *2*, e149. [CrossRef] [PubMed]

43. Demichelis, C.; Franciotta, D.; Cortese, A.; Callegari, I.; Serrati, C.; Mancardi, G.L.; Schenone, A.; Leonardi, A.; Benedetti, L. Remarkable Rituximab Response on Tremor Related to Acute-Onset Chronic Inflammatory Demyelinating Polyradiculoneuropathy in an Antineurofascin155 Immunoglobulin G4-Seropositive Patient. *Mov. Disord. Clin. Pr.* **2018**, *5*, 559–560. [CrossRef] [PubMed]

44. Cortese, A.; Lombardi, R.; Briani, C.; Callegari, I.; Benedetti, L.; Manganelli, F.; Luigetti, M.; Ferrari, S.; Clerici, A.M.; Marfia, G.A.; et al. Antibodies to neurofascin, contactin-1, and contactin-associated protein 1 in CIDP: Clinical relevance of IgG isotype. *Neurol. Neuroimmunol. Neuroinflammation* **2019**, *7*, e639. [CrossRef]

45. Stich, O.; Perera, S.; Berger, B.; Jarius, S.; Wildemann, B.; Baumgartner, A.; Rauer, S. Prevalence of neurofascin-155 antibodies in patients with multiple sclerosis. *J. Neurol. Sci.* **2016**, *364*, 29–32. [CrossRef] [PubMed]

46. Häusser-Kinzel, S.; Weber, M.S. The Role of B Cells and Antibodies in Multiple Sclerosis, Neuromyelitis Optica, and Related Disorders. *Front. Immunol.* **2019**, *10*, 201. [CrossRef] [PubMed]

47. Prineas, J.W.; Parratt, J.D. Multiple sclerosis: Serum anti-CNS autoantibodies. *Mult. Scler. J.* **2017**, *24*, 610–622. [CrossRef]

48. Willison, H.J.; Veitch, J.; Swan, A.V.; Baumann, N.; Comi, G.; Gregson, N.A.; Iiia, I.; Jacobs, B.C.; Zielasek, J.; Hughes, R.A.C. Inter-laboratory validation of an ELISA for the determination of serum anti-ganglioside antibodies. *Eur. J. Neurol.* **1999**, *6*, 71–77. [CrossRef]

49. Clark, A.; Kaller, M.; Galino, J.; Willison, H.J.; Rinaldi, S.; Bennett, D.L. Co-cultures with stem cell-derived human sensory neurons reveal regulators of peripheral myelination. *Brain* **2017**, *140*, 898–913. [CrossRef]

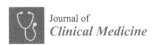

Article

Immunoadsorption for Treatment of Patients with Suspected Alzheimer Dementia and Agonistic Autoantibodies against Alpha1a-Adrenoceptor—Rationale and Design of the IMAD Pilot Study

Sylvia Stracke [1,*,†], Sandra Lange [2,†], Sarah Bornmann [3], Holger Kock [4], Lara Schulze [5], Johanna Klinger-König [5], Susanne Böhm [6], Antje Vogelgesang [3], Felix von Podewils [3], Agnes Föel [3,7], Stefan Gross [8,9], Katrin Wenzel [10], Gerd Wallukat [10], Harald Prüss [11,12], Alexander Dressel [13], Rudolf Kunze [14], Hans J. Grabe [5,7,†], Sönke Langner [2,15,†] and Marcus Dörr [8,9,*,†]

1   Department for Internal Medicine A, Nephrology, University Medicine Greifswald, Ferdinand-Sauerbruch-Straße, 17475 Greifswald, Germany
2   Institute of Diagnostic Radiology and Neuroradiology, University Medicine Greifswald, 17475 Greifswald, Germany; sandra.lange@uni-greifswald.de (S.L.); soenke.langner@med.uni-rostock.de (S.L.)
3   Department of Neurology, University Medicine Greifswald, 17475 Greifswald, Germany; bornmanns@uni-greifswald.de (S.B.); antje.vogelgesang@uni-greifswald.de (A.V.); Felix.vonPodewils@med.uni-greifswald.de (F.v.P.); agnes.floeel@med.uni-greifswald.de (A.F.)
4   Strategic Research Management, University Medicine Greifswald, 17475 Greifswald, Germany; holger.kock@uni-greifswald.de
5   Department of Psychiatry and Psychotherapy, University Medicine Greifswald, 17475 Greifswald, Germany; lara.schulze@uni-greifswald.de (L.S.); Johanna.Klinger-Koenig@med.uni-greifswald.de (J.K.-K.); Hans.Grabe@med.uni-greifswald.de (H.J.G.)
6   Coordinating Centre for Clinical Trials, University Medicine Greifswald, 17475 Greifswald, Germany; Susanne.Boehm@med.uni-greifswald.de
7   German Center for Neurodegenerative Diseases (DZNE), 17475 Rostock/Greifswald, partner site Greifswald, Germany
8   Department of Internal Medicine B, University Medicine Greifswald, Ferdinand-Sauerbruch-Straße, 17475 Greifswald, Germany; stefan.gross1@uni-greifswald.de
9   German Centre for Cardiovascular Research (DZHK), 17475 Greifswald, Germany
10 Berlin Cures GmbH, 13125 Berlin, Germany; wenzel@berlincures.de (K.W.); wallukat@berlincures.de (G.W.)
11 German Center for Neurodegenerative Diseases (DZNE) Berlin, 10117 Berlin, Germany; harald.pruess@charite.de
12 Department of Neurology and Experimental Neurology, Charité—Universitätsmedizin Berlin, 10117 Berlin, Germany
13 Department of Neurology, Carl-Thiem-Klinikum, 03048 Cottbus, Germany; a.dressel@ctk.de
14 Science Office, Hessenhagen 2, 17268 Flieth-Stegelitz, Germany; Rudolf.Kunze@gmx.de
15 Institute of Diagnostic and Interventional Radiology, University Medicine Rostock, 18057 Rostock, Germany
*   Correspondence: sylvia.stracke@med.uni-greifswald.de (S.S.); marcus.doerr@uni-greifswald.de (M.D.); Tel.: +49-(0)-3834-86-80752 (S.S.); +49-(0)-3834-86-80510 (M.D.); Fax: +49-(0)-3834-86-6662 (S.S.); +49-(0)-3834-86-80502 (M.D.)
†   Denotes equal contribution.

Received: 30 April 2020; Accepted: 15 June 2020; Published: 19 June 2020

Abstract: Background: agonistic autoantibodies (agAABs) against G protein-coupled receptors (GPCR) have been linked to cardiovascular disease. In dementia patients, GPCR-agAABs against the α1- and ß2-adrenoceptors (α1AR- and ß2AR) were found at a prevalence of 50%. Elimination of agAABs by immunoadsorption (IA) was successfully applied in cardiovascular disease. The IMAD trial (Efficacy of immunoadsorption for treatment of persons with Alzheimer dementia and agonistic autoantibodies against alpha1A-adrenoceptor) investigates whether the removal of α1AR-AABs by a 5-day IA procedure has a positive effect (improvement or non-deterioration) on changes of hemodynamic, cognitive, vascular and metabolic parameters in patients with suspected Alzheimer's clinical syndrome within a one-year follow-up period. Methods: the IMAD trial is designed as an exploratory monocentric interventional trial corresponding to a proof-of-concept phase-IIa study. If cognition capacity of eligible patients scores 19–26 in the Mini Mental State Examination (MMSE), patients are tested for the presence of agAABs by an enzyme-linked immunosorbent assay (ELISA)-based method, followed by a bioassay-based confirmation test, further screening and treatment with IA and intravenous immunoglobulin G (IgG) replacement. We aim to include 15 patients with IA/IgG and to complete follow-up data from at least 12 patients. The primary outcome parameter of the study is uncorrected mean cerebral perfusion measured in mL/min/100 gr of brain tissue determined by magnetic resonance imaging with arterial spin labeling after 12 months. Conclusion: IMAD is an important pilot study that will analyze whether the removal of α1AR-agAABs by immunoadsorption in α1AR-agAAB-positive patients with suspected Alzheimer's clinical syndrome may slow the progression of dementia and/or may improve vascular functional parameters.

Keywords: Alzheimer's clinical syndrome; dementia; immunoadsorption; autoantibodies; α1-Adrenergic receptor

1. Introduction

Nearly 50 million people worldwide suffer from Alzheimer's disease (AD) or other forms of dementia, and around 10 million new cases emerge every year, leading to a number of 150 million affected people expected in 2050 [1–3] Dementia has a lifetime prevalence ranging between 5% and 7% for those aged ≥60 years and is a major cause of disability among older adults [4,5] AD is the leading cause of dementia, responsible for two-thirds of all cases [6]. Since no causal treatment for AD is available yet, prevention strategies, psychosocial interventions and symptomatic pharmacological interventions are recommended and are central components of the treatment [7].

Up to now, research of causal therapies is focusing on the knowledge of typical neuropathological features of AD like amyloid plaques and neurofibrillary tangles which are associated with the tau-pathology [8,9]. In particular, the ß-amyloid hypothesis of AD has stimulated the development of therapy concepts directed against the amyloid protein and amyloid deposits in the brain of patients with AD.

One strategy is passive immunization with monoclonal antibodies which bind to ß-amyloid. Although it has been demonstrated that these antibodies may reduce the amyloid burden in the brain of AD patients, positive clinical effects were minimal or absent so far. Many promising compounds like Bapineuzumab, Gantenerumab or Solanezumab have failed in phase III of clinical trials or are still being evaluated (Aducanumab) [10–12].

Other ß-amyloid (Aß)-directed therapies focus on the enzymatic cleavage of the amyloid precursor protein (APP). It is known that ß-secretases contribute essentially to the production of Aß40/42 which is the toxic aggregating form of amyloid. Thus, ß-secretase inhibitors have been identified to be therapeutically beneficial. However, recently, a world-wide clinical trial on the secretase inhibitor Verubecestat was withdrawn because Verubecestat did not improve clinical ratings of dementia among patients with prodromal Alzheimer's disease. Some measures even suggested an impairment of cognition and daily function compared to placebo [13].

The focus on Aß also led to the concept of removing it from plasma by therapeutic plasma exchange (TPE). Aß is bound to serum albumin by >90% which in turn is removed and discarded by TPE [14,15]. TPE-treatment with albumin replacement favored the stabilization of cerebral perfusion in mild to moderate AD patients compared to non-treated controls [15]. The same Spanish group currently conducts a prospective multicenter, randomized, blinded and placebo-controlled, parallel-group, phase IIb/III trial in patients with mild to moderate AD ("Alzheimer's Management by Albumin Replacement (AMBAR)"). This study evaluates TPE with different replacement volumes of therapeutic albumin (5% and 20%), with or without intravenous immunoglobulins and is still ongoing [14]. Another group sought to remove Aß and developed an ex vivo adsorptive filtration system that resulted in an 80–100% reduction of Aßs within 30 min of circulation but has not yet been tested in humans [16].

In view of the numerous negative results, it seems to be necessary to shift attention to new therapeutic targets. In this respect, different pathologies of cognitive decline besides the Aß and the tau-pathologies may be considered. Importantly, clinical, pathological and epidemiological data point to a relevant overlap between cerebrovascular disease (CVD) and Alzheimer's clinical syndrome [17]. Furthermore, cerebral microvascular lesions that are detected as white matter hyperintensities (WMH) on magnetic resonance imaging (MRI) are associated with typical gray matter atrophy patterns of AD in a considerable number of patients [18]. Thus, factors that alter the microenvironment of the endothelium and the smooth muscle cells of blood vessels may compromise the molecular exchange between blood and brain.

Rationale of the Clinical Investigation

Naturally occurring agonistic autoantibodies (agAABs) against G protein-coupled receptors (GPCR) have been linked to cardiovascular disease such as dilated cardiomyopathy, myocarditis, malignant hypertension, vascular renal rejection, diabetes mellitus type 2 or dementia [19]. Agonistic AABs are functional antibodies that can activate the respective receptor. Agonistic AABs differ clearly from non-functional AABs. The latter trigger autoimmune disease in an Fc-receptor mediated manner whereas functional agAABs are able to bind cell receptors and activate intracellular signaling pathways that are normally triggered by endogenous ligands [20]. A pathological example of agAABs is Graves' hyperthyroidism with autoantibodies activating the thyroid-stimulating hormone (TSH)-receptor and with subsequent overproduction of thyroid hormones [21]. Other examples for GPCR-agAABs are AABs directed against adrenoceptors (AR; e.g., ß1AR and ß2AR, α1AR), the angiotensin (2) receptor type 1 (AT-R1) and the endothelin receptor type A (ETA) [19]. The agAABs against AR are directed against the first or second extracellular loop of the receptor. They bind to constant epitopes defined by the amino acid sequence in the respective loop. These AABs belong to the immunoglobulin class G (isotypes 1–3). GPCR-agAABs elicit a long-lasting dimerization of adrenoceptors and continuously activate cellular processes such as phosphorylation of intracellular proteins and modulation of calcium signaling that results e.g., in the case of agAABs against the α1AR in the proliferation of smooth muscle cells and thickening of vessel walls [22]. In response to their natural agonists, the receptor density on the cell membrane is regulated by receptor desensitization. This mechanism is inhibited by agAABs [22]. In an animal model, continuous stimulation triggered by α1AR-AABs leads to cerebrovascular remodeling and obliteration [23].

In a small clinical trial, treatment of Graves' disease with rituximab, a B-cell depleting monoclonal antibody specifically reduced the production of TSH-receptor antibodies [24]. In a case of thyreotoxic crisis, TPE is also used to remove agAABs against TSH-receptor and albumin-bound thyroid hormones [25].

Cerebrovascular remodeling may lead to disturbances in cerebral blood flow and a lack of outflow of Aß. A clearing defect for Aß rather than an Aß-overproduction has been proven experimentally for AD patients [26]. From this view, AABs against the α1AR may interfere with Aß clearance mechanisms and act as a risk factor and a modulating component of dementia in patients with Alzheimer's clinical syndrome.

In line with this, the GPCR-α1AR was also reported to be a target for agAABs in patients with essential and malignant hypertension [27]. In a pilot study in five α1AR-AAB-positive patients with resistant hypertension, removal of these AABs by immunoadsorption lowered the mean arterial blood pressure significantly by approximately 10 mmHg, and the effect was still present after 180 days [28]. In line with this, a recent study in 816 subjects showed that the occurrence of α1AR-AABs predicted arterial stiffness progression even in normotensives over a 5-year period [29].

A disease that has been very well investigated with regard to agAABs is dilated cardiomyopathy (DCM). Among others, agAABs against the GPCR-ß1-adrenoceptor (ß1R) seem to play an important role in DCM. Their elimination from the blood by immunoadsorption (IA) has been transferred to a therapeutic intervention in clinical praxis. Removal of circulating antibodies by IA with subsequent intravenous immunoglobulin G substitution (IA/IgG) has been shown to result in improvement of cardiac function, in better exercise capacity, and in decrease of myocardial inflammation in DCM [30–33]. Removal of functional AABs does not have to be a constant process as in non-functional AAB triggered disease. Already a one-week-course of IA seems to yield a so-called legacy effect that may persist for a long time [34]. In DCM, removal of the agAABs by a one-week-course of IA lasts for up to 12 months and even longer [35,36].

Noticeably, in dementia patients, agAABs against both the α1R- and ß2R-adrenoceptors were also found at a prevalence of approx. 50%. Thus, in a primary care cohort who screened positive for dementia, 40 out of 95 participants were also positive for agAAB (29 subjects with α1AR-AABs and 21 with ß2AR-AABs) [37]. However, agAABs could not discriminate between Alzheimer's Dementia and other forms of dementia. Patients with coronary heart disease were more likely (OR = 4.23) to have α1AR-AABs than those without coronary heart disease. The presence of agAAB against adrenoceptors, especially α1AR-agAABs, in persons suffering from dementia motivated a first pilot trial on the effects of IA on the course of dementia [38]. In this trial, in four out of eight patients an effective depletion of agAAB could be achieved by a 4-day per-protocol IA treatment, while another four patients received a less effective 2–3 day treatment due venous access problems. IA was safe to use in these patients, and the mean change in Mini Mental State Examination (MMSE) score of these patients remained constant over 12 to 18 months.

The IMAD trial (Efficacy of immunoadsorption for treatment of persons with Alzheimer dementia and agonistic autoantibodies against alpha1A-adrenoceptor) aims to ascertain whether the positive effects of IA on slowing down dementia progression can be replicated. Moreover, IMAD will comprehensively examine potential effects of this treatment in patients with Alzheimer's clinical syndrome by a combination of brain and vessel imaging along with cognitive tests and further cardiovascular, cerebrovascular and laboratory examinations.

2. Methods

2.1. Objectives

The IMAD trial is designed as an exploratory monocentric interventional trial corresponding to a proof-of-concept phase-IIa study. The aim of IMAD is to evaluate whether IA with subsequent IgG-substitution (IA/IgG) is related to an improved uncorrected mean brain perfusion after 12 months as a surrogate for potential beneficial effects on disease progression in patients with an Alzheimer's clinical syndrome and mild to moderate cognitive impairment. In addition, potential effects of IA/IgG on cognitive measures as well as cardiovascular, cerebrovascular and laboratory parameters will be investigated.

2.2. Patients

Potential participants for this trial need to have an Alzheimer's clinical syndrome, according to the definition as outlined in Jack et al. [39]. In patients without obvious exclusion criteria, cognitive capacity is again assessed before inclusion using the MMSE. If a mild to moderate impairment (defined by a MMSE score between 19 and 26) is confirmed, patients are tested for the presence of agAABs by an ELISA-based method, followed by a bioassay-based confirmation test (methodological details are given in Section 2.5.8). Patients with a positive test result by the bioassay are eligible for further screening. We aim to include in total 15 patients with IA/IgG and 12 patients with complete follow-up data.

2.3. Inclusion and Exclusion Criteria

Criteria that have to be fulfilled for all participants (inclusion criteria) and reasons that prevent inclusion into the study (exclusion criteria) are summarized in Table 1.

Table 1. Inclusion and exclusion criteria.

	Criteria
Inclusion	- Age 55–85
	- Previous or suspected diagnosis of Alzheimer's clinical syndrome
	- Presence of agAAB against alpha1-adrenoceptor (α1AR)
	- Mini mental state examination score between 19 and 26
	- Written informed consent
Exclusion	- Presence of autoantibodies against the NMDA receptor
	- Defective blood coagulation at time of inclusion
	- Severe protein deficiency disorders
	- Known manifest vitamin/folic acid deficiency (substitution allowed)
	- Active infectious disease, or sings of ongoing infection with CRP >10 mmol/L
	- Impaired renal function (serum creatinine >220 µmol/L)
	- Any disease requiring immunosuppressive drugs or therapeutic antibodies
	- Non-curative treated malignant disease or another life-threatening disease with poor prognosis (estimated survival less than 2 years), except for basal-cell carcinoma
	- Unstable angina pectoris, second or third degree atrioventricular block or symptomatic sick sinus syndrome without implanted pacemaker, history of myocardial infarction, bypass or other revascularization procedures, valvular heart defect (≥2. degree)
	- Severely reduced left ventricular systolic function (LVEF <30%) and/or heart failure symptoms according to NYHA class III/IV
	- Clinical manifestation of arterial disease, vascular surgery: ACl-Stenosis >60%; PAD > IIb, history of stroke, diffusion disorder or expired territorial stroke in MRI
	- Endocrine disorder excluding diabetes mellitus
	- Severe hepatic disorder (Child–Pugh score 5 or more)
	- Drug therapy against dementia since less than 3 months
	- Psychopharmacological drug therapy since less than 3 months
	- Dialysis requirement
	- MRI contraindications (e.g., pacemaker)
	- Legal tutelage
	- Previous treatments with IA or immunoglobulins
	- ACE-treatment during the IA
	- Severe mental disorder (bipolar disorder, schizophrenia, depression) requiring treatment
	- Alcohol or drug abuse
	- Inability to undergo the study procedure
	- Participation in any other clinical/interventional study within less than 30 days prior to screening

ACE, angiotensin converting enzyme; ACI, internal carotid artery; agAAB, agonistic autoantibodies; CRP, C reactive protein; IA, immunoadsorption LVEF, left ventricular systolic function; MRI, magnetic resonance imaging; NMDA, N-methyl-D-aspartate; NYHA, New York Heart Association; PAD, peripheral artery disease.

2.4. Study Design

During the screening phase, patients are checked for eligibility according the inclusion and exclusion criteria (Table 1). Patients fulfilling these criteria are comprehensively examined during a baseline visit, followed by IA/IgG treatment. All participants of the IMAD trial are followed up after 1, 6 and 12 months. The complete study flow is illustrated in Figure 1.

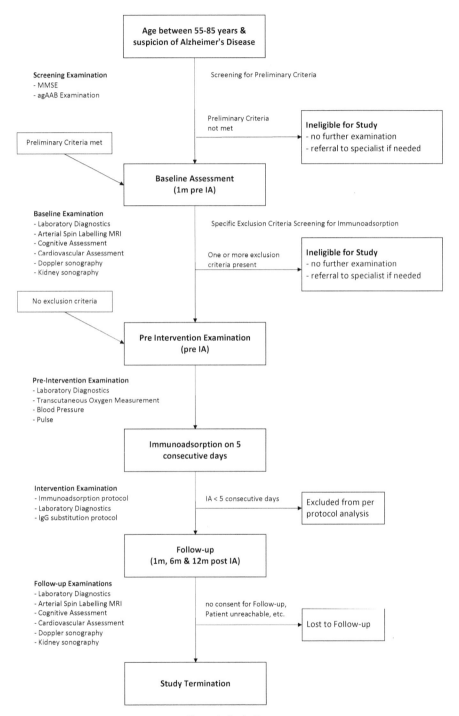

Figure 1. Study flow.

The IMAD trial is an interdisciplinary project which involves the departments and institutes of radiology, neurology, psychiatry, cardiology, nephrology and laboratory medicine of the University Medicine Greifswald. The study complies with the Declaration of Helsinki and it has been approved by the Ethics Committee of the University of Greifswald (MPG 02/16; MPG 02/16a). The trial is registered at ClinicalTrials.gov (NCT03132272).

2.5. Examinations and Assessments

Patients undergo a comprehensive examination program including brain perfusion assessment by MRI (primary outcome parameter: uncorrected mean brain perfusion assessed by arterial spin labeling [ASL]) and assessment of further structural and vascular brain MRI parameters. In addition, several cognitive, cardiovascular, cerebrovascular and laboratory parameters are assessed during baseline and all follow-up visits. Table 2 gives an overview about methods, main parameters and respective time points.

Table 2. Methods, main outcome parameters and time points.

Method	Parameter	Screening	Baseline	Follow-Ups	Comments
Arterial Spin Labelling MRI	Cerebral blood flow		X	X	
MRI Basic protocol	Brain Volume, WMH, CBM; MTA		X	X	
Time-of-flight MR angiography	Vessel anatomy and size		X	X	
Diffusion Tensor Imaging	Fractional anisotropy		X	X	
ADAS-Cog	Cognition		X	X	
MMSE	Cognition	X	X	X	
GDS	Depression		X	X	
VLMT	Cognition		X	X	
Benton Test	Cognition		X	X	
Brachial blood	Brachial blood pressure values	X	X	X	
Pulse wave analysis	Arterial stiffness, central hemodynamics		X	X	
Digital endothelial vascular function and stiffness	Endothelial function and vascular stiffness		X		
Echocardiography	Cardiac function and structure		X		
Transcutaneous oxygen measurement	Oxygenation		X	X	
Kidney sonography	Renal function		X	X	
Doppler Sonography	Carotid Arteria blood flow		X	X	
Liquor analytics	Tau/P-Tau		(X)	(X)	Optional
Liquor analytics	ß-A40/42		(X)	(X)	Optional

IA, immunoadsorption; MRI, magnetic resonance imaging; CBM, cerebral microbleeds; MTA, medial temporal lobe atrophy; DTI, diffusion tensor imaging; ADAS, Alzheimer's Disease Assessment Scale; MMSE, Mini-Mental State Examination; GDS, Geriatric Depression Scale; VLMT, Verbal Learning and Memory Test; LVEF, left ventricular ejection fraction; WMH, white matter hyperintensities; optional parameters are depending upon patient agreement; follow-up visits are conducted 1, 6 and 12 months after IA treatment.

For examinations with a high potential for an observer bias (e.g., MRI, echocardiography), images will be stored and the reading will be done offline in a blinded manner. Specifically, they will be assessed without knowledge of the respective patient and time point. All examinations and methods used are described in more detail in the following sections.

2.5.1. Brain Magnetic Resonance Imaging (MRI)

MR Imaging Protocol

All subjects undergo brain imaging at 1.5T (Magnetom Aera, Semens, Germany) using a 20-channel head coil for image acquisition. Structural MR imaging protocol includes a sagittal 3D T1-weighted sequence with an inplane resolution of 1×1 mm and a slice thickness of 1.3 mm (repetition time [TR] = 1860 ms, echo time [TE] = 3.88 ms, inversion time [TI] = 1000 ms, 160 slices); a sagittal 3D FLAIR dataset with 1×1 mm inplane spatial resolution and 1.1 mm slice thickness (TR = 5000 ms, TE = 214 ms, TI = 1800 ms, field of view [FoV] = 265×265 mm); a diffusion weighted imaging (DWI) sequence with b-values 0/1000 s/mm^2 (TR = 5600 ms, TE = 113 ms, 1.2 × 1.2 mm voxel size, 5 mm slice thickness) and a time-of-flight angiography of the circle of Willis with 0.5 × 0.5 mm spatial resolution with a slice thickness of 0.8 mm (TR = 31 ms, TE = 7.15 ms, FoV = 200 mm).

Cerebral perfusion is assessed using a 2D pseudo-continuous arterial spin-labeling sequence (PICORE Q2T) with 5 mm slice thickness and an in-plane spatial resolution of 4 mm with 64 slices. Other imaging parameters are a post labeling delay of 1.8 s, bolus duration of 700 ms, TR = 2500 ms and TE = 13 ms.

A diffusion tensor imaging (DTI) dataset is acquired in all patients (TR = 4700 ms, TE = 116 ms, b-value 0/1000 s/mm^2, 12 directions) with a slice thickness of 4 mm and an in-plane spatial resolution of 1.5 × 1.5 mm.

Total acquisition time is 42 min. All scans are checked by a board certified neuroradiologist for gross abnormalities.

MR Image Analysis

For structural image analysis, all MR datasets are transferred to a dedicated Horos workstation (www.horosproject.org). WMH are evaluated on axial reconstructions of the 3D FLAIR dataset with 3 mm slice thickness according to the Fazekas scale [40]. The Fazekas score are dichotomized into low (Fazekas grade 0–1) and high (Fazekas grade 2–3). Cerebral microbleeds are defined as hypointense lesions smaller than 10 mm on b = 0 diffusion weighted images. Lacunar lesions are defined as small lesions in the deep white and grey matter with a diameter between 3 and 10 mm and cerebrospinal fluid-like signal on all sequences. For quantitative analysis, lacunar lesions and microbleeds are counted by visual inspection and for further statistical analysis dichotomized in present or absent.

Medial temporal lobe atrophy (MTA) score is rated on coronal reformations of the 3D T1w dataset according to previously described criteria [41]. For statistical analysis, the mean MTA score of both sides is dichotomized into high (>1.5) and low (≤1.5) as described elsewhere [42].

Vessel diameter of the internal carotid artery (ICA), the anterior (ACA) and middle cerebral artery (MCA) and the basilar artery (BA) are evaluated by manual measurements. For the ICA, measurements are performed at the level of the cavernous sinus, for the MCA in the median M1 segment, for the ACA immediately distal the anterior communicating artery and for the basilar artery at the level of the origin of the superior cerebellar artery, respectively.

Brain volume estimation are performed using T1w images. Therefore, the measured raw DICOM data are converted into NIFTI (Neuroimaging Informatics Technology Initiative) format using dcm2nii, which is part of the neuroimaging tool MRIcron. Preprocessing using FSL (version 6.0, www.fsl.fmrib.ox.ac.uk/fsl) included correction for gradient nonlinearities, non-brain tissue removal, linear registration to standard space, and tissue segmentation [43]. Evaluation of the pseudo-continuous ASL images is performed as previously described by Binnewijzend et al. [43]. Therefore, ASL images are also corrected for gradient nonlinearities in all three directions and then linearly registered to the brain-extracted T1-weighted images. The brain mask is used to calculate uncorrected mean whole-brain cerebral blood flow (CBF). These volume estimates are then transformed to the ASL data space to correct partial volume-corrected cortical and white matter CBF maps [44]. CBF values are also extracted using regions of interest (ROIs) in the frontal, temporal, occipital and parietal brain areas and the hippocampus based on the MNI152 atlas and the Harvard–Oxford cortical atlas. The primary outcome parameter of the study is uncorrected mean cerebral perfusion measured in mL/min/100 gr of brain tissue determined by ASL.

Preprocessing of DTI data includes also conversion to NIFTI format. Then, the tool eddy correct, part of FSL, is used to correct the diffusion-weighted data with respect to subject motion and deformations introduced by eddy current artifacts of the MRI scanner. Fractional anisotropy (FA) images are created by fitting a tensor model to the raw diffusion data using FSL DTI-FIT. FA analyses was performed on a whole brain basis and using the ROI from CBF-analyses.

2.5.2. Cognitive Assessment

Mini-Mental State Examination (MMSE)

We use MMSE-2 which is a revised version of the original MMSE [45,46] routinely used to measure cognitive decline. The MMSE-2 consists of three versions: the standard version, the brief version and the expanded version of the MMSE. In this study, the standard version is used in order to maximize the benefit of the use of the scale while minimizing the duration of the cognitive assessment. The MMSE-2 shows a sufficient internal consistency (Cronbach's alpha 0.66–0.79) [46].

Alzheimer's Disease Assessment Scale - Cognition (ADAS-Cog)

The Alzheimer's Disease Assessment Scale (ADAS) is commonly used to assess cognitive dysfunction in individuals with Alzheimer's Disease and other types of dementia [47,48]. The ADAS-Cog was developed as a two-part scale: one that measures cognitive impairment and one that measures non-cognitive factors such as mood and behavior. In IMAD, only the cognitive scale of the ADAS-Cog is applied, which consists of 11 parts and measures the cognitive functioning, language, and memory in a 30-min test. Five parallel versions are available to avoid recall bias due to multiple testing. The final score ranges from 0 to 70 points, with higher scores indicating more serious cognitive impairment. The ADAS shows a good internal consistency (Cronbach's alpha 0.61–0.76) [49]. During the baseline visit, a cognitive profile over the 11 dimensions measured by the ADAS-Cog is created. The profile is compared to reference values provided by Graham et al. [48] (Figure 2). According to the reference values, the cognitive profile of patients with mild to moderate AD predominately shows higher impairment in memory, and to a lesser extent, in cognitive functioning. In contrast, language is hardly impaired in this stadium (Figure 2). Thus, patients with a different cognitive profile undergo further examinations to exclude differential diagnoses. For patients included into the IMAD trial, a cognitive change is estimated according to Stern et al. [50] to predict future cognitive decline during the follow-up period. The estimated cognitive change is later compared to the observed cognitive changes over 12 months after IA/IgG.

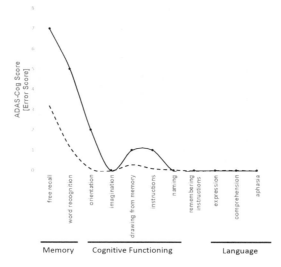

Figure 2. Example of a patient's cognitive profile of the Alzheimer's Disease Assessment Scale–Cognition (ADAS-Cog) with mild to moderate dementia from a patient included in the IMAD trial (own figure). Continuous line, cognitive profile with mild to moderate dementia; dashed line, cognitive profile with no cognitive impairment; grey area, 95% confidence interval for the cognitive profile. Without impairment according to Graham, Emery and Hodges [48].

Verbal Learning and Memory Test (VLMT)

The Verbal Learning and Memory Test (VLMT) allows a short and individual assessment of verbal learning and memory. The VLMT [51] uses 15 semantically independent words to assess verbal memory. In a second step, an interference list with 15 new words is learned and recalled to distract from the first, target list. After 20–30 min a delayed recall of the target list and a recognition test with a new list combining the 30 learned words with 20 semantically and phonemically similar words is done.

Benton Test

The Benton Test (first edition: Benton, 1946) is a visual retention test for clinical use testing the memory of visuo-spatial stimuli. The patient has to reproduce, draw or recognize presented graphic stimuli. In this trial, instruction A (10 figures shown for 10 s) and parallel forms C, D and E are used. The Benton Test has been shown to have a high internal consistency (Cronbach's alpha = 0.94–0.98) and validity [52].

Geriatric Depression Scale (GDS)

The Geriatric Depression Scale (GDS) is used to measure depressive symptoms in older persons. It is a 15-item questionnaire demanding a dichotomous (yes/no) evaluation of depressive symptoms. It was also shown to be applicable for persons with advanced cognitive impairment [53]. The GDS shows a high internal consistency (Cronbach's alpha 0.91).

The standardized questionnaires used in the IMAD trial as well as the respective cut-off values applied are summarized in Table 3.

Table 3. Assessments by standardized questionnaires.

Test	Abbreviation	No Impairment	Severe Impairment	Normal Range
Mini-Mental State Examination	MMSE	30	0	26–30
Alzheimer's Disease Assessment Scale—cognitive Scale	ADAS-Cog	0	70	0–4
Memory		0	22	-
Cognitive Functioning		0	28	-
Language		0	15	-
Verbal Learning and Memory Test	VLMT			
Learning		75	0	48–75
Loss after Interference		0	15	-
Loss after Delay		0	15	0–3
Recognition		0	15	-
Benton Test	Benton Test			
Number Correct Score		10	0	-
Error Score		0	-	-
Geriatric Depression Scale	GDS	0	15	0–5

ADAS-Cog, Alzheimer's Disease Assessment Scale–Cognition; VLMT, GDS, Geriatric Depression Scale; Verbal Learning and Memory Test.

2.5.3. Cardiovascular Examinations

All cardiovascular examinations are conducted according to standardized procedures by certified study nurses and physicians at the cardiovascular examination center of the German Centre for Cardiovascular Disease (DZHK) in Greifswald. The following examinations are part of the IMAD phenotyping:

Brachial Blood Pressure Measurement

Measurements of the brachial blood pressure are taken using an Omron 705 IT (OMRON Healthcare Europe) blood pressure monitor with appropriate cuff size after a resting period of at least 5 min in a sitting position. Accordingly, three measurements are taken on the right arm, with a 3-min break between each measurement [54]. All individual measurements (systolic blood pressure [mmHg], diastolic blood pressure [mmHg], heart rate [/min]) are recorded.

Pulse-Wave Analysis and Central Hemodynamics

To perform cuff-based non-invasive data capturing at the brachial artery, the invasively validated Mobil–O–Graph pulse-wave analysis (PWA) monitor (IEM GmbH, Stolberg, Germany) with inbuilt ARCSolver algorithm is used [55,56]. After conventional blood pressure measurements, the brachial cuff is inflated additionally to the diastolic blood pressure level and held for about 10 s to record pulse waves. Subsequently, central pressure curves are automatically obtained through a transfer function. In total, three measurements are taken, with a 3-min break between each measurement. The following parameters are assessed by this method: pulse-wave velocity (PWV [m/s]), augmentation index (Aix [%]), heart-rate corrected augmentation index (Alx@75 [%]), central systolic blood pressure (cSBP [mmHg]), and central diastolic (cDBP [mmHg]).

Digital Endothelial Vascular Function and Stiffness

Digital pulse amplitude is measured with a pulse amplitude tonometry device placed on the tip of the right index finger (Endo-PAT2000, Itamar Medical, Caesarea, Israel) [57]. This device comprises a pneumatic plethysmograph that applies uniform pressure to the surface of the distal finger, allowing measurement of pulse volume changes. Throughout the study, the inflation pressure of the digital device is electronically set to 10 mm Hg below diastolic blood pressure or 70 mm Hg (whichever is lower). Baseline pulse amplitude is measured for 2 min 20 s. Arterial flow is interrupted for 5 min by a cuff placed on a proximal forearm using an occlusion pressure of 200 mm Hg or 60 mm Hg above systolic blood pressure (whichever is higher). The pulse amplitude is recorded electronically and analyzed by the computerized, automated algorithm of the device that provides the average pulse amplitude for each 30-s interval after forearm cuff deflation up to 4 min [57]. The following parameters which are known markers of endothelial function and vascular stiffness is derived from these measurements: augmentation index (Aix [%]), heart-rate corrected augmentation index (AIx@75% [%]), reactive hyperemia index (RHI) [57].

Transcutaneous Oxygen Pressure (tcPO2)

Transcutaneous oxygen pressure (tcPO2) measurements are performed with the PRÉCISE 8008 device (medicap GmbH, Ulrichstein, Germany). After a resting period of at least 10 min in supine position, four probes are placed at the dorsum of the feet and at the back of both hands. Measurements are taken while patients are breathing ambient air, in a resting supine position at room temperature, between 22 °C and 25 °C. The site on the foot is carefully cleaned before the probes are applied to the skin, using adhesive rings and contact liquid, supplied by the manufacturer. The measurements are performed after calibration and preheating of the transducer to approximate 44 °C [58]. After termination of the procedure tcPO2 [mmHg] values for the four measurement sites are recorded.

Echocardiography

Transthoracic echocardiography as a non-invasive gold standard for the determination cardiac function and morphology is performed by certified physicians (Vingmed Vivid 9, 5S transducer 2.0–5.0 MHz, GE Medical Systems GmbH, Hamburg, Germany). All images and loops are stored digitally and are analyzed offline. The reading of the echocardiograms is performed according to current recommendations [59] includes parameters of left atrial and left ventricular (LV) structure (left atrial diameter in parasternal short axis [mm]; left atrial volume in 4 chamber view [cm^2], enddiastolic/endsystolic thickness of the intraventricular septum and posterial wall [mm], LV mass [g], enddiastolic/endsystolic LV volume [mL]) as well as LV systolic and diastolic function (biplane LV ejection fraction according to Simpsons rule [%], global longitudinal strain [%], peak velocity of the mitral E- and A-wave [cm/s], deceleration time of the mitral E-wave [ms], isovolumetric relaxation time [ms], peak velocity of the excursion of the lateral and septal mitral annulus in the early diastolic phase [cm/s], ratio between the peak velocity of the excursion of the mean lateral/septal mitral annulus in the early diastolic phase and the peak velocity of the mitral E-wave).

2.5.4. Kidney Function and Ultrasound

Kidney function is determined by blood and urinary laboratory tests: estimated glomerular filtration rate by serum creatine and urinary albumin–creatinine ratio.

Renal ultrasound is performed with a HITACHI EUB-7500 machine. Kidney length is determined as the maximum longitudinal dimension. Parenchymal thickness is measured as the shortest distance from the renal sinus fat to the renal capsule at three different points: at the upper and lower pole and at the middle. The parenchymal-pyelon-index is calculated as the sum of ventral and dorsal parenchymal thickness (in a cross-section of the kidney) divided by the width of the central echo complex. The following categories are generally assessed: location, anomalies as agenesis, hypo- or hyperplasia, horseshoe kidney; kidney length; kidney width; parenchymal thickness; surface roughness; echogenicity; parenchymal-pyelon-index; medullary or parenchymal calcification; number and size of cysts, stones, infraction zones and tumors [60].

2.5.5. Ultrasound of the Extracranial Arteries

Ultrasound of the extracranial arteries is performed with a Philips UI 22 machine. Extracranial carotid and vertebral arteries (VA) are examined with linear ultrasound transducers (bandwidth 3–13 MHz). Systolic, diastolic, and mean flow velocities in common carotid artery, internal carotid artery (ICA), and V2 segments of VA are documented after angle correction. We classify ICA stenosis uniformly according to current ultrasound criteria for grading internal carotid artery stenoses of the the German Society of Ultrasound in Medicine (DEGUM) and Transfer to grading system of the North American Symptomatic Carotid Endarterectomy Trial (NASCET) [61]: if peak systolic velocity (PSV) is ≥125 cm/s, ICA stenosis is defined as being equivalent to ≥50% according to North American Symptomatic Carotid Endarterectomy Trial criteria. Occlusion is defined by absence of Doppler and color signal, typical proximal biphasic Doppler spectra, and additional indirect criteria like crossflow. Carotid plaque is defined as any arterial wall irregularity thicker than 1.5 mm or exceeding >50% of the surrounding wall thickness that protruded into the vessel lumen.

VA measurements are taken in the V2 segment and considered abnormal if there is direct evidence of local or indirect evidence of proximal or distal flow abnormalities. Overall, abnormal flow characteristic of the posterior circulation is defined by at least unilateral (1) flow abnormality of the (extracranial) V2 segment of either VA, (2) intracranial VA stenosis or occlusion, or (3) basilar artery (BA) stenosis or occlusion.

2.5.6. Blood and Urine Samples

Blood and urine samples are obtained according to standard operating procedures. In total, 403.7 mL blood and 42.0 mL urine are obtained per participant (250.0 mL for serum analysis, 121.5 mL for plasma analytics, 16 mL EDTA, 16.2 mL Citrate). At the study center, samples are analyzed immediately after blood and urine sampling. Two aliquots of 0.5 mL serum are stored in a freezer (−80 °C) for further analysis.

For sample analyses at independent laboratories (see Section 2.5.8), blood samples (170.0 mL for serum analytics, 49.5 mL for plasma analytics) are collected at the study center. Further sample management is accomplished by biometec GmbH, Greifswald, Germany.

Blood samples are obtained according to standard operating procedures. In total, 29 mL were obtained per participant (8.5 mL for serum analysis, 8 mL for plasma analytics, 10 mL EDTA, 2.5 mL for blood RNA). At the study center they were stored in a freezer at −80 °C. For this analysis, 100 aliquots were available.

2.5.7. Laboratory Parameters

A complete list of the laboratory parameters can be found in the Appendix A (Table A1). Laboratory analytics of blood and urine are carried out in accordance with established standard operating procedures and preanalytical protocols follow the schemes of the GANI_MED (Greifswald Approach to Individualized Medicine) project [62].

2.5.8. Assessment of Autoantibodies

An enzyme-linked immunosorbent assay (ELISA) is used to detect agAAB as described previously [37,63]. Analyses are performed by an independent laboratory (E.R.D.E.-AAK-Diagnostik GmbH, Berlin, Germany) blinded to clinical patient data. In brief, peptides are directed against the ß1-adrenergic receptor loop 1 and ß2- adrenergic receptor loops 1 and 2. Modified peptides are bound to 96-well streptavidin-coated plates. Peptides are coupled to preblocked streptavidin-coated 96-well plates (Perbio Science, Bonn, Germany). Patient serum is added in a 1:100 dilution and incubated for 60 min. As detection antibody a horseradish peroxidase conjugated anti-human IgG antibody is used (Biomol, Hamburg, Germany). Antibody binding is visualized by the 1-Step Ultra TMB ELISA (Perbio Science, Bonn, Germany). The absorbance is measured at 450 nm against 650 nm with an SLT Spectra multiplate reader (TECAN, Crailsheim, Germany).

As confirmation test, a bioassay is used that has been established by Wallukat and Wollenberger for the identification and quantification of GPCR-AABs [64], and that has been modified and standardized as described previously [65,66]. Analyses are performed by an external laboratory (Berlin Cures GmbH, Berlin, Germany) without knowledge about any further patient characteristics or parameters. In this bioassay, the chronotropic response of spontaneously beating cultured neonatal rat cardiomyocytes to patients' IgG-containing GPCR-AABs is recorded [67].

Anti-NMDA (N-methyl-D-aspartate) autoantibodies are determined in the participant's sera by immunohistochemistry according to manufacturer's instruction (Anti-Glutamate-Receptor-IgG (Typ NMDA)–IFFT, EUROIMMUN, Lübeck, Germany).

Additional measurements are performed by biometec GmbH, Greifswald. This includes analyzes of antibodies against oxidized low-density lipoprotein (oxLDL) and β-amyloid, vasculitis marker (aab against myeloperoxidase (anti-MPO), proteinase 3 (anti-PR3), glomerular basement membrane (anti-GBM)), B-cell activity and antibody development (B-cell activating factor (BAFF)) and neurodegeneration (neurogranin).

2.6. Intervention

Immunoadsorption is performed with ADAsorb apheresis devices equipped with Globaffin adsorber columns in the dialysis department of the University Medicine Greifswald.

The Globaffin column is a regenerative twin adsorber system that utilizes peptide ligands (Peptid-GAM®; Fresenius Medical Care, Bad Homburg, Germany) covalently bound to sepharose. These peptide ligands have a strong affinity for Fc fragments of immunoglobulins from any source and selectively remove immunoglobulins and immune complexes from plasma without affecting other plasma proteins. The Globaffin adsorber system has previously been used in antibody mediated disorders, such as dilated cardiomyopathy and acute renal transplant rejection [68].

In contrast to unselective plasma exchange where all plasma components including albumin, clotting factors and immunoglobulins are discarded and replaced with a fluid containing either albumin and colloid or donor plasma, immunoadsorption is a semi-selective device. First, the patient's plasma is separated from blood cells by a membrane. Plasma is then passed over the Globaffin twin adsorber system which selectively remove IgG, IgA, and IgM before the plasma is re-infused to the patient.

Typically, approximately four column volumes (250 mL) are processed before the plasma stream is directed to the second column within the device and the first column undergoes a four-step regeneration, so that the apheresis cycle can be reiterated: (1) replacement of residual plasma by 0.9% NaCl solution; (2) elution of bound immunoglobulin by hydrochloric acid [glycine-HCl] buffer at pH 2.8; (3) neutralization by phosphate buffered saline [PBS] and 4. replacement of PBS by 0.9% NaCl (Figure 3).

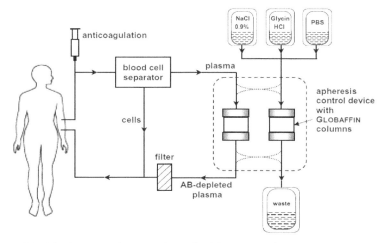

Figure 3. Principle of immunoadsorption. Principle of the immunoadsorption treatment. Reprinted from [68] with permission of John Wiley and Sons.

A separate twin-column pair is assigned to each patient. A total of approximately 2.0-fold of blood plasma volume is processed per day (approximately 4 to 6 h per session) on five consecutive days. After the immunoadsorption series, the patients receive 500 mg per kg body weight intravenous immunoglobulin substitution on day 6 (during approximately 6 h). The dose is determined based on body weight and amounts to 500 mg/kg, depending on the packaging size. The eluates of the regeneration of the columns are collected automatically and are used for detailed immunological analyses. The patients are hospitalized for the immunoadsorption procedures and Ig substitution period in the neurological department of the University Medicine Greifswald.

2.7. Statistical Considerations

The objective of this trial is to assess the effects of IA/IgG in patients with agAABs and dementia in patients with suspected Alzheimer's clinical syndrome. The primary target parameter is uncorrected mean cerebral brain perfusion as assessed by ASL 12 months after treatment.

2.7.1. Statistical Analyses

Analyses will follow an exploratory approach since we plan n = 15 subjects but do not consider a comparison group. Although the main focus of analysis is descriptive, there is an interest in comparing the development of outcomes of 1 month before and 12 months after IA/IgG.

Effect sizes will be estimated using appropriate (generalized) linear mixed regression models. If necessary non-parametric models will be used. To evaluate effect sizes, suggestions according to Cohen (1988) are used [69]. Analyses are performed as intention-to-treat (ITT) and per-protocol (PP).

2.7.2. Missing Data

Missing values are not replaced with substituted values. Due to the small sample size and the exploratory character of the investigation, imputation techniques are not recommended.

2.7.3. Effect Size Consideration

Assuming a prevalence of agAABs of 31.5% and a drop-out rate of 20%, 120 participants have to be checked for eligibility to reach the aim of 15 participants enrolled in the intervention. With a sample size of n = 12, an expected α-error of 5% and a power of 80%, standardized effect sizes of 0.766 can be detected (for one-sided paired *t*-tests), thus allowing a possible drop out of maximal 3 participants.

For data analyses, Stata (Version 14, StataCorp, College Station, TX, USA), SPSS statistics version 22 (IBM Corp., Armonk, NY, USA) or MATLAB (Version R2015a, Mathworks Inc., Natick, MA, USA) will be used.

3. Discussion

The IMAD study investigates a new pathophysiological and therapeutic aspect of Alzheimer's clinical syndrome, the removal of α1AR-agAABs by immunoadsorption in patients with cognitive impairment and suspected AD. Outcome parameters comprise cerebral blood flow measured by arterial spin labelling MRI (primary), cognition measured by validated cognitive tests and other questionnaires (ADAS-Cog, MMSE, VLMT, Benton Test, GDS) and vascular effects assessed by echocardiography, sonography, blood pressure, pulse wave velocity, plethysmography and transcutaneous oxygen measurement.

Extracorporeal therapies for dementia in Alzheimer's clinical syndrome and CVD are innovative therapeutic options. Recently, three different medical devices have been tested: dialysis, TPE and IA. The Spanish AMBAR study is currently examining whether the peripheral lowering of Aß by TPE and concurrent albumin substitution has an impact on cognitive performance [70]. Kitaguchi and colleagues use dialysis systems [71] and adsorptive double-filtration systems [8] to lower the plasma levels of Aß. Both groups are assuming that the removal of Aß may reduce the cerebral Aß load. By using IA, we contrary aim to target vascular effects of α1AR-agAABs and only secondarily at a probably better clearance of Aß. The IMAD study can profit from the experience of a previously performed open pilot trial [38]. In this earlier study, the applicability of apheresis to dementia patients and safety aspects were examined. The sustainability of the elimination of α1AR-agAABs was proven and the first indications of a stabilization of cognitive performance were observed. The IMAD study now investigates whether the removal of α1AR-AABs by a 5-day IA procedure has a positive effect (improvement or non-deterioration) on impairment-relevant hemodynamic, cognitive, neurological, vascular and metabolic parameters within a one-year follow-up period.

As an exploratory trial, the IMAD study has, owing to feasibility constraints, a small projected sample size in a monocentric, single-arm and unblinded design. Thus, only large effects can reach statistical significance and, even then, the absence of a control group and other trial site(s) will still confine the validity of the results. Nevertheless, this trial may provide important insights whether eliminating or reducing α1AR-agAABs as a contributing factor of dementia-related cerebrovascular impairment opens up a completely new treatment approach for α1AR-agAABs-positive persons along the course of dementia progression in patients with Alzheimer's clinical syndrome. It is of course possible that other agAABs also play a role in the disease course, e.g., ß2AR which has been found in dementia patients in previous studies [37,38].

In this respect, the comprehensive and extensive set of measured endpoints has the potential to indicate possible intervention effects on a broad (patho)physiological spectrum. Indeed, the trial protocol has been devised deliberately to comprise as many measurable physiological and metabolic parameters as possible besides the neurocognitive tests. Therefore, the IMAD trial results will allow to correlate intervention effects with potential physiological or functional mode(s) of action. Such correlations may form the basis of targeted, larger and statistically more robust trials to specifically and precisely uncover the effects of immunoadsorption on affected patients. In the future, the optimal intervention time during the disease progression and the determinants that predict and govern the response profile should be addressed in order to achieve a maximal beneficial effect of IA. In this regard, one challenge will be to pinpoint the actual pathomechanistically active autoantibodies or autoantibodies to delineate less-invasive specific depletion or inactivation schemes.

However, if the IA treatment approach does turn out to have a beneficial capacity for at least a well-defined subgroup of patients at risk of dementia progression in Alzheimer's clinical syndrome, its one-time character (a single week of hospitalization) will certainly be advantageous, discarding or at least attenuating the pharmacotherapeutic need for long-term compliance adherence. For reasons that have not yet been clarified, the GPCR-AABs seldom reoccur after being removed—both in DCM [36,72,73] and in dementia [38].

In the case of a positive outcome of the planned study, functional vascular improvement and cognitive stability or improvement over at least 12 months, knowledge and experience should have been gained to start a well-planned controlled, prospective, multicenter and randomized clinical study. Its data could then be used to prove that IA is suitable for the treatment of mild and moderate dementia with vascular pathological AABs and complements antidementive drug therapies with other targets.

Our study design has potential strengths and limitations that merit further discussion. We see the interdisciplinary approach where knowledge from different disciplines and viewpoints are combined as a unique strength. A further strength resulting directly from this is the comprehensive phenotyping with different end-points to generate a broad spectrum of results that may help design a subsequent multicenter pilot study. As a potential limitation we see the small sample size with low statistical power. For this reason, we are also not able to investigate other potential risk factors (e.g., genetic disposition). As we include patients with cognitive impairment without additional testing of CSF biomarkers we face limitations in the diagnostic classification of their syndromes. Thus, we prefer to label their impairments as suspected or probable AD. On the other hand, we use well-validated neuropsychological testing (MMSE, ADAS-cog, Benton Test, VLMT) and carefully exclude many medical conditions that could lead to secondary and potentially treatable dementia. Moreover, based on the MRI scans we can exclude patients with organic/structural brain damages from the study. In fact, our intention behind this patient selection was the inclusion of patients in their beginning or early phase of probable AD to detect possible changes due to immunoadsorption in physiological and cognitive parameters which might not occur in later states of dementia and to ensure the ability of collaboration and adherence throughout a 12-months follow-up period of the study. Furthermore, we may miss results in the long-term for future associations and detection of causalities due to the relatively short follow up time of 12 months. Additionally, knowledge about the prevalence of agonistic autoantibodies

J. Clin. Med. **2020**, *9*, 1919

in other forms of dementia and in the general population is limited. Keeping these limitations in mind, our study is designed as an exploratory study and aims at showing proof of principle.

4. Conclusions

IMAD is an important pilot study that will analyze whether the removal of α1AR-agAABs by immunoadsorption in α1AR-agAAB-positive persons slows the progression of dementia in Alzheimer's clinical syndrome and/or improves vascular functional parameters.

Author Contributions: Conceptualization, S.S., S.L. (Sandra Lange), H.K., J.K.-K., S.B., A.V., S.G., A.D., R.K., H.J.G., S.L. (Sönke Langner) and M.D.; Formal analysis, S.G.; Investigation, S.S., S.L. (Sandra Lange), S.B., L.S., J.K.-K., A.V., F.v.P., A.F., K.W., G.W., H.P., H.J.G., S.L. (Sönke Langner) and M.D.; Methodology, M.D.; Project administration, S.L. (Sandra Lange), H.K., S.B. and S.L. (Sönke Langner); Supervision, M.D.; Writing—original draft, S.S., S.L. (Sandra Lange) and M.D.; Writing—review and editing, S.S., S.L. (Sandra Lange), S.B., H.K., L.S., J.K.-K., S.B., A.V., F.v.P., A.F., S.G., K.W., G.W., H.P., A.D., R.K., H.J.G., S.L. (Sönke Langner) and M.D. All authors have read and agreed to the published version of the manuscript.

Funding: The University Medicine Greifswald has received unrestricted financial support by Fresenius Medical Care Deutschland GmbH (Bad Homburg, Germany) for carrying out the study. Fresenius Medical Care did not have any influence on design and conduct of the study as well as on data analyses and writing of the manuscript.

Acknowledgments: We would like to thank Kristin Werner for assisting the immunoadsorption procedure and study coordination and Bianca Ladwig for supporting the data acquisition and curation.

Conflicts of Interest: AF has received consulting fees from Bayer, Roche, Novartis, and Biogen Idec, and honoraria for oral presentations from Novartis, Böhringer-Ingelheim, Biogen Idec, Paul-Martini-Stiftung, and Daiichi-Sankyo. HP received research support from Diamed and speaker honoraria from Fresenius Medical Care. RK is scientific consultant in therapeutic apheresis for Fresenius Medical Deutschland GmbH, Bad Homburg, Germany. HJG has received travel grants and speakers' honoraria from Fresenius Medical Care, Neuraxpharm, Servier and Janssen Cilag as well as research funding from Fresenius Medical Care. MD has received travel grants and speakers' honoraria from Fresenius Medical Care. All other authors did not report any conflicts of interest related to this manuscript.

Appendix A

Table A1. Laboratory parameters.

Parameter	Screening	Baseline	d1 Pre-IA	d1 Post-IA	d2 Pre-IA	d2 Post-IA	d3 Pre-IA	d3 Post-IA	d4 Pre-IA	d4 Post-IA	d5 Pre-IA	d5 Post-IA	d6 Subst.	Follow-Ups
						Immunoadsorption								
agAB A1AR	X													X
anti oxLDL				X	X	X	X	X	X	X	X	X		X
anti MPO			X											X
anti PR3			X											X
anti GBM			X											X
anti NMDA		X												
anti Amyloid β		X	X	X	X	X	X	X	X	X	X	X		X
Neurogranin			X											X
Oxidized low density lipoprotein (oxLDL)			X											X
BAFF			X											X
Leucocytes		X	X		X		X		X		X		X	X
Erythrocytes		X	X		X		X		X		X		X	X
Hemoglobin		X	X		X		X		X		X		X	X
Hematocrit		X	X		X		X		X		X		X	X
Platelets		X	X		X		X		X		X		X	X
Mean Platelet Volume		X	X		X		X		X		X		X	X
Platelet Distribution Width		X	X		X		X		X		X		X	X
Lymphocytes		X	X		X		X		X		X		X	X
Prothrombin time (Quick)		X	X		X		X		X		X		X	X
International Normalized Ratio (INR)		X	X		X		X		X		X		X	X
Partial Thromboplastine Time (aPTT)		X	X		X		X		X		X		X	X
Mean Cell Volume (MCV)		X	X		X		X		X		X		X	X
Mean Cellular Hemoglobin (MCH)		X	X		X		X		X		X		X	X
Mean Cellular Hemoglobin Concentration (MCHC)		X	X		X		X		X		X		X	X
Red Blood Cell Distribution Curve		X	X		X		X		X		X		X	X
Red Blood Cell Distribution Width (RBCD)		X	X		X		X		X		X		X	X
Sodium		X	X		X		X		X		X		X	X
Potassium		X	X		X		X		X		X		X	X
Calcium		X	X		X		X		X		X		X	X
Phosphate		X	X		X		X		X		X		X	X
Glucose		X	X		X		X		X		X		X	X
Creatinine		X	X		X		X		X		X		X	X
Urea		X	X		X		X		X		X		X	X
Uric Acid		X	X		X		X		X		X		X	X
Total Cholesterol		X	X		X		X		X		X		X	X
High density lipoprotein (HDL)-Cholesterol		X	X		X		X		X		X		X	X
Low density lipoprotein (LDL)-Cholesterol		X	X		X		X		X		X		X	X
Total Triglyzeride		X	X		X		X		X		X		X	X
Alanine-Aminotransferase		X	X		X		X		X		X		X	X
Aspartate-Aminotransferase		X	X		X		X		X		X		X	X
γ-Glutamyl Transferase		X	X		X		X		X		X		X	X
Total Bilirubin		X	X		X		X		X		X		X	X

J. Clin. Med. **2020**, *9*, 1919

Table A1. *Cont.*

Parameter	Screening	Baseline	d1 Pre-IA	d1 Post-IA	d2 Pre-IA	d2 Post-IA	d3 Pre-IA	d3 Post-IA	d4 Pre-IA	d4 Post-IA	d5 Pre-IA	d5 Post-IA	d6 Subst.	Follow-Ups
							Immunoadsorption							
Lipase		X	X		X		X		X		X		X	X
C-reactive Protein (CRP)		X	X		X		X		X		X		X	X
Thyroid (TSH)		X	X		X		X		X		X		X	X
HbA1c		X	X		X		X		X		X		X	X
Albumin		X	X		X		X		X		X		X	X
Protein		X	X		X		X		X		X		X	X
Cystatin C		X	X		X		X		X		X		X	X
Fibrinogen		X	X		X		X		X		X		X	X
Complement C3		X	X		X		X		X		X		X	X
Complement C4		X	X		X		X		X		X		X	X
Factor VIII		X	X		X		X		X		X		X	X
Antithrombin		X	X		X		X		X		X		X	X
Immunoglobulin IgG1		X	X		X		X		X		X		X	X
Immunoglobulin IgG2		X	X		X		X		X		X		X	X
Immunoglobulin IgG3)		X	X		X		X		X		X		X	X
Immunoglobulin IgG4		X	X		X		X		X		X		X	X
Immunoglobulin M		X	X		X		X		X		X		X	X
Immunoglobulin A		X	X		X		X		X		X		X	X
Total Immunoglobulin G		X	X	X	X	X	X	X	X	X	X	X	X	X
Total Immunoglobulin		X	X		X		X		X		X		X	X
Vitamin B12		X	X		X		X		X		X		X	X
25-Hydroxy-Vitamin D		X	X		X		X		X		X		X	X
Folic Acid		X	X		X		X		X		X		X	X
Homocysteine		X	X		X									
Specific gravity (Urine)		X	X		X		X		X		X		X	X
pH (Urine)		X	X		X		X		X		X		X	X
Leucocytes (Urine)		X	X		X		X		X		X		X	X
Nitrite (Urine)		X	X		X		X		X		X		X	X
Protein (Urine)		X	X		X		X		X		X		X	X
Glucose (Urine)		X	X		X		X		X		X		X	X
Ketone (Urine)		X	X		X		X		X		X		X	X
Urobilinogen (Urine)		X	X		X		X		X		X		X	X
Bilirubin (Urine)		X	X		X		X		X		X		X	X
Erythrocytes/Blood (Urine)		X	X		X		X		X		X		X	X
U-Creatine (Urine)		X	X		X		X		X		X		X	X
U-Protein (Urine)		X	X		X		X		X		X		X	X
U-Albumin (Urine)		X	X		X		X		X		X		X	X

References

1. Prince, M. *World Alzheimer Report the Global Impact of Dementia. An Analysis of Prevalence, Incidence, Cost and Trends*; Alzheimer's Disease International: London, UK, 2015.
2. Eggink, E.; van Charante, E.P.M.; van Gool, W.A.; Richard, E. A Population Perspective on Prevention of Dementia. *J. Clin. Med.* **2019**, *8*, 834. [CrossRef] [PubMed]
3. World Health Organization (WHO). Dementia-Key Facts. Available online: https://www.who.int/news-room/fact-sheets/detail/dementia (accessed on 27 May 2020).
4. Vetrano, D.L.; Rizzuto, D.; Calderon-Larranaga, A.; Onder, G.; Welmer, A.K.; Bernabei, R.; Marengoni, A.; Fratiglioni, L. Trajectories of functional decline in older adults with neuropsychiatric and cardiovascular multimorbidity: A Swedish cohort study. *PLoS Med.* **2018**, *15*, e1002503. [CrossRef] [PubMed]
5. Vetrano, D.L.; Rizzuto, D.; Calderon-Larranaga, A.; Onder, G.; Welmer, A.K.; Qiu, C.; Bernabei, R.; Marengoni, A.; Fratiglioni, L. Walking Speed Drives the Prognosis of Older Adults with Cardiovascular and Neuropsychiatric Multimorbidity. *Am. J. Med.* **2019**, *132*, 1207–1215 e6. [CrossRef] [PubMed]
6. Alzheimer's Association. 2020 Alzheimer's Disease Facts and Figures. *Alzheimers Dement.* **2020**, *6*, 391–460.
7. Deutsche Gesellschaft für Psychiatrie, Psychotherapie und Nervenheilkunde (DGPPN); Deutsche Gesellschaft für Neurologie (DGN). S3-Leitlinie "Demenzen". 2016. Available online: https://www.awmf.org/uploads/tx_szleitlinien/038-013l_S3-Demenzen-2016-07.pdf (accessed on 27 May 2020).
8. Brier, M.R.; Gordon, B.; Friedrichsen, K.; McCarthy, J.; Stern, A.; Christensen, J.; Owen, C.; Aldea, P.; Su, Y.; Hassenstab, J.; et al. Tau and Abeta imaging, CSF measures, and cognition in Alzheimer's disease. *Sci. Transl. Med.* **2016**, *8*, 338ra66. [CrossRef] [PubMed]
9. Holtzman, D.M.; Carrillo, M.C.; Hendrix, J.A.; Bain, L.J.; Catafau, A.M.; Gault, L.M.; Goedert, M.; Mandelkow, E.; Mandelkow, E.M.; Miller, D.S.; et al. Tau: From research to clinical development. *Alzheimers Dement.* **2016**, *12*, 1033–1039. [CrossRef]
10. van Dyck, C.H. Anti-Amyloid-beta Monoclonal Antibodies for Alzheimer's Disease: Pitfalls and Promise. *Biol. Psychiatry* **2018**, *83*, 311–319. [CrossRef]
11. Doody, R.S.; Thomas, R.G.; Farlow, M.; Iwatsubo, T.; Vellas, B.; Joffe, S.; Kieburtz, K.; Raman, R.; Sun, X.; Aisen, P.S.; et al. Phase 3 trials of solanezumab for mild-to-moderate Alzheimer's disease. *N. Engl. J. Med.* **2014**, *370*, 311–321. [CrossRef]
12. Salloway, S.; Sperling, R.; Fox, N.C.; Blennow, K.; Klunk, W.; Raskind, M.; Sabbagh, M.; Honig, L.S.; Porsteinsson, A.P.; Ferris, S.; et al. Two phase 3 trials of bapineuzumab in mild-to-moderate Alzheimer's disease. *N. Engl. J. Med.* **2014**, *370*, 322–333. [CrossRef]
13. Egan, M.F.; Kost, J.; Tariot, P.N.; Aisen, P.S.; Cummings, J.L.; Vellas, B.; Sur, C.; Mukai, Y.; Voss, T.; Furtek, C.; et al. Randomized Trial of Verubecestat for Mild-To-Moderate Alzheimer's Disease. *N. Engl. J. Med.* **2018**, *378*, 1691–1703. [CrossRef]
14. Cuberas-Borros, G.; Roca, I.; Boada, M.; Tarraga, L.; Hernandez, I.; Buendia, M.; Rubio, L.; Torres, G.; Bittini, A.; Guzman-de-Villoria, J.A.; et al. Longitudinal Neuroimaging Analysis in Mild-Moderate Alzheimer's Disease Patients Treated with Plasma Exchange with 5% Human Albumin. *J. Alzheimers Dis.* **2018**, *61*, 321–332. [CrossRef] [PubMed]
15. Boada, M.; Lopez, O.; unez, L.N.; Szczepiorkowski, Z.M.; Torres, M.; Grifols, C.; Paez, A. Plasma exchange for Alzheimer's disease Management by Albumin Replacement (AMBAR) trial: Study design and progress. *Alzheimers Dement. (N. Y.)* **2019**, *5*, 61–69. [CrossRef] [PubMed]
16. Kitaguchi, N.; Kawaguchi, K.; Yamazaki, K.; Kawachi, H.; Sakata, M.; Kaneko, M.; Kato, M.; Sakai, K.; Ohashi, N.; Hasegawa, M.; et al. Adsorptive filtration systems for effective removal of blood amyloid beta: A potential therapy for Alzheimer's disease. *J. Artif. Organs.* **2018**, *21*, 220–229. [CrossRef] [PubMed]
17. Attems, J.K.; Jellinger, A. The overlap between vascular disease and Alzheimer's disease–lessons from pathology. *BMC Med.* **2014**, *12*, 206. [CrossRef] [PubMed]
18. Habes, M.; Erus, G.; Toledo, J.B.; Zhang, T.; Bryan, N.; Launer, L.J.; Rosseel, Y.; Janowitz, D.; Doshi, J.; van der Auwera, S.; et al. White matter hyperintensities and imaging patterns of brain ageing in the general population. *Brain* **2016**, *139*, 1164–1179. [CrossRef]
19. Wallukat, G.; Schimke, I. Agonistic autoantibodies directed against G-protein-coupled receptors and their relationship to cardiovascular diseases. *Semin. Immunopathol.* **2014**, *36*, 351–363. [CrossRef]

20. Cabral-Marques, O.; Riemekasten, G. Functional autoantibodies targeting G protein-coupled receptors in rheumatic diseases. *Nat. Rev. Rheumatol.* **2017**, *13*, 648–656. [CrossRef]

21. Nakatake, N.; Sanders, J.; Richards, T.; Burne, P.; Barrett, C.; Pra, C.D.; Presotto, F.; Betterle, C.; Furmaniak, J.; Smith, B.R. Estimation of serum TSH receptor autoantibody concentration and affinity. *Thyroid* **2006**, *16*, 1077–1084. [CrossRef]

22. Wallukat, G.; Fu, M.L.; Magnusson, Y.; Hjalmarson, A.; Hoebeke, J.; Wollenberger, A. Agonistic effects of anti-peptide antibodies and autoantibodies directed against adrenergic and cholinergic receptors: Absence of desensitization. *Blood Press. Suppl.* **1996**, *3*, 31–36.

23. Karczewski, P.; Pohlmann, A.; Wagenhaus, B.; Wisbrun, N.; Hempel, P.; Lemke, B.; Kunze, R.; Niendorf, T.; Bimmler, M. Antibodies to the alpha1-adrenergic receptor cause vascular impairments in rat brain as demonstrated by magnetic resonance angiography. *PLoS ONE* **2012**, *7*, e41602. [CrossRef]

24. El Fassi, D.; Banga, J.P.; Gilbert, J.A.; Padoa, C.; Hegedus, L.; Nielsen, C.H. Treatment of Graves' disease with rituximab specifically reduces the production of thyroid stimulating autoantibodies. *Clin. Immunol.* **2009**, *130*, 252–258. [CrossRef] [PubMed]

25. Beyer, G.; Kuster, I.; Budde, C.; Wilhelm, E.; Hoene, A.; Evert, K.; Stracke, S.; Friesecke, S.; Mayerle, J.; Steveling, A. Hyperthyroid and acute tonsillitis in a 23-year-old woman. *Internist (Berl.)* **2016**, *57*, 717–723. [CrossRef] [PubMed]

26. Mawuenyega, K.G.; Sigurdson, W.; Ovod, V.; Munsell, L.; Kasten, T.; Morris, J.C.; Yarasheski, K.E.; Bateman, R.J. Decreased clearance of CNS beta-amyloid in Alzheimer's disease. *Science* **2010**, *330*, 1774. [CrossRef] [PubMed]

27. Fu, M.L.; Herlitz, H.; Wallukat, G.; Hilme, E.; Hedner, T.; Hoebeke, J.; Hjalmarson, A. Functional autoimmune epitope on alpha 1-adrenergic receptors in patients with malignant hypertension. *Lancet* **1994**, *344*, 1660–1663.

28. Wenzel, K.; Haase, H.; Wallukat, G.; Derer, W.; Bartel, S.; Homuth, V.; Herse, F.; Hubner, N.; Schulz, H.; Janczikowski, M.; et al. Potential relevance of alpha(1)-adrenergic receptor autoantibodies in refractory hypertension. *PLoS ONE* **2008**, *3*, e3742. [CrossRef]

29. Li, G.; Cao, Z.; Wu, X.W.; Wu, H.K.; Ma, Y.; Wu, B.; Wang, W.Q.; Cheng, J.; Zhou, Z.H.; Tu, Y.C. Autoantibodies against AT1 and alpha1-adrenergic receptors predict arterial stiffness progression in normotensive subjects over a 5-year period. *Clin. Sci. (Lond.)* **2017**, *131*, 2947–2957. [CrossRef]

30. Felix, S.B.; Beug, D.; Dörr, M. Immunoadsorption therapy in dilated cardiomyopathy. *Expert. Rev. Cardiovasc. Ther.* **2015**, *13*, 145–152. [CrossRef]

31. Felix, S.B.; Staudt, A.; Dorffel, W.V.; Stangl, V.; Merkel, K.; Pohl, M.; Docke, W.D.; Morgera, S.; Neumayer, H.H.; Wernecke, K.D.; et al. Hemodynamic effects of immunoadsorption and subsequent immunoglobulin substitution in dilated cardiomyopathy: Three-month results from a randomized study. *J. Am. Coll. Cardiol.* **2000**, *35*, 1590–1598. [CrossRef]

32. Herda, L.R.; Trimpert, C.; Nauke, U.; Landsberger, M.; Hummel, A.; Beug, D.; Kieback, A.; Dörr, M.; Empen, K.; Knebel, F.; et al. Effects of immunoadsorption and subsequent immunoglobulin G substitution on cardiopulmonary exercise capacity in patients with dilated cardiomyopathy. *Am. Heart J.* **2010**, *159*, 809–816. [CrossRef]

33. Staudt, A.; Schaper, F.; Stangl, V.; Plagemann, A.; Bohm, M.; Merkel, K.; Wallukat, G.; Wernecke, K.D.; Stangl, K.; Baumann, G.; et al. Immunohistological changes in dilated cardiomyopathy induced by immunoadsorption therapy and subsequent immunoglobulin substitution. *Circulation* **2001**, *103*, 2681–2686. [CrossRef]

34. Staudt, A.; Hummel, A.; Ruppert, J.; Dörr, M.; Trimpert, C.; Birkenmeier, K.; Krieg, T.; Staudt, Y.; Felix, S.B. Immunoadsorption in dilated cardiomyopathy: 6-month results from a randomized study. *Am. Heart J.* **2006**, *152*, 712 e1-6. [CrossRef] [PubMed]

35. Winters, J.L. Apheresis in the treatment of idiopathic dilated cardiomyopathy. *J. Clin. Apher.* **2012**, *27*, 312–319. [CrossRef] [PubMed]

36. Dandel, M.; Wallukat, G.; Englert, A.; Lehmkuhl, H.B.; Knosalla, C.; Hetzer, R. Long-term benefits of immunoadsorption in beta(1)-adrenoceptor autoantibody-positive transplant candidates with dilated cardiomyopathy. *Eur. J. Heart Fail.* **2012**, *14*, 1374–1388. [CrossRef]

37. Thyrian, J.R.; Hertel, J.; Schulze, L.N.; Dörr, M.; Prüss, H.; Hempel, P.; Bimmler, M.; Kunze, R.; Grabe, H.J.; Teipel, S.; et al. Prevalence and Determinants of Agonistic Autoantibodies Against alpha1-Adrenergic

Receptors in Patients Screened Positive for Dementia: Results from the Population-Based DelpHi-Study. *J. Alzheimers Dis.* **2018**, *64*, 1091–1097. [CrossRef] [PubMed]

38. Hempel, P.; Heinig, B.; Jerosch, C.; Decius, I.; Karczewski, P.; Kassner, U.; Kunze, R.; Steinhagen-Thiessen, E.; Bimmler, M. Immunoadsorption of Agonistic Autoantibodies Against alpha1-Adrenergic Receptors in Patients With Mild to Moderate Dementia. *Ther. Apher. Dial.* **2016**, *20*, 523–529. [CrossRef]

39. Jack, C.R.; Bennett, D.A., Jr.; Blennow, K.; Carrillo, M.C.; Dunn, B.; Haeberlein, S.B.; Holtzman, D.M.; Jagust, W.; Jessen, F.; Karlawish, J.; et al. NIA-AA Research Framework: Toward a biological definition of Alzheimer's disease. *Alzheimers Dement.* **2018**, *14*, 535–562. [CrossRef]

40. Fazekas, F.; Chawluk, J.B.; Alavi, A.; Hurtig, H.I.; Zimmerman, R.A. MR signal abnormalities at 1.5 T in Alzheimer's dementia and normal aging. *AJR Am. J. Roentgenol.* **1987**, *149*, 351–356. [CrossRef]

41. Scheltens, P.; Launer, L.J.; Barkhof, F.; Weinstein, H.C.; van Gool, W.A. Visual assessment of medial temporal lobe atrophy on magnetic resonance imaging: Interobserver reliability. *J. Neurol.* **1995**, *242*, 557–560. [CrossRef]

42. Leijenaar, J.F.; Ivan Maurik, S.; Kuijer, J.P.A.; van der Flier, W.M.; Scheltens, P.; Barkhof, F.; Prins, N.D. Lower cerebral blood flow in subjects with Alzheimer's dementia, mild cognitive impairment, and subjective cognitive decline using two-dimensional phase-contrast magnetic resonance imaging. *Alzheimers Dement. (Amst.)* **2017**, *9*, 76–83. [CrossRef]

43. Binnewijzend, M.A.; Kuijer, J.P.; Benedictus, M.R.; van der Flier, W.M.; Wink, A.M.; Wattjes, M.P.; van Berckel, B.N.; Scheltens, P.; Barkhof, F. Cerebral blood flow measured with 3D pseudocontinuous arterial spin-labeling MR imaging in Alzheimer disease and mild cognitive impairment: A marker for disease severity. *Radiology* **2013**, *267*, 221–230. [CrossRef]

44. Asllani, I.; Borogovac, A.; Brown, T.R. Regression algorithm correcting for partial volume effects in arterial spin labeling MRI. *Magn. Reson. Med.* **2008**, *60*, 1362–1371. [CrossRef]

45. Folstein, M.F.; Folstein, S.E.; McHugh, P.R. Mini-mental state. A practical method for grading the cognitive state of patients for the clinician. *J. Psychiatr. Res.* **1975**, *12*, 189–198. [CrossRef]

46. Folstein, M.F.; Folstein, S.E.; White, T.; Messer, M.A. *MMSE-2. Mini-Mental State Examination*, 2nd ed.; PAR Inc.: Lutz, FL, USA, 2010.

47. Rosen, W.G.; Mohs, R.C.; Davis, K.L. A new rating scale for Alzheimer's disease. *Am. J. Psychiatry* **1984**, *141*, 1356–1364.

48. Graham, N.L.; Emery, T.; Hodges, J.R. Distinctive cognitive profiles in Alzheimer's disease and subcortical vascular dementia. *J. Neurol. Neurosurg. Psychiatry* **2004**, *75*, 61–71.

49. Ihl, R.; Mohs, R.; Weyer, G. *Alzheimer's Disease Assessment Scale: ADAS*; Beltz Test: Göttingen, Germany, 1990.

50. Stern, R.G.; Mohs, R.C.; Davidson, M.; Schmeidler, J.; Silverman, J.; Kramer-Ginsberg, E.; Searcey, T.; Bierer, L.; Davis, K.L. A longitudinal study of Alzheimer's disease: Measurement, rate, and predictors of cognitive deterioration. *Am. J. Psychiatry* **1994**, *151*, 390–396.

51. Helmstaedter, C.; Lendt, M.; Lux, S. *VLMT: Verbaler Lern-und Merkfähigkeitstest*; Beltz Test: Göttingen, Germany, 2001.

52. Yesavage, J.A. Geriatric depression scale. *Psychopharmacol. Bull.* **1988**, *24*, 709–711.

53. Yesavage, J.A.; Brink, T.L.; Rose, T.L.; Lum, O.; Huang, V.; Adey, M.; Leirer, V.O. Development and validation of a geriatric depression screening scale: A preliminary report. *J. Psychiatr. Res.* **1982**, *17*, 37–49. [CrossRef]

54. Volzke, H.; Alte, D.; Schmidt, C.O.; Radke, D.; Lorbeer, R.; Friedrich, N.; Aumann, N.; Lau, K.; Piontek, M.; Born, G.; et al. Cohort profile: The study of health in Pomerania. *Int. J. Epidemiol.* **2011**, *40*, 294–307. [CrossRef]

55. Weber, T.; Wassertheurer, S.; Rammer, M.; Maurer, E.; Hametner, B.; Mayer, C.C.; Kropf, J.; Eber, B. Validation of a brachial cuff-based method for estimating central systolic blood pressure. *Hypertension* **2011**, *58*, 825–832. [CrossRef]

56. Wassertheurer, S.; Kropf, J.; Weber, T.; van der Giet, M.; Baulmann, J.; Ammer, M.; Hametner, B.; Mayer, C.C.; Eber, B.; Magometschnigg, D. A new oscillometric method for pulse wave analysis: Comparison with a common tonometric method. *J. Hum. Hypertens* **2010**, *24*, 498–504. [CrossRef]

57. Hamburg, N.M.; Keyes, M.J.; Larson, M.G.; Vasan, R.S.; Schnabel, R.; Pryde, M.M.; Mitchell, G.F.; Sheffy, J.; Vita, J.A.; Benjamin, E.J. Cross-sectional relations of digital vascular function to cardiovascular risk factors in the Framingham Heart Study. *Circulation* **2008**, *117*, 2467–2474. [CrossRef]

58. Deng, W.; Dong, X.; Zhang, Y.; Jiang, Y.; Lu, D.; Wu, Q.; Liang, Z.; Yang, G.; Chen, B. Transcutaneous oxygen pressure (TcPO(2)): A novel diagnostic tool for peripheral neuropathy in type 2 diabetes patients. *Diabetes Res. Clin. Pract.* **2014**, *105*, 336–343. [CrossRef]

59. Recommendations for Cardiac Chamber Quantification by Echocardiography in Adults: An Update from the American Society of Echocardiography and the European Association of, Cardiovascular Imaging. *Eur. Heart J. Cardiovasc. Imaging* **2016**, *17*, 412. [CrossRef]

60. Schmidt, G.G.; Kursbuch, C. *Ultraschall Nach den Richtlinien der DEGUM und der KVR*, 6th ed.; Thieme: New York, NY, USA, 2015.

61. Arning, C.; Widder, B.; von Reutern, G.M.; Stiegler, H.; Gortler, M. Revision of DEGUM ultrasound criteria for grading internal carotid artery stenoses and transfer to NASCET measurement. *Ultraschall Med.* **2010**, *31*, 251–257. [CrossRef]

62. Grabe, H.J.; Assel, H.; Bahls, T.; Dörr, M.; Endlich, K.; Endlich, N.; Erdmann, P.; Ewert, R.; Felix, S.B.; Fiene, B.; et al. Cohort profile: Greifswald approach to individualized medicine (GANI_MED). *J. Transl. Med.* **2014**, *12*, 144. [CrossRef]

63. Karczewski, P.; Hempel, P.; Bimmler, M. Role of alpha1-adrenergic receptor antibodies in Alzheimer's disease. *Front. Biosci. (Landmark Ed.)* **2018**, *23*, 2082–2089.

64. Wallukat, G.A.W. Effects of the serum gamma globulin fraction of patients with allergic asthma and dilated cardiomyopathy on chronotropic beta adrenoceptor function in cultured neonatal rat heart myocytes. *Biomed. Biochim. Acta* **1987**, *46*, S634–S639.

65. Wallukat, G.; Saravia, S.G.M.; Haberland, A.; Bartel, S.; Araujo, R.; Valda, G.; Duchen, D.; Ramirez, I.D.; Borges, A.C.; Schimke, I. Distinct patterns of autoantibodies against G-protein-coupled receptors in Chagas' cardiomyopathy and megacolon. Their potential impact for early risk assessment in asymptomatic Chagas' patients. *J. Am. Coll. Cardiol.* **2010**, *55*, 463–468. [CrossRef]

66. Wallukat, G.; Prüss, H.; Muller, J.; Schimke, I. Functional autoantibodies in patients with different forms of dementia. *PLoS ONE* **2018**, *13*, e0192778.

67. Davideit, H.; Haberland, A.; Bartel, S.; Schulze-Rothe, S.; Muller, J.; Wenzel, K. Determination of Agonistically Acting Autoantibodies to the Adrenergic Beta-1 Receptor by Cellular Bioassay. *Methods Mol. Biol.* **2019**, *1901*, 95–102.

68. Ronspeck, W.; Brinckmann, R.; Egner, R.; Gebauer, F.; Winkler, D.; Jekow, P.; Wallukat, G.; Muller, J.; Kunze, R. Peptide based adsorbers for therapeutic immunoadsorption. *Ther. Apher. Dial.* **2003**, *7*, 91–97. [CrossRef] [PubMed]

69. Cohen, J. *Statistical Power Analysis for the Behavioral Sciences*; Academic Press: New York, NY, USA, 1988.

70. Boada, M.; Anaya, F.; Ortiz, P.; Olazaran, J.; Shua-Haim, J.R.; Obisesan, T.O.; Hernandez, I.; Munoz, J.; Buendia, M.; Alegret, M.; et al. Efficacy and Safety of Plasma Exchange with 5% Albumin to Modify Cerebrospinal Fluid and Plasma Amyloid-beta Concentrations and Cognition Outcomes in Alzheimer's Disease Patients: A Multicenter, Randomized, Controlled Clinical Trial. *J. Alzheimers Dis.* **2017**, *56*, 129–143. [CrossRef] [PubMed]

71. Kitaguchi, N.; Kawaguchi, K.; Nakai, S.; Murakami, K.; Ito, S.; Hoshino, H.; Hori, H.; Ohashi, A.; Shimano, Y.; Suzuki, N.; et al. Reduction of Alzheimer's disease amyloid-beta in plasma by hemodialysis and its relation to cognitive functions. *Blood Purif.* **2011**, *32*, 57–62. [CrossRef] [PubMed]

72. Trimpert, C.; Herda, L.R.; Eckerle, L.G.; Pohle, S.; Muller, C.; Landsberger, M.; Felix, S.B.; Staudt, A. Immunoadsorption in dilated cardiomyopathy: Long-term reduction of cardiodepressant antibodies. *Eur. J. Clin. Investig.* **2010**, *40*, 685–691. [CrossRef]

73. Muller, J.; Wallukat, G.; Dandel, M.; Bieda, H.; Brandes, K.; Spiegelsberger, S.; Nissen, E.; Kunze, R.; Hetzer, R. Immunoglobulin adsorption in patients with idiopathic dilated cardiomyopathy. *Circulation* **2000**, *101*, 385–391. [CrossRef]

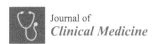

Article

Plasma Exchange or Immunoadsorption in Demyelinating Diseases: A Meta-Analysis

Mark Lipphardt, Manuel Wallbach and Michael J. Koziolek *

Department of Nephrology and Rheumatology, University Medical Center Göttingen, Robert-Koch-Str. 40, D-37075 Goettingen, Germany; mark.lipphardt@med.uni-goettingen.de (M.L.); manuel.wallbach@med.uni-goettingen.de (M.W.)
* Correspondence: mkoziolek@med.uni-goettingen.de; Tel.: +49-55-1396-5751; Fax: +49-55-1396-5752

Received: 11 May 2020; Accepted: 18 May 2020; Published: 25 May 2020

Abstract: Multiple sclerosis (MS) is an inflammatory disease mainly affecting the central nervous system. In MS, abnormal immune mechanisms induce acute inflammation, demyelination, axonal loss, and the formation of central nervous system plaques. The long-term treatment involves options to modify the disease progression, whereas the treatment for the acute relapse has its focus in the administration of high-dose intravenous methylprednisolone (up to 1000 mg daily) over a period of three to five days as a first step. If symptoms of the acute relapse persist, it is defined as glucocorticosteroid-unresponsive, and immunomodulation by apheresis is recommended. However, several national and international guidelines have no uniform recommendations on using plasma exchange (PE) nor immunoadsorption (IA) in this case. A systematic review and meta-analysis was conducted, including observational studies or randomized controlled trials that investigated the effect of PE or IA on different courses of MS and neuromyelitis optica (NMO). One thousand, three hundred and eighty-three patients were included in the evaluation. Therapy response in relapsing-remitting MS and clinically isolated syndrome was 76.6% (95%CI 63.7–89.8%) in PE- and 80.6% (95%CI 69.3–91.8%) in IA-treated patients. Based on the recent literature, PE and IA may be considered as equal treatment possibilities in patients suffering from acute, glucocorticosteroid-unresponsive MS relapses.

Keywords: multiple sclerosis; plasma exchange; immunoadsorption

---

1. Introduction

Multiple sclerosis (MS) is a disease which is defined as an inflammatory condition affecting the central nervous system. Its main course of damage is due to abnormal immune mechanisms, resulting in acute inflammation, demyelination, axonal loss, and the formation of central nervous system plaques consisting of inflammatory cells [1,2].

The epidemiology of MS differs greatly depending on the geographic regions with a prevalence from high levels in North America and Europe (>100/100,000 inhabitants) to low rates in Eastern Asia and sub-Saharan Africa (2/100,000 population). Women are generally more affected than men [3].

Symptoms that occur with the onset of MS are very unspecific, since MS can affect all regions of the central nervous system and can make it hard for a physician to make an early diagnosis. Symptoms of MS include vision problems with a decreased visual acuity (VA) and a prolonged visual evoked potential (VEP), weakness, fatigue, spasms, ataxia, cognitive dysfunction, or numbness [4]. The occurrence of an optic neuritis in its typical form is considered to be associated with MS. However, it is also regarded as a demyelinating clinically isolated syndrome (CIS) with the risk to convert to MS, especially in the white population [5]. With such a variety of symptoms a thorough medical history and examination is essential to make the right diagnosis of MS. Blood tests, lumbar punctures, magnetic resonance imaging, and evoked potential tests help in the process of differentiating between other diseases [6]. Based on the symptoms and the progression of the disease MS is divided in four types:

Relapsing-Remitting MS (RRMS), Secondary-Progressive MS (SPMS), Primary-Progressive MS (PPMS), and Progressive-Relapsing MS (PRMS).

MS can be characterized as a T-cell-driven disease with T helper (Th) cells, especially Th-1, Th-2, and Th-17 cells, as the main players in a various inflammatory cascade [7]. For instance, Th-1 cells are responsible for producing Interferon gamma (IFNγ) and tumor necrosis factor alpha (TNF-α) [8]. With the secretion of IFNy and TNF-α inflammation can be maintained by inhibiting Th-2 cell differentiation, since Th-2 cells produce anti-inflammatory cytokines like interleukin (IL)-4 and IL-13 [9,10]. Th-17 cells stimulate inflammation via secreting a vast number of various cytokines like IL-17, IL-21, IL-22, and IL-26 [11–13]. As a counterpart regulatory T (Treg) cells inhibit autoimmune responses [14]. In addition to that immunoglobulins (Ig) (especially IgG) are important in the pathogenesis of MS. Evidence of intrathecal Ig production and oligoclonal IgG bands contribute to the diagnosis of MS. Further differentiation shows various types of specific autoantibodies against myelin in subgroups of patients with MS, e.g., anti-myelin oligo-dendrocyte glycoprotein (anti-MOG) or anti-myelin basic protein (anti-MBP) [15]. Antibody-producing B-cells traveling between CNS, blood, and peripheral lymphatic organs clonally expanded B-cells and aggregated B-cells in meninges corroborate a pathophysiological role of B-cells and/or humoral immune answer in the pathogenesis of MS [16–19].

Based on the myelin protein loss, the geography and extension of plaques, the patterns of oligodendrocyte destruction, and the immunohistopathological evidence of complement activation Lucchinetti et al. described four different immunohistopathological patterns of demyelination in MS [20]. Patterns I and II showed close similarities to T-cell-mediated or T-cell plus antibody-mediated autoimmune encephalomyelitis. Patterns III and IV on the other hand were highly suggestive of a primary oligodendrocyte dystrophy.

Neuromyelitis optica (NMO) on the other hand is described as an idiopathic, severe, demyelinating disease of the central nervous system with the preference to affect the optic nerve and spinal cord. NMO has been considered as a variant of MS. However, with the analysis of clinical, laboratory, immunological, and pathological data the difference to MS is now acknowledged [21].

The treatment regime can be divided in treatment to modify the disease progression and treatment for the acute relapse. In the latter, the administration of high-dose intravenous methylprednisolone (up to 1000 mg daily) over a period of three to five days usually represents the first step in acute MS relapse treatment. A higher second high-dose intravenous methylprednisolone pulse with up to 2 g can be considered in unresponsive patients after an interval of 2 weeks [22–24]. Glucocorticoids may downregulate cellular cytotoxicity and lead to the death of activated B cells, but they will not modulate tissue destruction or conduction blockade by local antibody deposition [25]. If symptoms persist, the relapse is defined as glucocorticosteroid-unresponsive and immunomodulation by apheresis is recommended. However, several national and international guidelines have no uniform recommendations on using plasma exchange (PE) or immunoadsorption (IA) in this case. The American Society for Apheresis (ASFA) recommends PE for treatment to category II ("apheresis accepted as second-line therapy") and IA for treatment to category III ("optimum role of apheresis therapy is not established") [26]. The American Academy of Neurology also advises the use of PE for adjunctive treatment of relapsing forms of MS (Level B), while IA is not addressed [27,28]. The German guidelines are currently under reconstruction but formerly recommended both procedures as equivalent [29].

In this current issue, we review the use of IA and PE in treating, especially, the acute relapse of MS.

2. Effects of Apheresis Therapy

During PE, the patient's plasma, including all plasma proteins, is removed and substituted by human albumin solution or fresh frozen plasma. The concept of IA involves a selective elimination of plasma proteins, e.g., antibodies, while sparing other plasma proteins [30]. Both techniques include an extracorporeal circulation circuit with systemic and/or local anticoagulation, as well as the need of a vascular access. The latter can either be peripheral venous, if individual vascular situation allows it, or by a central venous catheter. In IA, a secondary circuit is established in which a defined physico-chemical interaction of selected plasma proteins with a defined matrix should theoretically guarantee selective removal of circulating pathogens. In praxis, a bandwidth of proteins are removed [31,32] which are responsible for therapeutic effects but also possible side effects of IA. These effects differ with regard to used matrix of the adsorber, which physicians should be aware.

The exact mechanism by which apheresis treatment works is actually not fully understood. MS patients may benefit by the immediate removal of plasma antibodies, immune complexes and cytokines, induction of a redistribution of antibodies from the extravascular space, and subsequent immunomodulatory changes [30]. Here, cell types with receptors for immunoglobulins (Fc receptors), such as monocytes, macrophages, and natural killer cells, are especially of interest [25]. Besides effects on humoral immune system, experimental data suggest a reduction of circulating autoantigens and regulatory proteins [32] and induction of a higher relative quantity of Treg to Th17 cells [33], as well as a silencing of cellular autoimmune response [32].

Early active MS lesions with an immunohistopathological type II pattern, which are selectively associated with Ig's and complement deposited along myelin sheaths, predict the best response to apheresis therapy in patients with steroid-unresponsive relapse [34], corroborating the hypothesis of effects on humoral immune response.

3. Plasma Exchange

3.1. Multiple Sclerosis (with Relapsing-Remitting and Progressive MS Sub-Sections)

The first study comparing the normal therapy regime with PE was performed by Khatri et al. in 1985 and included fifty-four patients with chronic progressive MS [35]. The results showed that patients with the additional PE have a higher improvement rate than patients with a "sham" PE. Following the study of Khatri et al., Weiner et al. enrolled 116 patients in a multicenter, randomized, double-blinded, controlled trial of 11 PE treatments in acute exacerbations of MS [36]. One of the main results showed patients treated with PE to have a significantly enhanced improvement after four weeks. In 1999, a study group of the Mayo Clinic conducted a randomized, sham-controlled, double-blinded study of PE in MS patients with severe neurological deficits after acute relapses, unresponsive to corticosteroids [37]. This study resulted in a moderate to greater improvement in neurological deficits in 42.1% of patients with true PE versus 5.9% of patients with sham PE. With the improved work with PE in the clinical setting, a variety of retrospective studies could demonstrate an improvement rate between 59–87.5% [38–40]. In a large study with 153 patients enrolled, Magana et al. identified 90 patients with moderate to marked functional neurological improvement within 6 months after treatment with PE [41].

An excellent and actual overview on apheresis in progressive MS forms is available in Reference [30]. So far, the ASFA recommends PE for treatment to category III: "Optimum role of apheresis therapy is not established. Decision making should be individualized" [26].

3.2. Clinically Isolated Syndrome

More recent studies set their focus not only on the relapsing-remitting and progressive MS sub-sections but also on the clinically isolated syndrome [42–44]. Therapy response rates ranged between 72–76%, therefore achieving a clinical response in the majority of patients.

3.3. Optic Neuritis

Studies analyzing the use of PE in the setting of for severe steroid unresponsive optic neuritis were performed by Ruprecht et al. and Deschamps et al. [45,46]. Ruprecht et al. al. demonstrated an improvement of visual acuity in 70% of patients. Out of these seven patients, three continued to improve with their visual acuity, two remained at a stable state, whereas two patients suffered from worsening symptoms during the follow-ups [46].

In the study performed by Deschamps et al., thirty-four patients with a remaining visual acuity of 0.1 were treated with PE. Afterwards, the median visual acuity was 0.8 [45].

Studies on PE are summarized in Table 1. However, the reader must be aware that the comparability of the studies is limited by the different technical implementation of PE. This varied in frequency, treated plasma volume, and total number of PEs. As a result, the ASFA defined a corridor of technical implementation that recommended treatment of 1–1.5-fold plasma volume per session for a number of 5 to 7 treatments over a period of 10 to 14 days [26].

Table 1. Studies on plasma exchange (PE) in treatment of relapsing-remitting multiple sclerosis (RRMS), clinically isolated syndrome (CIS), progressive MS, isolated optic neuritis, and neuromyelitis optica (NMO). EDSS = Expanded Disability Status Scale.

"Relapsing-Remitting Multiple Sclerosis" and "Clinically Isolated Syndrome"							
Citation	Year	*n*	Design	No. of Treatments	Treated Plasma Volume (mL)	Outcome	Limitation
[36]	1989	116	Double-blind, multi-center, randomized	11	n.a.	Significant improvement after 4 weeks	No plasmapheresis protocol specifications
[37]	1999	36	Double-blind	7	3000	Therapy response in 42% of patients	Patient collective with heterogenous MS-types
[39]	2005	13	Retrospective	5	3000	Therapy response in 71% of patients	Small number of subjects
[47]	2007	6	Retrospective	4	1.0-fold plasma volume	Therapy response in 100% of patients	Small number of subjects
[40]	2009	20	Retrospective	3–7	1.5-fold plasma volume	Therapy response in 76% of patients regarding visual acuity	Small number of subjects
[38]	2010	4	Retrospective	5	2750	Therapy response in 75% of patients	no placebo, Small number of subjects, the study was observational in character
[41]	2011	153	Retrospective	7	n.a.	Therapy response in 59% of patients	Patient collective with heterogenous MS-types
[48]	2013	15	Retrospective	≥7	1.0-fold plasma volume	Therapy response in 93.3% of patients	RRMS + CIS
[49]	2014	11	Retrospective	Median 7 (3–8)	3000 (2200–3500)	Therapy response in 91% of patients	CIS only
[43]	2015	90	Retrospective	3–8	1.0-fold plasma volume	Therapy response in 72% of patients	The lack of a control group
[50]	2016	16	Retrospective	n.a.	2000	Therapy response in 91% of patients regarding visual evoked potential	Small number of subjects and a higher expanded disability status scale in patients in the PE only group
[51]	2018	46	Retrospective	Mean 7.39 sessions	n.a.	Complete therapy response in 41% of patients and partial therapy response in 39% of patients	Patient collective with heterogenous MS-types
[44]	2019	42	Retrospective	4–11	Mean 2930 median 2000	Therapy response in 73% of patients	patients without sufficient follow-up data had a significantly higher patient age and longer duration of disease
[42]	2019	30	Double-blind, randomized, uni-center	On 5 days	0.69 ± 0.12-fold individual total plasma volume	Therapy response in 76% of patients	Lack of blinding and small number of subjects

Table 1. *Cont.*

"Progressive Multiple Sclerosis"							
Citation	**Year**	**n**	**Design**	**No. of Treatments**	**Treated Plasma Volume (mL)**	**Outcome**	**Limitation**
[52]	1983	18	Prospective, randomized	4–5	n.a.	Therapy response in 27.8% of patients	Small number of subjects, no plasmapheresis protocol specifications
[35]	1985	54	Double-blind controlled	20	n.a.	Therapy response in 54% of patients	No plasmapheresis protocol specifications
[53]	1994	24	Prospective	8	n.a.	Therapy response in 87.5% of patients	Small number of subjects, no plasmapheresis protocol specifications
[41]	2011	10	Retrospective	7	n.a.	Therapy response in 30% of patients	Small number of subjects
[54]	2015	6	open-label, single-center proof of concept study	4	2000–2500	Therapy response in 66.7% of patients	Small number of subjects
"Isolated Optic Neuritis"							
Citation	**Year**	**n**	**Design**	**No. of Treatments**	**Treated Plasma Volume (mL)**	**Outcome**	**Limitation**
[46]	2004	10	Retrospective	n.a.	n.a.	Therapy response in 70% of patients	Small number of subjects
[55]	2012	23	Retrospective	5	~3000	Therapy response in 70% of patients	heterogenous
[56]	2012	16	Retrospective	5	1.0-fold plasma volume	Therapy response in 87.5% of patients	Small number of subjects
[45]	2016	34	Retrospective	Median 5, range 5–10	1.5-fold body mass volume	Therapy response in 56% of patients regarding visual acuity	The lack of a control group
"Neuromyelitis Optica"							
Citation	**Year**	**n**	**Design**	**No. of Treatments**	**Treated Plasma Volume (mL)**	**Outcome**	**Limitation**
[57]	2007	6	Retrospective	3–5	2000–3000	Therapy response in 50% of patients	Small number of subjects
[58]	2011	5	Retrospective	≥5	1.0-fold plasma volume	Therapy response in 80% of patients	Small number of subjects
[41]	2011	26	Retrospective	7	n.a.	Therapy response in 42.3% of patients	Historical cohort study
[59]	2013	31	Retrospective	n.a.	n.a.	Therapy response in 65% of patients	No study controlled treatment regimes
[60]	2013	15	Retrospective	6	1.0–1.5-fold plasma volume	Therapy response in 78% of patients	Small number of subjects
[61]	2016	65	Retrospective	5–7	1.5-fold plasma volume	Therapy response in 65% of patients	Selection bias; use of EDSS scores as the primary outcome measure
[62]	2017	21	Retrospective	5	n.a.	Therapy response in 81% of patients	Use of EDSS scores as the primary outcome measure
[63]	2018	28	Retrospective	5	1000	Therapy response in 42.9% of patients	Use of EDSS scores as the primary outcome measure
[64]	2018	29	Retrospective	2–7	1.0-fold plasma volume	Therapy response in 82.8% of patients	Heterogenous treatment protocols
[65]	2018	9	Retrospective	7	1.0-fold plasma volume	Therapy response in 75% of patients	Small number of subjects

Table 1. *Cont.*

					"Neuromyelitis Optica"		
Citation	Year	*n*	Design	No. of Treatments	Treated Plasma Volume (mL)	Outcome	Limitation
[66]	2018	5	Retrospective	5 (3–7)	1.0-fold plasma volume	Therapy response in 80% of patients	Small number of subjects
[67]	2018	146	Retrospective	≥3	n.a.	Therapy response in 86% of patients	Heterogenous treatment protocols
[68]	2019	15	Retrospective	2–3	n.a	Therapy response in 100% of patients	Small number of subjects

4. Immunoadsorption

4.1. Multiple Sclerosis (with Relapsing-Remitting and Progressive MS Sub-Sections)

IA was firstly introduced in the treatment of MS by de Andres et al. in 2000 [69]. They managed a prompt and unequivocal clinical response with a parallel decrease in IgG, fibrinogen, and C3 complement plasma levels in all three patients treated with IA. In the following years, retrospective studies confirmed the initial results of de Andres et al., showing improvement rates from 85–88.3% in MS patients receiving an IA therapy [70,71].

4.2. Clinically Isolated Syndrome

Studies incorporating patients with clinically isolated syndrome showed marked to moderate clinical response with a total gain of function in 66–100% of patients after treatment with immunoadsorption [42,72].

4.3. Neuromyelitis Optica

The first prospective study investigating effects of IA therapy in patients with MS with steroid-refractory optical neuritis showed an improvement of the mean visual acuity in 8 from 11 patients at day 180 ± 10 after IA [32]. A more recent study confirmed the efficacy and good tolerance of IA in relapses of MS patients with failure to respond to a steroid pulse therapy adequately. Moreover, the study established IA as first-line relapse treatment during pregnancy and breastfeeding [73].

The most commonly used column was a tryptophane-linked polyvinyl alcohol adsorber, but also a Sepharose-conjugated sheep antibodies to human IgG, as well as protein A column, have been used. Table 2 gives an overview about IA-studies in acute relapses of MS.

5. Plasma Exchange vs. Immunoadsorption

5.1. Multiple Sclerosis (with Relapsing-Remitting and Progressive MS Sub-Sections)

Recently, studies have been designed to compare the efficacy of PE versus IA. The most impressive work is that of Dorst et al. [42]. Sixty-one patients with acute relapse of multiple sclerosis or clinically isolated syndrome and without complete clinical remission of symptoms after at least one cycle of high-dose intravenous methylprednisolone were randomly assigned to receive IA ($n = 31$) or PE ($n = 30$). In the IA group (using a protein A adsorber), the 2.0-fold individual total plasma volume was processed on day 1, and the 2.5-fold on days 2–5. In the PE group, 2 L of plasma (corresponding to the 0.69 ± 0.12-fold individual total plasma volume) were removed each day and substituted by 5% human albumin solution. The median improvement of Multiple Sclerosis Functional Composite after 4 weeks compared to baseline was 0.385 (interquartile range (IQR) 0.200–0.675; $p < 0.001$) in the IA group and 0.265 (IQR 0.100–0.408; $p < 0.001$) in the PE group. Improvement in the IA group was significantly larger ($p = 0.034$) compared to PE. Response rates after 4 weeks were 86.7% in the IA group and 76.7% in the PE group. One deep venous thrombosis occurred in each group. One limitation in interpretation of this study, however, is that the apheresis dose applied was quite different in the two treatment arms and the observation period was relatively short.

Hohenstein et al. reported the successful use of IA with regenerating adsorbers in MS patients as a single center experience [78]. Faissner et al. compared PE and IA directly and demonstrated in a grouped analysis of patients treated with combined PE/ IA, PE, or IA alone, that all groups presented with a better result of visual evoked potentials, providing a valid treatment option in steroid-refractory MS-relapses [50].

5.2. Clinically Isolated Syndrome

Dorst et al. [42] also enrolled patients suffering from a clinically isolated syndrome in their recent study. The results are discussed above.

5.3. Neuromyelitis Optica

In a small cohort study, Faissner et al. showed equivalent results treating patients with neuromyelitis optica spectrum disorder with IA instead of PE, constituting IA as a valid therapeutic option [77]. Studies of our own also indicate PE and IA to be of equal efficacy and treatment safety [44,79]. We assessed 140 adult patients treated with PE (n = 73) or IA (n = 67) in steroid refractory multiple sclerosis or neuromyelitis optica. During our studies, we became aware of the fact that differences in body-mass-index, duration of disease, number of treatments, vascular access and treated plasma volumes between IA - and PE cohorts are a main concern for possible bias in the assessment of IA and PE as a treatment for MS patients. We also performed a retrospective single-center cohort study of pediatric patients with inflammatory CNS demyelinating disorders showing excellent tolerance and favorable outcomes of PE and IA in all pediatric patients [31].

6. Meta-Analysis on Apheresis Effects on Demyelinating Diseases

6.1. Search Strategy and Inclusion Criteria

A systematic search was performed using Medline and Cochrane Library with combinations of the search terms "plasma exchange" OR "immunoadsorption" in combination with the terms "multiple sclerosis" OR "clinical isolated syndrome" OR "neuromyelitis optica" between 1980 and January 2020. Reports were screened independently for relevance based on title and abstract content by two authors (M.L. and M.J.K.). Randomized-controlled trials, as well as prospective cohort studies and retrospective studies and case series, were included if sufficient information on therapy response of PE or IA was provided. Studies with heterogeneous mixing MS, CIS, and/or NMO patients regarding therapy response were excluded if the treatment response was not specified separately in the individual indications. Moreover, case series with a case number less than five in the individual indication were also excluded. It should be mentioned as a limitation that there was no uniform definition of the term "therapy response" in the selected works and, with the exception of a few studies, the majority was retrospective data collection. The flow chart in Figure 1 summarizes the selection of studies in the meta-analysis.

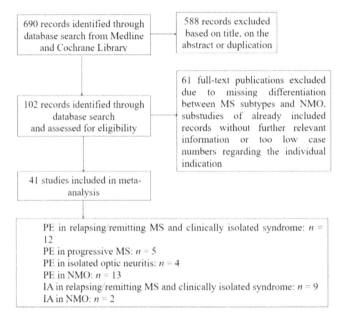

Figure 1. Flow chart of study selection. MS = multiple sclerosis, NMO = neuromyelitis optica, PE = plasma exchange, IA = immunoadsorption.

6.2. Statistical Analysis

Analysis was performed using RevMan V.5.3 (Nordic Cochrane Centre, Copenhagen, Denmark, the Cochrane Collaboration, 2014). Data were quantitatively synthesized by an inverse-variance-weighted meta-analysis using a random-effect model because of the presence of heterogeneity. The normal approximation interval (sqrt($p(1-p)/n$)) was used to generate the confidence interval for the therapy response rate. For studies where the normal approximation interval was zero, the confidence interval was set to one to calculate the random effect model. The 95% normal approximation confidence interval is provided in the meta-analyses.

7. Results

With the present search strategy and assessment of full-texts 690 studies, 40 observational and 1 randomized with a total of 1.383 patients could be analyzed. Figure 1 shows the flow chart of study selection.

Effects of PE can be summarized as follows: in relapsing-remitting MS and clinically isolated syndrome (12 studies and 398 patients) therapy response of 76.6% (95%CI 63.7–89.8%) (Figure 2A), in progressive MS (5 studies and 112 patients) therapy response of 53.9% (95%CI 29.5–78.4) (Figure 2B), in isolated optic neuritis (4 studies and 83 patients) therapy response of 71.5% (95%CI 56.4–86.6%) (Figure 2C), and in NMO (13 studies and 401 patients) therapy response of 72.5% (95%CI 61.0–83.9%) (Figure 2D).

Effects of IA can be summarized as follows: in relapsing-remitting MS and clinically isolated syndrome (9 studies and 352 patients), therapy response of 80.6% (95%CI 69.3–91.8%) (Figure 2E); and in NMO (2 studies and 37 patients), therapy response of 100% (95%CI 98.6–101.4%) (Figure 2F).

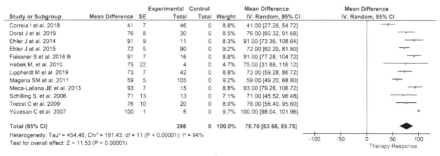

(A)

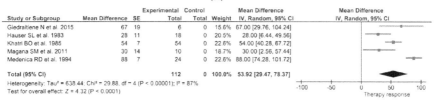

(B)

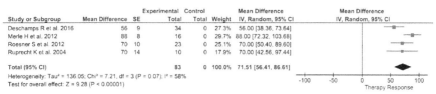

(C)

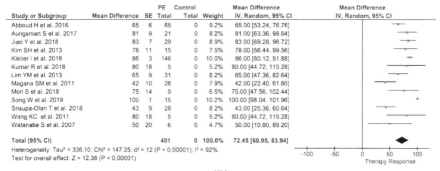

(D)

Figure 2. *Cont.*

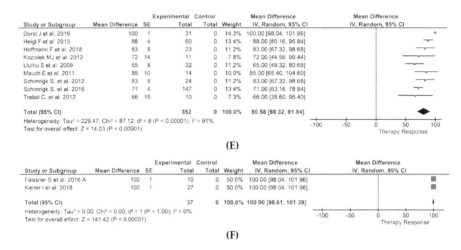

Figure 2. The 95% normal approximation confidence interval is provided in the meta-analyses. The given SE correspond to normal approximation confidence interval (sqrt(*p*(1-*p*)/*n*)). (**A**) Effects of PE in RRMS and CIS. (**B**) Effects of PE in PMS. (**C**) Effects of PE in opticus neuritis. (**D**) Effects of PE in NMO. (**E**) Effects of IA in RRMS and CIS. (**F**) Effects of IA in NMO. RRMS = relapsing-remitting multiple sclerosis, CIS = clinically isolated syndrome, PMS = progressive multiple sclerosis, SE = standard error, IV = instrumental variables. Figure 2A: Correia et al. [51], Dorst et al. [42], Ehler et al. [49], Ehler at al. [43], Faissner et al. [50], Habek et al. [38], Lipphardt et al. [44], Magana et al. [41], Meca-Lallana et al. [48], Schilling et al. [39], Trebst et al. [40], Yücesan et al. [47]. Figure 2B: Giedraitiene et al. [54], Hauser et al. [52], Khatri et al. [35], Magana et al. [41], Medenica et al. [53]. Figure 2C: Deschamps et al. [45], Merle et al. [56], Roesner et al. [55], Ruprecht et al. [46]. Figure 2D: Abboud et al. [61], Aungsmart et al. [62], Jiao et al. [64], Kim et al. [60], Kleiter et al. [67], Kumar et al. [66], Lim et al. [59], Magana et al. [41], Mori et al. [65], Song et al. [68], Srisupa-Olan et al. [63], Wang et al. [58], Watanabe et al. [57]. Figure 2E: Dorst et al. [42], Heigl et al. [70], Hoffmann et al. [73], Koziolek et al. [32], Llufriu et al. [80], Mauch et al. [71], Schimrigk et al. [75], Schimrigk et al. [76], Trebst et al. [72]. Figure 2F: Faissner et al. [77], Kleiter et al. [67].

Table 2. Studies on immunoadsorption in treatment of relapsing-remitting multiple sclerosis (RRMS), clinically isolated syndrome (CIS) and neuromyelitis optica (NMO).

Citation	Year	*n*	Design	No. of Treatments	Treated Plasma Volume (mL)	Matrix of Adsorber	Outcome	Limitation
					"RRMS" and "CIS"			
[69]	2000	3	Retrospective	5–6	n.a.	n.a.	Therapy response in 100% of patients	small number of subjects
[74]	2005	12	Prospective	14	1.5-fold plasma volume	Sepharose-conjugated sheep antibodies to human immunoglobulin (IgG)	No significant therapy response	small number of subjects and patient collective with heterogenous MS-types
[71]	2011	14	Retrospective	5–6	n.a.	Tryptophan	Therapy response in 85% of patients	small number of subjects
[75]	2012	24	Retrospective	Mean 5 (range 3–6)	2000–2500	Tryptophan	Therapy response in 83% of patients	small number of subjects and patient collective with heterogenous MS-types
[72]	2012	10	Retrospective	5–7	2500	Tryptophan	Therapy response in 66% of patients	small number of subjects
[32]	2012	11	Prospective	5	2500	Tryptophan	Therapy response in 72% of patients	small number of subjects

Table 2. *Cont.*

Citation	Year	n	Design	No. of Treatments	Treated Plasma Volume (mL)	Matrix of Adsorber	Outcome	Limitation
					"RRMS" and "CIS"			
[70]	2013	60	Retrospective	6	2000	Tryptophan	Therapy response in 88% of patients	only qualitative data regarding the therapeutic success and clinical data on tolerability were available
[76]	2016	147	Retrospective	n.a.	2000–2500	Tryptophan	Therapy response in 71% of patients	Expanded Disability Status Scale was used to measure a change in relapse-related disability
[73]	2018	23	Retrospective	Mean 5.8	2031 ± 230	Tryptophan	Therapy response in 83% of patients	Lack of a control group; use of immunoadsorption was limited in some study centers
[44]	2019	32	Retrospective	5–7	2000–2500	Tryptophan	Therapy response in 65% of patients	patients without sufficient follow-up data had a significantly higher patient age and longer duration of disease
[42]	2019	31	Prospective, double-blind, randomized, uni-center	On 5 days	2.0-fold total plasma volume on day 1, and the 2.5-fold total plasma volume on day 2–5	protein A	Therapy response in 100% of patients	Lack of blinding and small number of subjects

Citation	Year	n	Design	No. of Treatments	Treated Plasma Volume (mL)	Matrix of Adsorber	Outcome	Limitation
					"NMO"			
[77]	2016	10	Retrospective	Mean 5.2 (3–7)	2000–2500	Tryptophan	Therapy response in 100% of patients	Small number of subjects
[67]	2018	27	Retrospective	≥3	n.a.	Tryptophan or Protein A	Therapy response in 100% of patients	Heterogenous treatment protocols

8. Safety Profile

8.1. General

Another important fact to consider is the treatment safety. The noted rates of side effects during those apheresis treatments are very heterogeneous. In the literature one can find complication rates from 4.2% until 25.6% [81–84]. In 2011, Köhler et al. postulated lower side effects using IA in patients suffering from myasthenia gravis [85]. They claim that a possible reason for the difference was due to the absence of albumin-substitution. Zoellner et al. designed a study to investigate the fibrinogen level and the occurrence of bleeding complications [86]. They demonstrated IA to have a lower degree of fibrinogen reduction as PE. Bleeding complications occurred in 1.3–3.1% of treatments. Schneider-Gold et al. reported allergic reactions, hypocoagulability, and bronchorespiratory infections with a significant higher frequency in the PE-only group as compared to the IA-only group or the both combined [87].

8.2. Multiple Sclerosis (with Relapsing-Remitting and Progressive MS Sub-Sections) and Clinically Isolated Syndrome

In the recent study performed by Dorst et al. [42], a general well tolerance was observed with 5 mild infections in the PE group and 4 mild allergic reactions in the IA group. Furthermore, courses of anemia and thrombocytopenia were documented with anemia being more frequent in the PE group and thrombocytopenia being more frequent in the IA group.

8.3. Multiple Sclerosis (with Relapsing-Remitting and Progressive MS Sub-Sections) and Neuromyelitis Optica

In our studies the complication rate was about 3.7% in over 780 apheresis cycles. Furthermore, we could not detect any differences regarding the safety profile of IA versus PE [44,79].

All in all, both IA and PE have a high tolerability regarding the safety profile. It should be added that the majority of the documented side effects are to be considered as mild. However, the use of IA and PE should be reserved to specialized centers familiar with technical procedure and experienced with this specialized patient population to ensure a high quality of treatment with low complication rates.

9. Treatment Predictors

9.1. General

One major predicting factor is the time to initiate apheresis treatment. Early initiation of apheresis correlates with a higher response rate as was shown by several study groups [44,60,80,88]. In the onset of sudden hearing loss, the early initiation of apheresis treatment was also beneficial [89].

Comparing the cumulative corticosteroid doses in apheresis-responders versus non-responders, no significant difference was shown, which makes a synergistic effect of apheresis and corticosteroids unlikely [44].

9.2. Multiple Sclerosis (with Relapsing-Remitting and Progressive MS Sub-Sections)

Magana et al. postulated the duration of the disease and preserved deep tendon reflexes as important clinical predictors [41]. A different approach was followed by the study group of Stork et al., who conducted a single-center cohort study with 69 MS patients, evaluating treatment response in relation to histopathologically defined immunopathological patterns of MS [34]. As early active demyelinating MS lesions can be divided in 3 different immunopathological patterns of demyelination, Stork et al. demonstrated that patients with pattern 1 and 2 are most likely to benefit from apheresis treatment, especially in patients with pattern 2 who show signs of a humoral immune response in particular. Patients with pattern 3 most likely do not benefit from apheresis treatment. During our studies, we also became aware of the fact that patients having a good response to apheresis treatment were significantly younger than non-responders [44]. This observation may be due to a decrease in remyelination efficiency, as proposed by Sim et al. [90]. A gender-related treatment benefit towards the female gender was identified in sub-groups of MS patients [44,91].

9.3. Neuromyelitis Optica

In a large study performed by Kleiter et al., it was shown that PE or IA exerts a better recovery from acute relapses in patients suffering from neuromyelitis optica if they had isolated myelitis [92]. More recent studies focused on the plasma anti-aquaporin-4 immunoglobulin G antibody as a positive predictor for treatment success with PE or IA in patients suffering from neuromyelitis optica spectrum disorder [12]. In both studies, particularly, patients with a positive anti-aquaporin-4 immunoglobulin G antibody responded well to the treatment with PE and IA. In addition to that, no advantage was revealed for either PE or IA. The disease specificity of anti-aquaporin-4 immunoglobulin G antibody is almost at 100% and clinical studies with immunohistochemical evidence suggest that this antibody plays a central role in the pathogenesis of neuromyelitis optica spectrum disorder [93].

These predictors can thus be summarized according to various variables. Table 3 provides a compilation.

Table 3. Predictors of apheresis response. EDSS = Expanded Disability Status Scale; MRI = magnetic resonance imaging. * Pediatric patients only.

"Multiple Sclerosis" (with Relapsing-Remitting and Progressive MS Sub-Sections)			
Classification	Predictor	Citation	Meaning
Clinical signs and symptoms	EDSS ≤ 5	[43]	Indicates good apheresis response
	Preserved deep tendon reflexes	[41]	Indicates good apheresis response
Demographics	Younger age	[44]	Indicates good apheresis response
	Female	[37,91]	Indicates good apheresis response
Histological classification and localization	Gadolinium positive MRI lesions	[43]	Indicates good apheresis response
	Histological type 1 and 2 pattern	[34]	Indicates good apheresis response
	Histological type 3 pattern	[34]	Indicates poor apheresis response
Pre-treatment	No disease modifying drugs	[43]	Indicates good apheresis response
	Short duration of disease	[41]	Indicates good apheresis response

"Neuromyelitis Optica"			
Classification	Predictor	Citation	Meaning
Histological classification and localization	Isolated myelitis	[85]	Indicates good apheresis response
Laboratory values	Anti-aquaporin-4 IgG positive	[12]	Indicates good apheresis response

"Mixed"			
Classification	Predictor	Citation	Meaning
Apheresis	Early initiation	[44,60,80,88]	Indicates good apheresis response
Clinical signs and symptoms	Lower baseline scores on the EDSS, visual outcome, and gait scales	[94] *	Indicates good apheresis response
Pre-treatment	Cumulative corticosteroid doses	[44]	Irrelevant for apheresis response

10. Therapeutic Efficacy and Time Course

As for the time course of the therapeutic effect, the current literature agrees on regular neurological follow-ups after 6 months, manifesting a continuous and maximal clinical effect of the apheresis treatment [41,44,60,80]. Therapeutic effects over such a long period of time suggest immunomodulatory actions of apheresis rather than antibody removal on its own [95]. Those immunomodulatory actions happen most likely at the level of Th-cells and CNS-associated proteins, like the myelin basic protein. The prolonged therapeutic effect can be thought of as a clinical correlate of the immunomodulatory components of therapeutic apheresis. Furthermore, the duration of the apheresis induced therapeutic effect can be involved in the treatment process of initiating or changing disease-modifying drugs.

11. Conclusions

The focus of this current issue is the use and comparison of immunoadsorption and plasma exchange in the treatment of multiple sclerosis with the main concern of acute relapses.

Based on the studies of the current literature and performance of a meta-analysis, including 690 studies, 40 observational and 1 randomized with a total of 1383 patients, plasma exchange and immunoadsorption are treatment options of equal effectivity for acute glucocorticosteroid-unresponsive multiple sclerosis relapses.

For the meta-analysis randomized-controlled trials, prospective cohort studies, retrospective studies, and case series with sufficient information on therapy response of plasma exchange or immunoadsorption were included. Studies with heterogeneous mixing multiple sclerosis, clinically isolated syndrome, and/or neuromyelitis optica patients regarding therapy response were not included if the treatment response was not specified separately in the individual indications.

Plasma exchange has a therapy response of 76.6% in relapsing-remitting multiple sclerosis (RRMS) and clinically isolated syndrome (CIS), 53.9% in progressive multiple sclerosis (PMS), 71.5% in isolated optic neuritis, and 72.5% in neuromyelitis optica (NMO). Immunoadsorption (IA) has a therapy

J. Clin. Med. **2020**, 9, 1597

response of 80.6% in relapsing-remitting multiple sclerosis and clinically isolated syndrome and 100% in neuromyelitis optica.

Early treatment initiation with a median of 2–3 weeks and a patient age below 50 are considered to be beneficial regarding a treatment success. In addition to that, a treatment count of 5 to 7 with one plasma volume is also beneficial for treatment success, whereas patients suffering from progressive multiple sclerosis have a lower beneficial rate of apheresis therapy. Both immunoadsorption and plasma exchange have a high safety profile and a high tolerability regarding side effects.

Nevertheless, data situation is too heterogeneous regarding procedures and technical implementation to be finally assessed.

Author Contributions: Conceptualization, M.J.K.; Formal analysis, M.W.; Methodology, M.W.; Supervision, M.J.K.; Validation, M.L. and M.J.K.; Visualization, M.L.; Writing—original draft, M.L.; Writing—review & editing, M.W. and M.J.K. All authors have read and agreed to the published version of the manuscript.

Acknowledgments: This publication is dedicated to the work of G. A. Müller, who always promoted apheresis therapy during his time as a full professor at the chair of Nephrology Göttingen, Germany.

Conflicts of Interest: The authors declare no conflict of interest.

Abbreviations

ASFA	American society for apheresis
CIS	Clinical isolated syndrome
Ig	Immunoglobulin
IL	Interleukin
IFNγ	Interferon gamma
NMO	Neuromyelitis optica
MS	Multiple Sclerosis
PE	Plasma exchange
PPMS	Primary-Progressive MS
PRMS	Progressive-Relapsing MS
RRMS	Relapsing remitting MS
SPMS	Secondary-Progressive MS
Th	T helper
Treg	T regulatory
TNF-α	Tumor necrosis factor alpha
VA	Visual acuity
VEP	Visual evoked potential

References

1. Brucklacher-Waldert, V.; Stuerner, K.; Kolster, M.; Wolthausen, J.; Tolosa, E. Phenotypical and functional characterization of T helper 17 cells in multiple sclerosis. *Brain A J. Neurol.* **2009**, *132 Pt 12*, 3329–3341. [CrossRef]
2. Loma, I.; Heyman, R. Multiple sclerosis: Pathogenesis and treatment. *Curr. Neuropharmacol.* **2011**, *9*, 409–416. [CrossRef]
3. Leray, E.; Moreau, T.; Fromont, A.; Edan, G. Epidemiology of multiple sclerosis. *Rev. Neurol.* **2016**, *172*, 3–13. [CrossRef]
4. Compston, A.; Coles, A. Multiple sclerosis. *Lancet* **2008**, *372*, 1502–1517. [CrossRef]
5. Toosy, A.T.; Mason, D.F.; Miller, D.H. Optic neuritis. *Lancet Neurol.* **2014**, *13*, 83–99. [CrossRef]
6. Thompson, A.J.; Banwell, B.L.; Barkhof, F.; Carroll, W.M.; Coetzee, T.; Comi, G.; Correale, J.; Fazekas, F.; Filippi, M.; Freedman, M.S.; et al. Diagnosis of multiple sclerosis: 2017 revisions of the McDonald criteria. *Lancet Neurol.* **2018**, *17*, 162–173. [CrossRef]
7. Correale, J.; Villa, A. Role of CD8+ CD25+ Foxp3+ regulatory T cells in multiple sclerosis. *Ann. Neurol.* **2010**, *67*, 625–638. [CrossRef]

8.   Schoenborn, J.R.; Wilson, C.B. Regulation of interferon-gamma during innate and adaptive immune responses. *Adv. Immunol.* **2007**, *96*, 41–101.

9.   Minty, A.; Chalon, P.; Derocq, J.M.; Dumont, X.; Guillemot, J.C.; Kaghad, M.; Labit, C.; Leplatois, P.; Liauzun, P.; Miloux, B.; et al. Interleukin-13 is a new human lymphokine regulating inflammatory and immune responses. *Nature* **1993**, *362*, 248–250. [CrossRef]

10.   Zhu, J.; Paul, W.E. CD4 T cells: Fates, functions, and faults. *Blood* **2008**, *112*, 1557–1569. [CrossRef]

11.   Ghasemi, N.; Razavi, S.; Nikzad, E. Multiple Sclerosis: Pathogenesis, Symptoms, Diagnoses and Cell-Based Therapy. *Cell J.* **2017**, *19*, 1–10.

12.   Nishimura, H.; Enokida, H.; Sakamoto, T.; Takahashi, T.; Hayami, H.; Nakagawa, M. Immunoadsorption plasmapheresis treatment for the recurrent exacerbation of neuromyelitis optica spectrum disorder with a fluctuating anti-aquaporin-4 antibody level. *J. Artif. Organs* **2018**, *21*, 378–382. [CrossRef]

13.   Ouyang, W.; Kolls, J.K.; Zheng, Y. The biological functions of T helper 17 cell effector cytokines in inflammation. *Immunity* **2008**, *28*, 454–467. [CrossRef]

14.   Lee, G.R. The Balance of Th17 versus Treg Cells in Autoimmunity. *Int. J. Mol. Sci.* **2018**, *19*, 730. [CrossRef]

15.   Egg, R.; Reindl, M.; Deisenhammer, F.; Linington, C.; Berger, T. Anti-MOG and anti-MBP antibody subclasses in multiple sclerosis. *Mult. Scler. J.* **2001**, *7*, 285–289. [CrossRef]

16.   Dendrou, C.A.; Fugger, L.; Friese, M.A. Immunopathology of multiple sclerosis. *Nat. Rev. Immunol.* **2015**, *15*, 545–558. [CrossRef]

17.   Grigoriadis, N.; van Pesch, V. A basic overview of multiple sclerosis immunopathology. *Eur. J. Neurol.* **2015**, *22*, 3–13. [CrossRef]

18.   Howell, O.W.; Reeves, C.A.; Nicholas, R.; Carassiti, D.; Radotra, B.; Gentleman, S.M.; Serafini, B.; Aloisi, F.; Roncaroli, F.; Magliozzi, R.; et al. Meningeal inflammation is widespread and linked to cortical pathology in multiple sclerosis. *Brain A J. Neurol.* **2011**, *134*, 2755–2771. [CrossRef]

19.   Stern, J.N.H.; Yaari, G.; Vander Heiden, J.A.; Church, G.; Donahue, W.F.; Hintzen, R.Q.; Huttner, A.J.; Laman, J.D.; Nagra, R.M.; Nylander, A.; et al. B cells populating the multiple sclerosis brain mature in the draining cervical lymph nodes. *Sci. Transl. Med.* **2014**, *6*, 248ra107. [CrossRef]

20.   Lucchinetti, C.; Bruck, W.; Parisi, J.; Scheithauer, B.; Rodriguez, M.; Lassmann, H. Heterogeneity of multiple sclerosis lesions: Implications for the pathogenesis of demyelination. *Ann. Neurol.* **2000**, *47*, 707–717. [CrossRef]

21.   Wingerchuk, D.M.; Lennon, V.A.; Lucchinetti, C.F.; Pittock, S.J.; Weinshenker, B.G. The spectrum of neuromyelitis optica. *Lancet Neurol.* **2007**, *6*, 805–815. [CrossRef]

22.   Bevan, C.; Gelfand, J.M. Therapeutic Management of Severe Relapses in Multiple Sclerosis. *Curr. Treat. Options Neurol.* **2015**, *17*, 17. [CrossRef] [PubMed]

23.   Sellebjerg, F.; Barnes, D.; Filippini, G.; Midgard, R.; Montalban, X.; Rieckmann, P.; Selmaj, K.; Visser, L.H.; Sorensen, P.S. EFNS guideline on treatment of multiple sclerosis relapses: Report of an EFNS task force on treatment of multiple sclerosis relapses. *Eur. J. Neurol.* **2005**, *12*, 939–946. [CrossRef] [PubMed]

24.   Wiendl, H.; Toyka, K.V.; Rieckmann, P.; Gold, R.; Hartung, H.P.; Hohlfeld, R. Basic and escalating immunomodulatory treatments in multiple sclerosis: Current therapeutic recommendations. *J. Neurol.* **2008**, *255*, 1449–1463. [PubMed]

25.   Schroder, A.; Linker, R.A.; Gold, R. Plasmapheresis for neurological disorders. *Expert Rev. Neurother.* **2009**, *9*, 1331–1339. [CrossRef]

26.   Padmanabhan, A.; Connelly-Smith, L.; Aqui, N.; Balogun, R.A.; Klingel, R.; Meyer, E.; Pham, H.P.; Schneiderman, J.; Witt, V.; Wu, Y.; et al. Guidelines on the Use of Therapeutic Apheresis in Clinical Practice—Evidence-Based Approach from the Writing Committee of the American Society for Apheresis: The Eighth Special Issue. *J. Clin. Apher.* **2019**, *34*, 171–354. [CrossRef]

27.   Cortese, I.; Chaudhry, V.; So, Y.T.; Cantor, F.; Cornblath, D.R.; Rae-Grant, A. Evidence-based guideline update: Plasmapheresis in neurologic disorders: Report of the Therapeutics and Technology Assessment Subcommittee of the American Academy of Neurology. *Neurology* **2011**, *76*, 294–300. [CrossRef]

28.   Paroder-Belenitsky, M.; Pham, H. *Immunoadsorption, Transfusion Medicine and Hemostasis*, 3rd ed.; Stacy Masucci: Cambridge, UK, 2019; pp. 497–500.

29.   Available online: https://www.kompetenznetz-multiplesklerose.de/wp-content/uploads/2016/02/dgn-kknms_ms-ll_20140813.pdf (accessed on 20 May 2020).

30. Navarro-Martinez, R.; Cauli, O. Therapeutic Plasmapheresis with Albumin Replacement in Alzheimer's Disease and Chronic Progressive Multiple Sclerosis: A Review. *Pharmaceuticals* **2020**, *13*, 28. [CrossRef]
31. Koziolek, M.; Muhlhausen, J.; Friede, T.; Ellenberger, D.; Sigler, M.; Huppke, B.; Gartner, J.; Muller, G.A.; Huppke, P. Therapeutic apheresis in pediatric patients with acute CNS inflammatory demyelinating disease. *Blood Purif.* **2013**, *36*, 92–97. [CrossRef]
32. Koziolek, M.J.; Tampe, D.; Bahr, M.; Dihazi, H.; Jung, K.; Fitzner, D.; Klingel, R.; Muller, G.A.; Kitze, B. Immunoadsorption therapy in patients with multiple sclerosis with steroid-refractory optical neuritis. *J. Neuroinflamm.* **2012**, *9*, 80. [CrossRef]
33. Jamshidian, A.; Kazemi, M.; Shaygannejad, V.; Salehi, M. The Effect of Plasma Exchange on the Expression of FOXP3 and RORC2 in Relapsed Multiple Sclerosis Patients. *Iran. J. Immunol.* **2015**, *12*, 311–318. [PubMed]
34. Stork, L.; Ellenberger, D.; Beissbarth, T.; Friede, T.; Lucchinetti, C.F.; Bruck, W.; Metz, I. Differences in the Reponses to Apheresis Therapy of Patients With 3 Histopathologically Classified Immunopathological Patterns of Multiple Sclerosis. *JAMA Neurol.* **2018**, *75*, 428–435. [CrossRef] [PubMed]
35. Khatri, B.O.; McQuillen, M.P.; Harrington, G.J.; Schmoll, D.; Hoffmann, R.G. Chronic progressive multiple sclerosis: Double-blind controlled study of plasmapheresis in patients taking immunosuppressive drugs. *Neurology* **1985**, *35*, 312–319. [CrossRef]
36. Weiner, H.L.; Dau, P.C.; Khatri, B.O.; Petajan, J.H.; Birnbaum, G.; McQuillen, M.P.; Fosburg, M.T.; Feldstein, M.; Orav, E.J. Double-blind study of true vs. sham plasma exchange in patients treated with immunosuppression for acute attacks of multiple sclerosis. *Neurology* **1989**, *39*, 1143–1149. [CrossRef]
37. Weinshenker, B.G.; O'Brien, P.C.; Petterson, T.M.; Noseworthy, J.H.; Lucchinetti, C.F.; Dodick, D.W.; Pineda, A.A.; Stevens, L.N.; Rodriguez, M. A randomized trial of plasma exchange in acute central nervous system inflammatory demyelinating disease. *Ann. Neurol.* **1999**, *46*, 878–886. [CrossRef]
38. Habek, M.; Barun, B.; Puretic, Z.; Brinar, V.V. Treatment of steroid unresponsive relapse with plasma exchange in aggressive multiple sclerosis. *Ther. Apher. Dial.* **2010**, *14*, 298–302. [CrossRef]
39. Schilling, S.; Linker, R.A.; Konig, F.B.; Koziolek, M.; Bahr, M.; Muller, G.A.; Paulus, W.; Gartner, J.; Bruck, W.; Chan, A.; et al. Plasma exchange therapy for steroid-unresponsive multiple sclerosis relapses: Clinical experience with 16 patients. *Der Nervenarzt* **2006**, *77*, 430–438. [CrossRef]
40. Trebst, C.; Reising, A.; Kielstein, J.T.; Hafer, C.; Stangel, M. Plasma exchange therapy in steroid-unresponsive relapses in patients with multiple sclerosis. *Blood Purif.* **2009**, *28*, 108–115. [CrossRef]
41. Magana, S.M.; Keegan, B.M.; Weinshenker, B.G.; Erickson, B.J.; Pittock, S.J.; Lennon, V.A.; Rodriguez, M.; Thomsen, K.; Weigand, S.; Mandrekar, J.; et al. Beneficial plasma exchange response in central nervous system inflammatory demyelination. *Arch. Neurol.* **2011**, *68*, 870–878. [CrossRef]
42. Dorst, J.; Fangerau, T.; Taranu, D.; Eichele, P.; Dreyhaupt, J.; Michels, S.; Schuster, J.; Ludolph, A.C.; Senel, M.; Tumani, H. Safety and efficacy of immunoadsorption versus plasma exchange in steroid-refractory relapse of multiple sclerosis and clinically isolated syndrome: A randomised, parallel-group, controlled trial. *EClinicalMedicine* **2019**, *16*, 98–106. [CrossRef]
43. Ehler, J.; Koball, S.; Sauer, M.; Mitzner, S.; Hickstein, H.; Benecke, R.; Zettl, U.K. Response to Therapeutic Plasma Exchange as a Rescue Treatment in Clinically Isolated Syndromes and Acute Worsening of Multiple Sclerosis: A Retrospective Analysis of 90 Patients. *PLoS ONE* **2015**, *10*, e0134583. [CrossRef]
44. Lipphardt, M.; Muhlhausen, J.; Kitze, B.; Heigl, F.; Mauch, E.; Helms, H.J.; Muller, G.A.; Koziolek, M.J. Immunoadsorption or plasma exchange in steroid-refractory multiple sclerosis and neuromyelitis optica. *J. Clin. Apher.* **2019**, *34*, 381–391. [CrossRef]
45. Deschamps, R.; Gueguen, A.; Parquet, N.; Saheb, S.; Driss, F.; Mesnil, M.; Vignal, C.; Aboab, J.; Depaz, R.; Gout, O. Plasma exchange response in 34 patients with severe optic neuritis. *J. Neurol.* **2016**, *263*, 883–887. [CrossRef]
46. Ruprecht, K.; Klinker, E.; Dintelmann, T.; Rieckmann, P.; Gold, R. Plasma exchange for severe optic neuritis: Treatment of 10 patients. *Neurology* **2004**, *63*, 1081–1083. [CrossRef]
47. Yucesan, C.; Arslan, O.; Arat, M.; Yucemen, N.; Ayyildiz, E.; Ilhan, O.; Mutluer, N. Therapeutic plasma exchange in the treatment of neuroimmunologic disorders: Review of 50 cases. *Transfus. Apher. Sci.* **2007**, *36*, 103–107. [CrossRef]
48. Meca-Lallana, J.E.; Hernandez-Clares, R.; Leon-Hernandez, A.; Genoves Aleixandre, A.; Cacho Perez, M.; Martin-Fernandez, J.J. Plasma exchange for steroid-refractory relapses in multiple sclerosis: An observational, MRI pilot study. *Clin. Ther.* **2013**, *35*, 474–485. [CrossRef]

49. Ehler, J.; Koball, S.; Sauer, M.; Hickstein, H.; Mitzner, S.; Benecke, R.; Zettl, U.K. Therapeutic plasma exchange in glucocorticosteroid-unresponsive patients with Clinically Isolated Syndrome. *Ther. Apher. Dial.* **2014**, *18*, 489–496. [CrossRef]

50. Faissner, S.; Nikolayczik, J.; Chan, A.; Hellwig, K.; Gold, R.; Yoon, M.S.; Haghikia, A. Plasmapheresis and immunoadsorption in patients with steroid refractory multiple sclerosis relapses. *J. Neurol.* **2016**, *263*, 1092–1098. [CrossRef]

51. Correia, I.; Ribeiro, J.J.; Isidoro, L.; Batista, S.; Nunes, C.; Macario, C.; Borges, C.; Tomaz, J.; Sousa, L. Plasma exchange in severe acute relapses of multiple sclerosis—Results from a Portuguese cohort. *Mult. Scler. Relat. Disord.* **2018**, *19*, 148–152. [CrossRef]

52. Hauser, S.L.; Dawson, D.M.; Lehrich, J.R.; Beal, M.F.; Kevy, S.V.; Weiner, H.L. Immunosuppression and plasmapheresis in chronic progressive multiple sclerosis. Design of a clinical trial. *Arch. Neurol.* **1983**, *40*, 687–690. [CrossRef]

53. Medenica, R.D.; Mukerjee, S.; Huschart, T.; Corbitt, W. Interferon inhibitor factor predicting success of plasmapheresis in patients with multiple sclerosis. *J. Clin. Apher.* **1994**, *9*, 216–221. [CrossRef]

54. Giedraitiene, N.; Kaubrys, G.; Kizlaitiene, R.; Bagdonaite, L.; Griskevicius, L.; Valceckiene, V.; Stoskus, M. Therapeutic Plasma Exchange in Multiple Sclerosis Patients with Abolished Interferon-beta Bioavailability. *Med. Sci. Monit.* **2015**, *21*, 1512–1519.

55. Roesner, S.; Appel, R.; Gbadamosi, J.; Martin, R.; Heesen, C. Treatment of steroid-unresponsive optic neuritis with plasma exchange. *Acta Neurol. Scand.* **2012**, *126*, 103–108. [CrossRef]

56. Merle, H.; Olindo, S.; Jeannin, S.; Valentino, R.; Mehdaoui, H.; Cabot, F.; Donnio, A.; Hage, R.; Richer, R.; Smadja, D.; et al. Treatment of optic neuritis by plasma exchange (add-on) in neuromyelitis optica. *Arch. Ophthalmol.* **2012**, *130*, 858–862. [CrossRef]

57. Watanabe, S.; Nakashima, I.; Misu, T.; Miyazawa, I.; Shiga, Y.; Fujihara, K.; Itoyama, Y. Therapeutic efficacy of plasma exchange in NMO-IgG-positive patients with neuromyelitis optica. *Mult. Scler.* **2007**, *13*, 128–132. [CrossRef]

58. Wang, K.C.; Wang, S.J.; Lee, C.L.; Chen, S.Y.; Tsai, C.P. The rescue effect of plasma exchange for neuromyelitis optica. *J. Clin. Neurosci.* **2011**, *18*, 43–46. [CrossRef]

59. Lim, Y.M.; Pyun, S.Y.; Kang, B.H.; Kim, J.; Kim, K.K. Factors associated with the effectiveness of plasma exchange for the treatment of NMO-IgG-positive neuromyelitis optica spectrum disorders. *Mult. Scler.* **2013**, *19*, 1216–1218. [CrossRef]

60. Kim, S.H.; Kim, W.; Huh, S.Y.; Lee, K.Y.; Jung, I.J.; Kim, H.J. Clinical efficacy of plasmapheresis in patients with neuromyelitis optica spectrum disorder and effects on circulating anti-aquaporin-4 antibody levels. *J. Clin. Neurol.* **2013**, *9*, 36–42. [CrossRef]

61. Abboud, H.; Petrak, A.; Mealy, M.; Sasidharan, S.; Siddique, L.; Levy, M. Treatment of acute relapses in neuromyelitis optica: Steroids alone versus steroids plus plasma exchange. *Mult. Scler.* **2016**, *22*, 185–192. [CrossRef]

62. Aungsumart, S.; Apiwattanakul, M. Clinical outcomes and predictive factors related to good outcomes in plasma exchange in severe attack of NMOSD and long extensive transverse myelitis: Case series and review of the literature. *Mult. Scler. Relat. Disord.* **2017**, *13*, 93–97. [CrossRef]

63. Srisupa-Olan, T.; Siritho, S.; Kittisares, K.; Jitprapaikulsan, J.; Sathukitchai, C.; Prayoonwiwat, N. Beneficial effect of plasma exchange in acute attack of neuromyelitis optica spectrum disorders. *Mult. Scler. Relat. Disord.* **2018**, *20*, 115–121. [CrossRef]

64. Jiao, Y.; Cui, L.; Zhang, W.; Zhang, Y.; Wang, W.; Zhang, L.; Tang, W.; Jiao, J. Plasma Exchange for Neuromyelitis Optica Spectrum Disorders in Chinese Patients and Factors Predictive of Short-term Outcome. *Clin. Ther.* **2018**, *40*, 603–612. [CrossRef]

65. Mori, S.; Kurimoto, T.; Ueda, K.; Nakamura, M. Short-term effect of additional apheresis on visual acuity changes in patients with steroid-resistant optic neuritis in neuromyelitis optica spectrum disorders. *Jpn. J. Ophthalmol.* **2018**, *62*, 525–530. [CrossRef]

66. Kumar, R.; Paul, B.S.; Singh, G.; Kaur, A. Therapeutic Efficacy of Plasma Exchange in Neuromyelitis Optica. *Ann. Indian Acad. Neurol.* **2018**, *21*, 140–143.

67. Kleiter, I.; Gahlen, A.; Borisow, N.; Fischer, K.; Wernecke, K.D.; Hellwig, K.; Pache, F.; Ruprecht, K.; Havla, J.; Kumpfel, T.; et al. Apheresis therapies for NMOSD attacks: A retrospective study of 207 therapeutic interventions. *Neurol. Neuroimmunol. Neuroinflamm.* **2018**, *5*, e504. [CrossRef]

68. Song, W.; Qu, Y.; Huang, X. Plasma exchange: An effective add-on treatment of optic neuritis in neuromyelitis optica spectrum disorders. *Int. Ophthalmol.* **2019**, *39*, 2477–2483. [CrossRef]

69. De Andres, C.; Anaya, F.; Gimenez-Roldan, S. Plasma immunoadsorption treatment of malignant multiple sclerosis with severe and prolonged relapses. *Rev. Neurol.* **2000**, *30*, 601–605.

70. Heigl, F.; Hettich, R.; Arendt, R.; Durner, J.; Koehler, J.; Mauch, E. Immunoadsorption in steroid-refractory multiple sclerosis: Clinical experience in 60 patients. *Atheroscler. Suppl.* **2013**, *14*, 167–173. [CrossRef]

71. Mauch, E.; Zwanzger, J.; Hettich, R.; Fassbender, C.; Klingel, R.; Heigl, F. Immunoadsorption for steroid-unresponsive multiple sclerosis-relapses: Clinical data of 14 patients. *Der Nervenarzt* **2011**, *82*, 1590–1595. [CrossRef]

72. Trebst, C.; Bronzlik, P.; Kielstein, J.T.; Schmidt, B.M.; Stangel, M. Immunoadsorption therapy for steroid-unresponsive relapses in patients with multiple sclerosis. *Blood Purif.* **2012**, *33*, 1–6. [CrossRef]

73. Hoffmann, F.; Kraft, A.; Heigl, F.; Mauch, E.; Koehler, J.; Harms, L.; Kumpfel, T.; Kohler, W.; Ehrlich, S.; Bayas, A.; et al. Tryptophan immunoadsorption during pregnancy and breastfeeding in patients with acute relapse of multiple sclerosis and neuromyelitis optica. *Ther. Adv. Neurol. Disord.* **2018**, *11*. [CrossRef] [PubMed]

74. Moldenhauer, A.; Haas, J.; Wascher, C.; Derfuss, T.; Hoffmann, K.T.; Kiesewetter, H.; Salama, A. Immunoadsorption patients with multiple sclerosis: An open-label pilot study. *Eur. J. Clin. Investig.* **2005**, *35*, 523–530. [CrossRef] [PubMed]

75. Schimrigk, S.; Adibi, I.; Eberl, A.; Selka, I.; Galle, J.; Schmidt, S.; Fritz, H.G.; Fassbender, C.; Klingel, R.; Fuchtemann, D.; et al. Immunoadsorption as Relapse Escalation Therapy for Multiple Sclerosis. *Aktuel. Neurol.* **2012**, *39*, 174–179.

76. Schimrigk, S.; Faiss, J.; Kohler, W.; Gunther, A.; Harms, L.; Kraft, A.; Ehrlich, S.; Eberl, A.; Fassbender, C.; Klingel, R.; et al. Escalation Therapy of Steroid Refractory Multiple Sclerosis Relapse with Tryptophan Immunoadsorption—Observational Multicenter Study with 147 Patients. *Eur. Neurol.* **2016**, *75*, 300–306. [CrossRef] [PubMed]

77. Faissner, S.; Nikolayczik, J.; Chan, A.; Gold, R.; Yoon, M.S.; Haghikia, A. Immunoadsorption in patients with neuromyelitis optica spectrum disorder. *Ther. Adv. Neurol. Disord.* **2016**, *9*, 281–286. [CrossRef]

78. Hohenstein, B.; Passauer, J.; Ziemssen, T.; Julius, U. Immunoadsorption with regenerating systems in neurological disorders –A single center experience. *Atheroscler. Suppl.* **2015**, *18*, 119–123. [CrossRef]

79. Muhlhausen, J.; Kitze, B.; Huppke, P.; Muller, G.A.; Koziolek, M.J. Apheresis in treatment of acute inflammatory demyelinating disorders. *Atheroscler. Suppl.* **2015**, *18*, 251–256. [CrossRef]

80. Llufriu, S.; Castillo, J.; Blanco, Y.; Ramio-Torrenta, L.; Rio, J.; Valles, M.; Lozano, M.; Castella, M.D.; Calabia, J.; Horga, A.; et al. Plasma exchange for acute attacks of CNS demyelination: Predictors of improvement at 6 months. *Neurology* **2009**, *73*, 949–953. [CrossRef]

81. Bramlage, C.P.; Schroder, K.; Bramlage, P.; Ahrens, K.; Zapf, A.; Muller, G.A.; Koziolek, M.J. Predictors of complications in therapeutic plasma exchange. *J. Clin. Apher.* **2009**, *24*, 225–231. [CrossRef]

82. Mokrzycki, M.H.; Kaplan, A.A. Therapeutic plasma exchange: Complications and management. *Am. J. Kidney Dis.* **1994**, *23*, 817–827. [CrossRef]

83. Samtleben, W.; Blumenstein, M.; Liebl, L.; Gurland, H.J. Membrane plasma separation for treatment of immunologically mediated diseases. *Trans. Am. Soc. Artif. Intern. Organs* **1980**, *26*, 12–16. [PubMed]

84. Sprenger, K.B.; Rasche, H.; Franz, H.E. Membrane plasma separation: Complications and monitoring. *Artif. Organs* **1984**, *8*, 360–363. [PubMed]

85. Kohler, W.; Bucka, C.; Klingel, R. A randomized and controlled study comparing immunoadsorption and plasma exchange in myasthenic crisis. *J. Clin. Apher.* **2011**, *26*, 347–355. [CrossRef] [PubMed]

86. Zollner, S.; Pablik, E.; Druml, W.; Derfler, K.; Rees, A.; Biesenbach, P. Fibrinogen reduction and bleeding complications in plasma exchange, immunoadsorption and a combination of the two. *Blood Purif.* **2014**, *38*, 160–166. [CrossRef]

87. Schneider-Gold, C.; Krenzer, M.; Klinker, E.; Mansouri-Thalegani, B.; Mullges, W.; Toyka, K.V.; Gold, R. Immunoadsorption versus plasma exchange versus combination for treatment of myasthenic deterioration. *Ther. Adv. Neurol. Disord.* **2016**, *9*, 297–303. [CrossRef]

88. Keegan, M.; Pineda, A.A.; McClelland, R.L.; Darby, C.H.; Rodriguez, M.; Weinshenker, B.G. Plasma exchange for severe attacks of CNS demyelination: Predictors of response. *Neurology* **2002**, *58*, 143–146. [CrossRef]

89. Heigl, F.; Hettich, R.; Suckfuell, M.; Luebbers, C.W.; Osterkorn, D.; Osterkorn, K.; Canis, M. Fibrinogen/LDL apheresis as successful second-line treatment of sudden hearing loss: A retrospective study on 217 patients. *Atheroscler. Suppl.* **2009**, *10*, 95–101. [CrossRef]

90. Sim, F.J.; Zhao, C.; Penderis, J.; Franklin, R.J. The age-related decrease in CNS remyelination efficiency is attributable to an impairment of both oligodendrocyte progenitor recruitment and differentiation. *J. Neurosci.* **2002**, *22*, 2451–2459. [CrossRef]

91. Freedman, M.S.; De Stefano, N.; Barkhof, F.; Polman, C.H.; Comi, G.; Uitdehaag, B.M.; Casset-Semanaz, F.; Hennessy, B.; Lehr, L.; Stubinski, B.; et al. Patient subgroup analyses of the treatment effect of subcutaneous interferon beta-1a on development of multiple sclerosis in the randomized controlled REFLEX study. *J. Neurol.* **2014**, *261*, 490–499. [CrossRef]

92. Kleiter, I.; Gahlen, A.; Borisow, N.; Fischer, K.; Wernecke, K.D.; Wegner, B.; Hellwig, K.; Pache, F.; Ruprecht, K.; Havla, J.; et al. Neuromyelitis optica: Evaluation of 871 attacks and 1153 treatment courses. *Ann. Neurol.* **2016**, *79*, 206–216. [CrossRef]

93. Zekeridou, A.; Lennon, V.A. Aquaporin-4 autoimmunity. *Neurol. Neuroimmunol. Neuroinflamm.* **2015**, *2*, e110. [CrossRef] [PubMed]

94. Savransky, A.; Rubstein, A.; Rios, M.H.; Vergel, S.L.; Velasquez, M.C.; Sierra, S.P.; Marcarian, G.; Alba, R.; Pugliese, A.M.; Tenembaum, S. Prognostic indicators of improvement with therapeutic plasma exchange in pediatric demyelination. *Neurology* **2019**, *93*, 2065–2073. [CrossRef] [PubMed]

95. Goto, H.; Matsuo, H.; Nakane, S.; Izumoto, H.; Fukudome, T.; Kambara, C.; Shibuya, N. Plasmapheresis affects T helper type-1/T helper type-2 balance of circulating peripheral lymphocytes. *Ther. Apher.* **2001**, *5*, 494–496. [CrossRef] [PubMed]

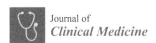

Article

Comparing Plasma Exchange to Escalated Methyl Prednisolone in Refractory Multiple Sclerosis Relapses

Steffen Pfeuffer [1,*,†]**, Leoni Rolfes** [1,†]**, Eike Bormann** [2]**, Cristina Sauerland** [2]**, Tobias Ruck** [1]**,
Matthias Schilling** [1]**, Nico Melzer** [1]**, Marcus Brand** [3]**, Refik Pul** [4]**, Christoph Kleinschnitz** [4]**,
Heinz Wiendl** [1] **and Sven G. Meuth** [1]

[1] Neurology Clinic and Institute for Translational Neurology, University of Muenster, 48149 Münster,
Germany; leoni.rolfes@ukmuenster.de (L.R.); tobias.ruck@ukmuenster.de (T.R.);
matthias.schilling@ukmuenster.de (M.S.); nico.melzer@ukmuenster.de (N.M.);
heinz.wiendl@ukmuenster.de (H.W.); sven.meuth@ukmuenster.de (S.G.M.)
[2] Institute of Biostatistics and Clinical Research, University of Muenster, 48149 Münster, Germany;
eike.bormann@ukmuenster.de (E.B.); cristina.sauerland@ukmuenster.de (C.S.)
[3] Department of Internal Medicine D, University of Muenster 48149 Münster, Germany;
marcus.brand@ukmuenster.de
[4] Department of Neurology, University Duisburg-Essen, 45147 Essen, Germany; refik.pul@uk-essen.de (R.P.);
christoph.kleinschnitz@uk-essen.de (C.K.)
* Correspondence: steffen.pfeuffer@ukmuenster.de; Tel.: +49-(0)-251-83-44463; Fax: +49-(0)-251-83-46812
† Both authors contributed equally.

Received: 3 December 2019; Accepted: 18 December 2019; Published: 22 December 2019

Abstract: Intravenous methyl prednisolone (IVMPS) represents the standard of care for multiple
sclerosis (MS) relapses, but fail to improve symptoms in one quarter of patients. In this regard,
apart from extending steroid treatment to a higher dose, therapeutic plasma exchange (TPE) has been
recognized as a treatment option. The aim of this retrospective, monocentric study was to investigate
the efficacy of TPE versus escalated dosages of IVMPS in refractory MS relapses. An in-depth
medical chart review was performed to identify patients from local databases. Relapse recovery
was stratified as "good/full", "average" and "worst/no" according to function score development.
In total, 145 patients were analyzed. Good/average/worst recovery at discharge was observed in
60.9%/32.6%/6.5% of TPE versus 15.2%/14.1%/70.7% of IVMPS patients, respectively. A total of
53.5% of IVMPS patients received TPE as rescue treatment and 54.8% then responded satisfactorily.
The multivariable odds ratio (OR) for worst/no recovery was 39.01 (95%–CI: 10.41–146.18; $p \leq 0.001$),
favoring administration of TPE as first escalation treatment. The effects were sustained at three-month
follow-ups, as OR for further deterioration was 6.48 (95%–CI: 2.48–16.89; $p \leq 0.001$), favoring TPE.
In conclusion, TPE was superior over IVMPS in the amelioration of relapse symptoms at discharge
and follow-up. This study provides class IV evidence supporting the administration of TPE as the
first escalation treatment to steroid-refractory MS relapses.

Keywords: multiple sclerosis; optic neuritis; plasma exchange; relapse; class IV; steroids

---

1. Introduction

The treatment of acute multiple sclerosis (MS) relapses has remained unaltered for decades.
The use of high-dose short-term intravenous (methyl-) prednisolone (IVMPS; 500–1000 mg per day for
three to five days) is the accepted treatment for relapses [1,2]. Of note, adrenocorticotropic hormone
(ACTH) gel is an alternative for patients who do not tolerate corticosteroids. Moreover, although it
has been suggested that intravenous immunoglobulins (IVIG) may be a therapeutic option if steroids

are contraindicated, two well conducted randomized controlled trials showed that IVIG as an add-on treatment with IVMPS did not confer additional benefit [3,4].

Interestingly, around 25% of patients remain with significant disability 14 days after IVMPS treatment initiation [5]. For these patients, one option is IVMPS treatment escalation (up to 2000 mg daily) for a further three to five days, as recommended by the national guidelines [2,6]. An alternative option is therapeutic plasma exchange (TPE), which has been proven effective in one small randomized trial that showed the superiority of TPE over sham treatment [7]. The effectiveness of TPE has been reported for all demyelinating disorders of the CNS, including optic neuritis (ON), clinically-isolated syndrome (CIS) and relapsing-remitting MS (RRMS) [8–10]. Consequently, several guidelines recommend TPE as an adjunctive treatment for increasing the chances of recovery for steroid-refractory relapses [11,12]. However, most studies evaluating TPE lacked an active comparator (such as escalated IVMPS) and comprised heterogeneous treatment regimens. Also, patients with demyelinating diseases other than RRMS were included in the study populations [7–9]. Evidence for IVMPS treatment escalation is to a large part based on a single study that compared MRI endpoints but not clinical endpoints [6]. Furthermore, IVMPS treatment escalation exhibited additional, non-genomic effects in animal models [13]. Robust clinical evidence for the currently recommended treatment sequence (initiation treatment with IVMPS, first escalation treatment with IVMPS, second escalation treatment with TPE) is still lacking [6,11,12].

We here analyzed patients with acute relapses of RRMS, CIS or isolated ON who were treated with escalated IVMPS, TPE, or a combination of both.

2. Experimental Section

2.1. Patients

Between January 2013 and December 2017, all of the in-patients in our department were screened. We identified patients diagnosed with RRMS, CIS, or isolated ON, who received a full course of IVMPS (1000 mg daily for five days without an oral taper) as initial treatment (referred to as "initiation treatment" throughout the manuscript). In a second step, we selected patients who received further relapse treatments (referred to as "escalation treatment" throughout the manuscript) and reviewed their medical chart in detail, using a standardized electronic case report form. All patients included in our analysis were hospitalized in our clinic for both the initiation as well as the escalation treatment.

The inclusion criteria for final analysis were:

(i)   established diagnosis of RRMS or CIS according to 2017 revised McDonald criteria [14] or optic neuritis in absence of any other infectious or inflammatory disease of the CNS (especially neuromyelitis optica spectrum disorders)

(ii) significant relapse with an increase of the Expanded Disability Status Scale (EDSS) score [15] of at least 1.0 in MS/CIS patients or a decrease of the best-corrected visual acuity (VA) in patients with isolated ON in analogy to a decrease of at least 1 according to the visual function system score (FSS) derived from the EDSS, as inclusion criteria for both initiation and escalation treatment

(iii) escalation therapy with either 2000 mg methylprednisolone per day for five days, five cycles of therapeutic plasma exchange or a combination thereof following initiation therapy with 1000 mg per day over 5 days

(iv) completion of escalation treatment within six weeks from relapse onset

Therapeutic plasma exchange was performed with a COM.TEC cell separator (Fresenius Hemo-Care GmbH, Bad Homburg, Germany). All patients received treatment via central venous catheters every other day, for a total of five sessions. Per session, one plasma volume was processed, while human albumin solution (5%) was used for substitution. The blood flow rates were 50–70 mL per min. All patients underwent regional pre-centrifugal anticoagulation with citrate, followed by post-centrifugal calcium application. In four cases, the treatment-free interval was extended by another day due to excessive hypofibrinogenemia.

Patients with the following criteria were excluded:

(i) pregnancy, as determined by pregnancy test
(ii) diagnosis of other systemic inflammatory disorders within the observation period
(iii) onset of relapse symptoms more than one month prior to initiation treatment with IVMPS
(iv) documentation of a secondary progressive disease course within the observation period

For the patients who received more than one escalation treatment within the observation period, we only evaluated the first relapse to avoid preselection bias.

2.2. Assessment of Effectiveness

To overcome limitations of the EDSS in depicting acute, relapse-associated disability, we decided to classify our patients into different response categories. For statistical analysis we applied FSS-based stratification as proposed by Conway and colleagues, which stratifies treatment responses based on peak- and recovery-FSS distances into "good/full", "partial", or "worst/no" recovery [16]. We show a modified matrix, as previously used, with outcome stratification in Figure S1 [17]. The outcomes were evaluated after treatment completion and at follow-up (3 months after discharge).

Relapses were considered as monosymptomatic when Kurtzke's FSS of the affected system exceeded the other FSS by at least 1 point. Consequently, if this condition was not given, the relapse was regarded as polysymptomatic. In this regard, patients that either showed similar relapse FSSs for pyramidal and cerebellar functions (3 patients) or pyramidal and sensory functions (5 patients), were assigned to their FSS that was EDSS-defining at follow-up. In addition, 4 patients with spinal lesions displayed a similar FSS for bowel and bladder function and pyramidal function. These patients were subjected to the FSS group "pyramidal", as no patients were identified with bowel and bladder dysfunction as monosymptomatic relapse.

2.3. Assessment of Safety

We also screened patients' medical charts for severe adverse events and graded the identified events according to recommendations made in the "Common Terminology Criteria for Adverse Events". The CTCAE classification is as follows: I: asymptomatic testing or mild symptoms without necessity for specific intervention; II: local or noninvasive intervention indicated; III: severe, but not immediately life-threatening event, hospitalization or prolongation of hospitalization necessary; IV: life-threatening event; V: death related to event. The study conduct was ethically approved by the local institutional review board of the University of Muenster, Germany (2017-298-f-S).

2.4. Statistical Analysis

The continuous variables are presented as median and interquartile range and compared between groups using a Kruskal–Wallis test. The categorical variables are presented as absolute and relative frequencies and compared using Fisher's exact test.

To evaluate the influence of multiple variables on the occurrence and outcome of serious adverse events, we applied logistic regression. The results are described with odds ratios (OR), the respective 95% confidence intervals (CI), and Wald-test p-values. Either "worst or no treatment response following first escalation treatment" or "stable course versus further deterioration at follow-up" or "development of severe adverse events" were used as dependent variables.

All analyses are explorative and should be interpreted accordingly. p-values below 0.05 are considered significant; no adjustment for multiple testing was applied. Statistical analysis was conducted with SPSS Version 25 (International Business Machines Corporation (IBM), Armonk, USA).

2.5. Data Availability Statement

Anonymized data will be shared upon request from qualified investigators.

3. Results

3.1. Patients

Between January 2013 and December 2017, a total of 541 patients received initiation treatment for MS relapses. Of those, 193 (35.7%) patients were admitted for escalation treatment and all had a persistent functional deficit as defined above. A total of 127 (65.8%) patients received a second course of IVMPS as a first escalation treatment, while 66 (34.2%) patients were directly subjected to TPE. For our final analysis we could include a total of 145 patients: 99 out of 127 patients who received a second course of IVMPS, and 46 out of 66 patients who were directly subjected to TPE. Of note, 53 out of 99 (53.5%) patients were subjected to TPE as the second escalation treatment. None of the TPE patients were re-exposed to increased doses of IVMPS (for consort plot see Figure 1).

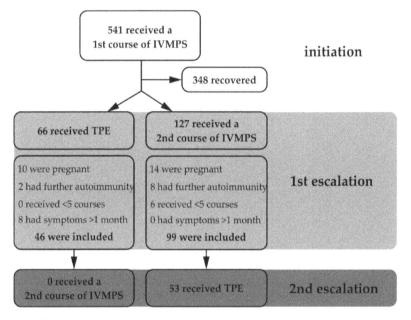

Figure 1. RRMS in-patients who were treated at the study site between January 2013 and December 2017 are described here. The data focus on those patients who received a full course of intravenous methyl prednisolone (5 × 1 g IVMPS) as the first escalation treatment after relapse. Patients who received a lower dosage (e.g., 3 × 1 g IVMPS) were excluded from the primary analysis.

Baseline characteristics of all treatment groups (IVMPS, TPE, and IVMPS + TPE) are shown in Table 1. Patients who did not receive additional TPE presented with lower peak relapse EDSS (median: IVMPS: 2.0; TPE: 3.0; IVMPS+TPE: 3.0; $p = 0.003$). Otherwise, patient characteristics showed no significant differences. The patients were, on average, young and early in their disease course, with only one patient being above 60 years old. The median time from retrospectively identified disease manifestation to current presentation was 1 year, and for 40% of patients it was their first demyelinating event.

Table 1. Rescue therapy patient baseline and follow-up characteristics compared between treatment groups.

	TPE	IVMPS	IVMPS+TPE	p
Patients, No.	46	46	53	-
Age, yr, median (IQR)	33 (29–45)	36 (27–43)	31.5 (27–41)	0.410 *
Male sex, No. (%)	13 (28.3)	14 (30.4)	14 (26.4)	0.922 #
MS duration, yr, median (IQR)				
- since onset	1 (0–3)	1 (0–4)	1 (0–4)	0.574 *
- since diagnosis	0 (0–2)	0 (0–2)	1 (0–3)	0.322 *
Relapses during last two years, median (IQR)	0.5 (0–1)	0 (0–1)	0 (0–1)	0.765 *
first demyelinating event, No. (%)	19 (41.3)	20 (43.48)	18 (33.96)	0.636 #
Baseline EDSS, median (IQR)	0 (0–1)	0 (0–1)	0 (0–2)	0.397 *
Relapse EDSS, median (IQR)	3 (2–3)	2 (2–3)	3 (2–3)	0.003 *
Affected function system, No. (%)				
- visual	25 (54.4)	25 (47.2)	19 (41.3)	
- pyramidal	4 (8.7)	4 (7.6)	8 (17.4)	
- brainstem	8 (17.4)	13 (24.5)	10 (21.8)	0.236 #
- cerebellar	3 (6.5)	7 (13.2)	1 (2.2)	
- sensory	6 (13.0)	3 (5.7)	8 (17.4)	
- cerebral	0 (0.0)	1 (1.9)	0 (0.0)	
Time to initiation treatment, d, median (IQR)	3 (1–7)	3 (1–5.25)	3 (1–5)	0.650*
Time to escalation treatment, d, median (IQR)	12.5 (8.75–16)	12 (10–15.25)	11 (8.5–14)	0.087*

Patient baseline characteristics compared between the different treatment groups. No.: Number; yr.: years; IQR: interquartile range. * Significance levels were calculated using a Kruskal–Wallis test. # Significance levels were calculated using Fisher's exact test.

One hundred and thirty-two patients fulfilled the 2017 revised McDonald criteria for the diagnosis of RRMS at relapse onset, whereas eight patients presented with isolated optic neuritis and five patients fulfilled the criteria for CIS. There were no differences in distribution between escalation treatment groups ($p = 0.756$).

Accordingly, the majority of patients did not receive disease modifying treatment (DMT) at relapse onset (62.1%). The treatment approved for mild to moderate courses of RRMS was administered to 22.8% of patients, whereas 15.2% received substances approved for the treatment of active RRMS (for a detailed description of administered DMT, see Table S1). The DMT subset use was evenly distributed between groups ($p = 0.793$). In 137 out of 145 patients the relapse was considered monosymptomatic. The most common relapse presentation was optic neuritis (69 patients; 47.6%). Generally, the frequencies of affected functional systems did not differ significantly between treatment groups ($p = 0.236$). Polysymptomatic relapses occurred in eight patients with infratentorial or spinal lesions and were assigned as outlined in the methods, according to their FSS that was EDSS-defining at follow-up.

3.2. Immediate Effects of Escalation Treatment

According to the previously described FSS-distance related analysis matrix, 28 (60.9%) patients showed good/full recovery following TPE, while 15 (15.2%) patients showed good/full recovery following escalation treatment with IVMPS. Partial recovery was observed in 12 (32.6%) TPE treated patients and in 15 (15.2%) IVMPS treated patients. Finally, no or worst recovery was documented in three (6.5%) TPE treated patients and in 69 (69.7%) IVMPS treated patients ($p < 0.001$, see Figure 2A). Next, 53 (53.5%) patients underwent rescue therapy with TPE following IVMPS, whereas the other patients received no further treatment prior to discharge irrespective of their response. Precise information on why no further treatment was given was not always available; patients' refusal of apheresis treatment was documented as reason in at least eight cases.

J. Clin. Med. **2020**, *9*, 35

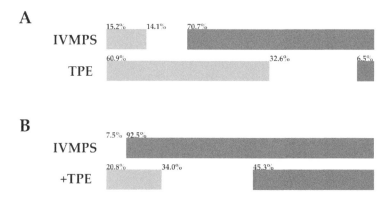

Figure 2. Different response groups following escalation treatment regimens are illustrated (green: good response; yellow: average response; red: worst response). (**A**) Upper bar represents patients who received IVMPS as the first escalation treatment (*n* = 99). Lower bar represents patients who received TPE as the first escalation treatment (*n* = 46). (**B**) Subgroup of patients who received two courses of escalation treatment (*n* = 53). Upper bar shows treatment response after first escalation with IVMPS and lower bar represents results following second escalation with TPE.

After the second escalation treatment with TPE, 25 (47.2%) patients showed a full response and 17 (32.1%) patients remitted partially, while 11 (20.7%) patients were unresponsive to the treatment (see Figure 2B). We performed regression analyses in order to evaluate the possible confounders and to check whether the higher proportion of treatment-resistant patients following IVMPS+TPE versus TPE alone was systematically influenced by different factors/confounders. Logistic regression analysis included "sex", "age", "affected function system (visual vs. other)", "disease duration", "baseline EDSS", and "time to treatment initiation". The adjusted odds ratio for "worst/no" treatment response was 39.01 (95%–CI: 10.42–142.71; *p*<0.001), favoring TPE treatment as the first escalation treatment (for full regression model see Table S2).

3.3. Sustained Effects of Escalation Treatment

Most patients were revisited at our outpatient clinic three months after discharge in order to re-evaluate the outcomes of relapse treatment and to initiate immunomodulatory treatment. A total of 135 (93.1%) patients were evaluated, with no significant differences between groups in terms of attendance (IVMPS: 93.0%; TPE: 90.5%; IVMPS+TPE: 91.8%; *p* = 1.000). The median follow-up duration was 95.5 days (IQR: 86–112), with again no relevant differences between treatment groups (*p* = 0.379). Eight patients reported further relapses with symptoms distinct from previous ones (6 patients/IVMPS group, one patient/TPE group, and one patient/IVMPS+TPE group); and three of these relapses affected the same functional system (optic nerve: two; brainstem: one; onset 53, 64, and 82 days after discharge, respectively). After excluding these patients, we re-evaluated the FSS according to the Conway model. In the IVMPS group, we found a significantly larger proportion of deteriorating patients (41.9%; vs. 12.2% for IVMPS+TPE and 7.1% for TPE; *p* = 0.001). The multivariable odds ratio for further deterioration of relapse symptoms at follow-up was 6.65, favoring the conduction of TPE (95%–CI: 2.52–17.54; *p*<0.001; for full regression model see Table S3).

3.4. Safety

Out of 145 patients, 116 (80.0%) experienced at least one single adverse event (Table 2). IVMPS treatment was frequently associated with hypertension, hyperglycemia, and hypokalemia, making it necessary to regularly substitute potassium (orally). Temporary insulin treatment was necessary in 14 patients (IVMPS: 6; IVMPS+TPE: 8; TPE: 0). Conversely, coagulopathy was associated with apheresis treatment. However, those events were mostly considered °II according to CTCAE. Infections were observed more often in patients who received two courses of IVMPS and among those, four were considered CTCAE °III due to the prolongation of hospitalization. In particular, one case of central venous catheter-associated septicemia required 14 days of vancomycin treatment until full recovery. Hypotension and coagulopathy each resulted in at least one treatment interruption in 28 TPE treated patients, whereas treatment interruption due to hypertension occurred in two IVMPS treated patients (systolic blood pressure>180mmHg each). Notably, we observed thromboembolic events in four out of the 99 patients exposed to escalated IVMPS, including one case of cerebral venous sinus thrombosis.

Table 2. Overview of documented adverse events during hospitalization.

	TPE (*n* = 46)	IVMPS (*n* = 46)	IVMPS+TPE (*n* = 53)
Hypertension (>135 mmHg SBP)	1 (2.2)	11 (19.6)	17 (32.1)
Hyperglycemia (>7.2 mmol/L)	1 (2.2)	20 (43.5)	32 (60.4)
Hypokalemia (<3.5 mmol/L)	4 (8.7)	29 (63.0)	43 (81.1)
Coagulopathy (aPTT>50 s or INR>1.7)	16 (34.8)	2 (4.4)	14 (32.1)
Thrombosis			
- Cerebral venous sinus	-	-	**1 (1.9)**
- Femoral veins	-	**1 (2.2)**	**1 (1.9)**
- Jugular veins/CVC	-	-	**1 (1.9)**
Infection			
- Thrombophlebitis	1 (2.2)	3 (6.6)	1 (1.9)
- Urinary Tract	4 (8.7)	8 (17.6)	9 (17.0)
- Respiratory Tract	-	2 (4.4)	**1 (1.9)**
- CVC infection/septicemia	-	-	**1 (1.9)**
(Temporary) treatment interruption			
- Coagulopathy	**4 (8.7)**	-	**7 (13.2)**
- Hypotension	**5 (10.9)**	-	**7 (13.2)**
- Hypertension	-	**1 (2.2)**	**1 (1.9)**
- Psychosis	-	**2 (4.4)**	-
- CVC dislocation	1 (2.2)	-	2 (3.8)
Pneumothorax	**1 (2.2)**	-	-
Patients with at least 1 event	29 (63.0)	38 (82.6)	49 (92.5)

Overview of adverse events documented during hospital stay. Numbers in brackets represent percentages. Numbers in bold indicate CTCAE °III events. TPE: therapeutic plasma exchange, IVMPS: intravenous (methyl-) prednisolone, SBP: systolic blood pressure; aPTT: activated partial thromboplastin time; INR: international normalized ratio; CVC: central venous catheter.

We evaluated whether the amount of previously administered IVMPS (initiation treatment with IVMPS and first escalation treatment with TPE vs. initiation and first escalation treatment with IVMPS and second escalation treatment with TPE) influenced the risk for serious adverse events (defined as CTCAE °III) during TPE treatment. The model resulted in an adjusted odds ratio of 4.63, favoring early treatment with TPE (95%–CI: 1.35–15.91; p = 0.015). However, severe adverse events were also more abundant in patients with longer disease duration, higher baseline EDSS, or longer time to treatment initiation (for full regression model see Table S4).

4. Discussion

Several studies have documented the beneficial effects of TPE treatment in acute relapsing MS, but virtually all study designs suffered from significant limitations. Studies were either one-armed, had varying treatment regimens, or consisted of a heterogeneous study population in terms of age, pre-treatment, disability, and disease subgroups (CIS, RRMS, and ON; but also neuromyelitis optica-spectrum disorders and other non-specified entities of CNS-demyelination) [8,9,18,19].

Moreover, a relevant proportion of studies on apheresis treatment solely included ON patients and only a few studies with diverse RRMS patient populations described the affected function systems or acute lesion localization in detail. Consequently, next to escalated IVMPS, the international guidelines recommend TPE as one option for treatment escalation following relapse, while refraining from recommending a specific treatment sequence [11].

Our retrospective cohort is well-defined and representative of more than 500 MS in-patients treated for acute relapses in our hospital within the past 5 years. These MS patients were young and mostly at the beginning of their symptomatic phase and therefore of special interest. Effective therapeutic interventions in this early phase of MS may positively influence long-term outcomes, as both relapse frequency and residual disability can be significantly impacted [20,21].

In our cohort, early apheresis treatment resulted in significantly higher response rates compared to escalation treatment with IVMPS. Interestingly, patients who underwent two courses of IVMPS prior to TPE showed poorer response at discharge compared to patients who only had one course of IVMPS prior to TPE. One explanation could be the longer time to apheresis treatment when conducted as the second instead of as the first escalation treatment. Notably, previous studies recommended the initiation of apheresis no later than six weeks after relapse onset in order to allow for the maximum efficacy of TPE, and all patients in this study were below this threshold [22–24]. We also hypothesize that the restitution of blood–brain barrier function, as induced by excessive doses of corticosteroids, might hamper the drainage of immunoglobulins and further inflammatory factors towards the blood, where they are ultimately cleared by TPE [25]. Ultimately, MS lesion pathology could have differed between patient groups. A so-called "type-2 lesion pattern", which is defined by the presence of immunoglobulins within MS lesions, was identified as a strong predictor for the success of TPE [24]. However, this information is usually not available in clinical routines and markers that have been supposed to be associated therewith, such as the presence of ring-enhancing lesions, could not be evaluated here, as MRI data were not regularly available.

As revealed by follow-up data three months after discharge, patients who underwent apheresis treatment exhibit a lower risk for further deterioration, which is in accordance with a previous report [22]. A likely explanation is the higher capacity of apheresis treatment to stop neuroinflammation and consecutive neuroaxonal degeneration, while IVMPS reverts the conduction block but fails to prevent nerve cell death [26]. This hypothesis is supported by the higher frequency of new relapses in patients who did not receive apheresis treatment, although in the short- and mid-term IVMPS treatment has been associated with a reduction in relapse frequency [27]. However, treatment outcomes after three months were supposed to be representative of long-term residuals, as further recovery was less likely beyond this time point in previous studies [28].

In terms of safety, there are some disadvantages of combining escalated IVMPS and TPE. Patients are exposed to high doses of IVMPS, including all the possible side-effects, without having a demonstrable benefit compared to TPE treatment alone. In line with this; we observed a significant increase of complications for the IVMPS escalation group, including several serious adverse events such as thromboembolism or severe infections.

As is typical for retrospective analyses, potentially unknown confounders that might have guided treatment decisions, such as the personal preferences of the treating consultant as well as the patient, health behaviors, comorbidity and MRI characteristics, challenge our study. In this context, we are not able to retrospectively address the criteria underlying the decision to treat a patient with TPE directly in the first escalation, rather than with escalated doses of IVMPS. Moreover, we have to deal with several limitations, such as bias from the selection and availability of data, recall bias, choice of relevant outcome and the methods of analysis. Furthermore, we have to be aware of limitations concerning the validity of our findings, as it is likely that adverse events are probably underestimated, since it was not known that this information was going to be of interest.

However, a large number of patients in our cohort experienced their first demyelinating event and we analyzed only the first relapse per patient, even though intra-individual differences in steroid-responsiveness over time have recently been described [29]. Furthermore, the previously known poor response to steroids used for relapse treatment was not documented anywhere in our medical charts.

In summary, our study found particular advantages of TPE over escalated IVMPS in escalation treatment of MS relapses. We recommend the rapid admission of steroid-refractory patients to apheresis treatment without escalated IVMPS treatment and identify the need to prospectively evaluate this approach in a contemporary patient cohort.

Supplementary Materials: The following are available online at http://www.mdpi.com/2077-0383/9/1/35/s1, Figure S1: Figure S2: Functional systems score (FSS) based relapse recovery model., Table S1: Results table from multivariable regression analysis with "worst or no treatment response following first escalation treatment" as dependent variable., Table S2: Results table from multivariable regression analysis with "stable course vs. further deterioration at follow-up" as dependent variable., Table S3: Results table from multivariable regression analysis with "development of severe adverse events" as dependent variable.

Author Contributions: S.P.: study concept and design, acquisition of data, analysis and interpretation of data, writing of the manuscript; L.R.: analysis and interpretation of data, writing and critical revision of manuscript for intellectual content; E.B.: analysis and interpretation of data, critical revision of manuscript for intellectual content; C.S.: analysis and interpretation of data, critical revision of manuscript for intellectual content; T.R.: analysis and interpretation of data, critical revision of manuscript for intellectual content; M.S.: acquisition of data, critical revision of manuscript for intellectual content; N.M.: critical revision of manuscript for intellectual content; Marcus Brand: critical revision of manuscript for intellectual content; R.P.: critical revision of manuscript for intellectual content; C.K.: critical revision of manuscript for intellectual content; H.W.: critical revision of manuscript for intellectual content; S.G.M.: study concept and design, critical revision of manuscript for intellectual content. All authors have read and agreed to the published version of the manuscript.

Funding: This research was supported financially by the German Multiple Sclerosis Society (S. Pfeuffer and S.G. Meuth) and the Deanery of the Medical Faculty, University of Muenster (S. Pfeuffer).

Conflicts of Interest: S.P.: received travel grants from Sanofi Genzyme and Merck Serono, lecturing honoraria from Sanofi Genzyme, Mylan Healthcare and Biogen and research support from Diamed and Merck Serono. L.R.: received travel reimbursements from Merck Serono, Roche and Sanofi Genzyme. E.B.: declares no conflicts of interest. C.S.: declares no conflicts of interest. T.R.: received travel grants and financial research support from Sanofi Genzyme and Novartis and received honoraria for lecturing from Roche, Merck, Genzyme, Biogen, and Teva. MS: received honoraria for lecturing and travel expenses for attending meetings from CSL Behring, Genzyme, Pfizer and TEVA. N.M.: received honoraria for lecturing and travel expenses for attending meetings from Biogen Idec, GlaxoSmith Kline, Teva, Novartis Pharma, Bayer Healthcare, Genzyme, Alexion Pharamceuticals, Fresenius Medical Care, Diamed, and BIAL, and has received financial research support from Euroimmun, Fresenius Medical Care, Diamed, Alexion Pharamceuticals, and Novartis Pharma. M.B.: received honoraria for lecturing and travel expenses for attending meetings from Fresenius Medical Care, Diamed, Alexion Pharamceuticals. R.P.: received honoraria for lecturing and consulting from Alexion, Bayer HealthCare, Biogen, Celgene, Merck, Mylan, Novartis, Roche, Sanofi Genzyme, and Teva. Refik Pul also received research grants from Merck and Novartis. C.K.: received honoraria for lecturing and consulting as well as financial research support from Ablynx, Almirall, Amgen, Bayer Vital, Bristol-Mayers Squibb, Biotronik, Boehringer Ingelheim, Biogen, Celgene, CSL Behring, Daiichi-Sankyo, Desitin, Eisai, Ever Pharma, Sanofi Genzyme, Merck Serono, Mylan, Medday, Novartis, Omniamed, Pfizer, Roche, Siemens, Stago and Teva. H.W.: received compensation for serving on Scientific Advisory Boards/Steering Committees, for Bayer Healthcare, Biogen Idec, Sanofi Genzyme, Merck Serono and Novartis. He has received speaker honoraria and travel support from Bayer Vital GmbH, Bayer Schering AG, Biogen, CSL Behring, EMD Serono, Fresenius Medical Care, Genzyme, Merck Serono, Omniamed, Novartis and Sanofi Aventis. He has received compensation as a consultant from Biogen Idec, Merck Serono, Novartis, Roche and Sanofi-Genzyme. Heinz Wiendl also received research support from Bayer Healthcare, Bayer Vital, Biogen Idec, Merck Serono, Novartis, Sanofi Genzyme, Sanofi US and TEVA Pharma, Merck Serono and Novartis. S.G.M.: received honoraria for lecturing, and travel expenses for attending meetings from Almirall, Amicus Therapeutics Germany, Bayer Health Care, Biogen, Celgene, Diamed, Genzyme, MedDay Pharmaceuticals, Merck Serono, Novartis, Novo Nordisk, ONO Pharma, Roche, Sanofi-Aventis, Chugai Pharma, QuintilesIMS and Teva. His research is funded by the German Ministry for Education and Research (BMBF), Deutsche Forschungsgemeinschaft (DFG), Else Kröner Fresenius Foundation, German Academic Exchange Service, Hertie Foundation, Interdisciplinary Center for Clinical Studies (IZKF) Muenster, German Foundation for Neurology and Almirall, Amicus Therapeutics Germany, Biogen, Diamed, Fresenius Medical Care, Genzyme, Merck Serono, Novartis, ONO Pharma, Roche, and Teva.

References

1. National Institute for Health and Care Excellence. Multiple Sclerosis: Management of Multiple Sclerosis in Primary and Secondary Care. Available online: www.nice.org.uk/guidance/cg186 (accessed on 3 December 2019).
2. Gold, R.; Chan, A.; Flachenecker, P.; Haghikia, A.; Hellwig, K.; Kappos, L. *DGN/KKNMS Leitlinie zur Diagnose und Therapie der MS*; German Society of Neurology: Berlin, Germany, 2012.
3. Sorensen, P.S.; Haas, J.; Sellebjerg, F.; Olsson, T.; Ravnborg, M.; TARIMS Study Group. IV immunoglobulins as add-on treatment to methylprednisolone for acute relapses in MS. *Neurology* **2004**, *63*, 2028–2033. [CrossRef] [PubMed]
4. Visser, L.H.; Beekman, R.; Tijssen, C.C.; Uitdehaag, B.M.; Lee, M.L.; Movig, K.L.; Lenderink, A.W. A randomized, double-blind, placebo-controlled pilot study of i.v. immunoglobulins in combination with i.v. methylprednisolone in the treatment of relapses in patients with MS. *Mult. Scler.* **2004**, *10*, 89–91. [CrossRef] [PubMed]
5. Stoppe, M.; Busch, M.; Krizek, L.; Then Bergh, F. Outcome of MS relapses in the era of disease-modifying therapy. *BMC Neurol.* **2017**, *17*, 151. [CrossRef]
6. Oliveri, R.L.; Valentino, P.; Russo, C.; Sibilia, G.; Aguglia, U.; Bono, F.; Fera, F.; Gambardella, A.; Zappia, M.; Pardatscher, K.; et al. Randomized trial comparing two different high doses of methylprednisolone in MS: A clinical and MRI study. *Neurology* **1998**, *50*, 1833–1836. [CrossRef] [PubMed]
7. Weinshenker, B.G.; O'Brien, P.C.; Petterson, T.M.; Noseworthy, J.H.; Lucchinetti, C.F.; Dodick, D.W.; Pineda, A.A.; Stevens, L.N.; Rodriguez, M.; et al. A randomized trial of plasma exchange in acute central nervous system inflammatory demyelinating disease. *Ann. Neurol.* **1999**, *46*, 878–886. [CrossRef]
8. Deschamps, R.; Gueguen, A.; Parquet, N.; Saheb, S.; Driss, F.; Mesnil, M.; Vignal, C.; Aboab, J.; Depaz, R.; Gout, O. Plasma exchange response in 34 patients with severe optic neuritis. *J. Neurol.* **2016**, *263*, 883–887. [CrossRef] [PubMed]
9. Ehler, J.; Koball, S.; Sauer, M.; Mitzner, S.; Hickstein, H.; Benecke, R.; Zettl, U.K. Response to Therapeutic Plasma Exchange as a Rescue Treatment in Clinically Isolated Syndromes and Acute Worsening of Multiple Sclerosis: A Retrospective Analysis of 90 Patients. *PLoS ONE* **2015**, *10*, 134583. [CrossRef]
10. Faissner, S.; Nikolayczik, J.; Chan, A.; Hellwig, K.; Gold, R.; Yoon, M.S.; Haghikia, A. Plasmapheresis and immunoadsorption in patients with steroid refractory multiple sclerosis relapses. *J. Neurol.* **2016**, *263*, 1092–1098. [CrossRef]
11. Cortese, I.; Chaudhry, V.; So, Y.T.; Cantor, F.; Cornblath, D.R.; Rae-Grant, A. Evidence-based guideline update: Plasmapheresis in neurologic disorders: Report of the Therapeutics and Technology Assessment Subcommittee of the American Academy of Neurology. *Neurology* **2011**, *76*, 294–300. [CrossRef]
12. Sellebjerg, F.; Barnes, D.; Filippini, G.; Midgard, R.; Montalban, X.; Rieckmann, P.; Selmaj, K.; Visser, L.H.; Sørensen, P.S. EFNS guideline on treatment of multiple sclerosis relapses: Report of an EFNS task force on treatment of multiple sclerosis relapses. *Eur. J. Neurol.* **2005**, *12*, 939–946. [CrossRef]
13. Schmidt, J.; Gold, R.; Schonrock, L.; Zettl, U.K.; Hartung, H.P.; Toyka, K.V. T-cell apoptosis in situ in experimental autoimmune encephalomyelitis following methylprednisolone pulse therapy. *Brain* **2000**, *123*, 1431–1441. [CrossRef] [PubMed]
14. Thompson, A.J.; Banwell, B.L.; Barkhof, F.; Carroll, W.M.; Coetzee, T.; Comi, G.; Correale, J.; Fazekas, F.; Filippi, M.; Freedman, M.S.; et al. Diagnosis of multiple sclerosis: 2017 revisions of the McDonald criteria. *Lancet Neurol.* **2018**, *17*, 162–173. [CrossRef]
15. Kurtzke, J.F. Rating neurologic impairment in multiple sclerosis: An expanded disability status scale (EDSS). *Neurology* **1983**, *33*, 1444–1452. [CrossRef] [PubMed]
16. Conway, B.L.; Zeydan, B.; Uygunoglu, U.; Novotna, M.; Siva, A.; Pittock, S.J.; Atkinson, E.J.; Rodriguez, M.; Kantarci, O.H. Age is a critical determinant in recovery from multiple sclerosis relapses. *Mult. Scler.* **2018**, *25*, 1754–1763. [CrossRef] [PubMed]
17. Rolfes, L.; Pfeuffer, S.; Ruck, T.; Melzer, N.; Pawlitzki, M.; Heming, M.; Brand, M.; Wiendl, H.; Meuth, S.G. Therapeutic Apheresis in Acute Relapsing Multiple Sclerosis: Current Evidence and Unmet Needs—A Systematic Review. *J. Clin. Med.* **2019**, *8*, 1623. [CrossRef] [PubMed]
18. Trebst, C.; Reising, A.; Kielstein, J.T.; Hafer, C.; Stangel, M. Plasma exchange therapy in steroid-unresponsive relapses in patients with multiple sclerosis. *Blood Purif.* **2009**, *28*, 108–115. [CrossRef]

19. Ruprecht, K.; Klinker, E.; Dintelmann, T.; Rieckmann, P.; Gold, R. Plasma exchange for severe optic neuritis: Treatment of 10 patients. *Neurology* **2004**, *63*, 1081–1083. [CrossRef]

20. Scalfari, A.; Neuhaus, A.; Degenhardt, A.; Rice, G.P.; Muraro, P.A.; Daumer, M.; Ebers, G.C. The natural history of multiple sclerosis: A geographically based study 10: Relapses and long-term disability. *Brain* **2010**, *133*, 1914–1929. [CrossRef]

21. Novotna, M.; Paz Soldan, M.M.; Abou Zeid, N.; Kale, N.; Tutuncu, M.; Crusan, D.J.; Atkinson, E.J.; Siva, A.; Keegan, B.M.; Pirko, I.; et al. Poor early relapse recovery affects onset of progressive disease course in multiple sclerosis. *Neurology* **2015**, *85*, 722–729. [CrossRef]

22. Keegan, M.; Pineda, A.A.; McClelland, R.L.; Darby, C.H.; Rodriguez, M.; Weinshenker, B.G. Plasma exchange for severe attacks of CNS demyelination: Predictors of response. *Neurology* **2002**, *58*, 143–146. [CrossRef]

23. Llufriu, S.; Castillo, J.; Blanco, Y.; Ramio-Torrenta, L.; Rio, J.; Valles, M.; Lozano, M.; Castella, M.D.; Calabia, J.; Horga, A.; et al. Plasma exchange for acute attacks of CNS demyelination: Predictors of improvement at 6 months. *Neurology* **2009**, *73*, 949–953. [CrossRef] [PubMed]

24. Keegan, M.; Konig, F.; McClelland, R.; Bruck, W.; Morales, Y.; Bitsch, A.; Panitch, H.; Lassmann, H.; Weinshenker, B.; Rodriguez, M.; et al. Relation between humoral pathological changes in multiple sclerosis and response to therapeutic plasma exchange. *Lancet* **2005**, *366*, 579–582. [CrossRef]

25. Gold, R.; Buttgereit, F.; Toyka, K.V. Mechanism of action of glucocorticosteroid hormones: Possible implications for therapy of neuroimmunological disorders. *J. Neuroimmunol.* **2001**, *117*, 1–8. [CrossRef]

26. Lee, J.M.; Yan, P.; Xiao, Q.; Chen, S.; Lee, K.Y.; Hsu, C.Y.; Xu, J. Methylprednisolone protects oligodendrocytes but not neurons after spinal cord injury. *J. Neurosci.* **2008**, *28*, 3141–3149. [CrossRef] [PubMed]

27. Then Bergh, F.; Kumpfel, T.; Schumann, E.; Held, U.; Schwan, M.; Blazevic, M.; Wismüller, A.; Holsboer, F.; Yassouridis, A.; Uhr, M.; et al. Monthly intravenous methylprednisolone in relapsing-remitting multiple sclerosis - reduction of enhancing lesions, T2 lesion volume and plasma prolactin concentrations. *BMC Neurol.* **2006**, *6*, 19. [CrossRef] [PubMed]

28. Lublin, F.D.; Baier, M.; Cutter, G. Effect of relapses on development of residual deficit in multiple sclerosis. *Neurology* **2003**, *61*, 1528–1532. [CrossRef] [PubMed]

29. Ehler, J.; Blechinger, S.; Rommer, P.S.; Koball, S.; Mitzner, S.; Hartung, H.P.; Leutmezer, F.; Sauer, M.; Zettl, U. Treatment of the First Acute Relapse Following Therapeutic Plasma Exchange in Formerly Glucocorticosteroid-Unresponsive Multiple Sclerosis Patients-A Multicenter Study to Evaluate Glucocorticosteroid Responsiveness. *Int. J. Mol. Sci.* **2017**, *18*, 1749. [CrossRef]

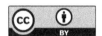

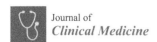

Review

Selective Apheresis of C-Reactive Protein for Treatment of Indications with Elevated CRP Concentrations

Stefan Kayser [1], Patrizia Brunner [2], Katharina Althaus [3], Johannes Dorst [3] and Ahmed Sheriff [1,4,*]

1   Pentracor GmbH, 16761 Hennigsdorf, Germany; kayser@pentracor.de
2   iAdsorb GmbH, 10787 Berlin, Germany; patrizia.brunner@gmx.de
3   Department of Neurology, University of Ulm, 89081 Ulm, Germany; katharina.althaus@uni-ulm.de (K.A.);
     johannes.dorst@uni-ulm.de (J.D.)
4   Medizinische Klinik m.S. Gastroenterologie/Infektiologie/Rheumatologie, Charité Universitätsmedizin,
     12203 Berlin, Germany
*   Correspondence: ahmed.sheriff@charite.de; Tel.: +49-3302-20-94-49-35

Received: 26 August 2020; Accepted: 10 September 2020; Published: 12 September 2020

Abstract: Almost every kind of inflammation in the human body is accompanied by rising C-reactive protein (CRP) concentrations. This can include bacterial and viral infection, chronic inflammation and so-called sterile inflammation triggered by (internal) acute tissue injury. CRP is part of the ancient humoral immune response and secreted into the circulation by the liver upon respective stimuli. Its main immunological functions are the opsonization of biological particles (bacteria and dead or dying cells) for their clearance by macrophages and the activation of the classical complement pathway. This not only helps to eliminate pathogens and dead cells, which is very useful in any case, but unfortunately also to remove only slightly damaged or inactive human cells that may potentially regenerate with more CRP-free time. CRP action severely aggravates the extent of tissue damage during the acute phase response after an acute injury and therefore negatively affects clinical outcome. CRP is therefore a promising therapeutic target to rescue energy-deprived tissue either caused by ischemic injury (e.g., myocardial infarction and stroke) or by an overcompensating immune reaction occurring in acute inflammation (e.g., pancreatitis) or systemic inflammatory response syndrome (SIRS; e.g., after transplantation or surgery). Selective CRP apheresis can remove circulating CRP safely and efficiently. We explain the pathophysiological reasoning behind therapeutic CRP apheresis and summarize the broad span of indications in which its application could be beneficial with a focus on ischemic stroke as well as the results of this therapeutic approach after myocardial infarction.

Keywords: CRP; apheresis; stroke; inflammation

1. General Introduction

Inflammatory processes involve a plethora of signaling pathways and affect the whole body, even if their origin is most often locally restricted in an acute setting. Mounting an inflammatory response is the body's strategy to primarily eliminate any cause of tissue damage and subsequently repair the injury [1]. This is rooted in the evolutionary background that damage is mainly caused by pathogens or at least exacerbated by them within an external wound. In this case the elicited inflammation is beneficial in fighting infiltrating bacteria or viruses as well as restoring tissue homeostasis. However, healing of injured tissue often happens at the cost of still healthy tissue/cells and involves additional cell death as collateral damage [2]. In specific situations, these negative effects outweigh the positive aspects of the inflammatory reaction. Whenever an injury is "sterile", meaning it occurred internally without pathogen involvement, inflammation aggravates deterioration by elimination of additional cells, which were either vital or only slightly and reversibly impaired. This happens for example after ischemic injury like stroke or myocardial infarction, leading to a larger extent of organ damage, increased scarring and thereby worsening clinical outcome [3,4]. Likewise, negative effects dominate in situations when the immune system produces an excessive general reaction that is not justified by the trigger [5]. For example, during acute pancreatitis, a systemic inflammatory response syndrome (SIRS), or an acute bacterial or viral infection (Sepsis) the inflammation might cause widespread tissue injury, which might result in multiple organ failure [6].

Although a plentitude of proteins is involved in inflammation, many of them are cytokines or modulators that do not actively participate in the elimination of pathogens or cells [1]. Several mediator proteins play a key role.

One of the acute-phase mediators directly involved in these pro-inflammatory processes is C-reactive protein (CRP) which was discovered by Tillett and Francis in 1930 [7]. CRP is well-established as one of the most reliable markers of inflammation, rising dramatically during any type of inflammation. It has been shown that CRP as an inflammatory mediator not only reflects tissue damage, but also aggravates the severity of damage and contributes causally to course and outcome of various diseases [8]. Therefore, CRP has to be regarded not only as a marker, but also as an active pro-inflammatory protein.

2. Role of CRP

CRP is a sensitive, reliable and early indicator of inflammation and infection. Evolutionarily highly conserved, this pentameric molecule is part of the ancient humoral immune response and involved in various immunological pathways as a key mediator [9,10]. It is predominantly synthesized and secreted into the blood circulation by hepatic cells as a response to trauma, inflammation, or infection. In these situations, the proinflammatory cytokines interleukin 6 (IL-6) and, to a lesser extent, interleukin 1β (IL-1β) as well as tumor necrosis factor @(TNF@) induce CRP expression on the transcriptional level [11–14]. Following an acute phase stimulus, serum CRP values increase up to levels a few thousand times higher than the normal (healthy) concentration of human CRP (0.05 to 3000 mg/L) [15,16]. The half-life in plasma is about 19 h [17,18].

After secretion, CRP efficiently detects and opsonizes bacteria upon their infiltration and initiates their phagocytosis by activation of complement [19,20]. This is probably its original purpose as one of the most ancient proteins within the humoral immune system.

However, CRP also detects and binds to endogenous cells [21,22]. Cells, which are either apoptotic, energy-depleted, or simply exposed to stressors like the acidic and often ischemic environment of inflammation display conformational and biochemical changes of their membrane [23]. One of these changes is the formation of lyso-phosphatidylcholine (LPC) by partial hydrolyzation of phosphatidylcholine (PC). To this end, one of its two fatty acid groups is removed by the secretory phospholipase A2 type IIa (sPLA2 IIa) [24,25]. This phospholipase is secreted and activated by inflammation (IL-6) and marks the beginning of detrimental destruction of still viable tissue after e.g., ischemia [26–29]. LPC is thereby accessible in the plasma membrane of dead, damaged, or inflamed cells. The CRP pentamer binds to LPC with high avidity in a so-called cooperative manner and subsequently mediates the elimination of these cells, similarly to infiltrating pathogens, by activating the classical complement pathway [30–35]. Complement C1q binds to CRP directly and mediates the binding of C2–C4 [36]. Thus, these cells are irreversibly marked for phagocytes which dispose the marked cells. Phagocytes in turn secrete IL-6 which induces the synthesis of additional CRP by the liver, subsequently amplifying the immune response. This way, more cells become marked by CRP (Figure 1).

Importantly, this mechanism facilitates binding of CRP to actually still vital cells, which may potentially regenerate with more CRP-free time. By interacting with complement, CRP triggers the destruction and therefore negatively affects the regeneration of tissue. By now, a large body of data obtained from animal experiments demonstrates that this CRP-mediated mechanism plays an active role in exacerbating ischemia and reperfusion-induced damage [37–43].

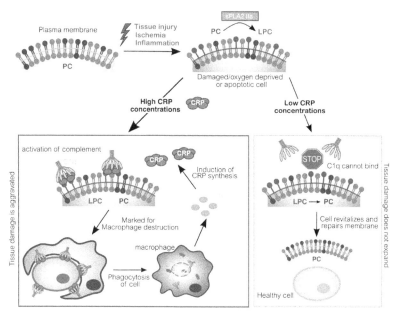

Figure 1. Molecular pathomechanism of CRP-mediated tissue damage. Upon inflammation or acute oxygen-deprivation, cells display a dramatic shortage of adenosine triphosphate (ATP). ATP is essential to prevent apoptosis which manifests in the outer cell membrane: Phosphatidylcholine (PC) is converted into lyso-phosphatidylcholine (LPC) by phospholipase (sPLA2 IIa). Due to the lack of ATP, this alteration cannot be reversed. CRP subsequently binds to LPC on anaerobic cells and recruits complement factors (C1q-C4). These opsonized cells will be disposed by phagocytes, which in turn induce CRP synthesis. Without CRP or in situations with low CRP concentrations (e.g., after CRP apheresis), energy deprived-cells are spared and may switch back to aerobic metabolism, repair molecular changes and revitalize again, leading to an overall reduced tissue damage [41,43–45]. CRP C-reactive protein; C1q Complement component 1q; IL-6 Interleukin 6; LPC Lysophosphatidylcholine; PC Phosphatidylcholine; sPLA2 IIa secretory phospholipase A2 type IIa.

On the molecular level it is not fully elucidated yet whether pro-inflammatory signaling is mediated by the pentameric, native form of CRP, or if CRP dissociates into its non-covalently bound monomers upon binding to LPC, which then exhibit novel binding capacities and other specific functions [46–48]. Publications which described anti-inflammatory actions of pentameric CRP hypothesized that CRP switches functions by undergoing structural changes. Although various quaternary structures of CRP are still not well proven in the physiological context, it might well be possible that CRP monomers exist in specific inflammatory microenvironments and represent different stages of inflammation [47,49]. It has been clearly shown that CRP is secreted in its native, pentameric form by the liver and-if at all-only dissociates locally within inflamed tissue. Hence, therapeutic interventions are more efficient targeting pentameric CRP as high circulating levels are the actual source for its detrimental action [50,51]. Its known physiological function is the disposal of cells (bacteria, necrotic and apoptotic cells).

To date, no pharmacologic inhibitor of inflammation has been proven to be successful in ischemia-related injuries, since they all featured unfavorable pharmacokinetic profiles or serious side effects. Therefore, a different strategy is needed to target the detrimental inflammatory response [43,52]. Specifically, targeting avoidable organ damage caused by the action of CRP represents a promising therapeutic option [43,53]. Decreasing CRP levels could potentially protect salvageable cells and give them more time to recover. Therefore, removing CRP from the blood circulation interrupts the innate cascade and reduces tissue damage [44]. Accordingly, CRP apheresis may potentially present a promising, highly efficient, and well-tolerated therapeutic option.

3. CRP Apheresis

Extracorporeal apheresis refers to the physical removal of substances from the blood by means of filtration, precipitation or adsorption. Immunoadsorption defines the specific binding of an immunologic protein by an adsorber matrix. The elimination of pathogenic substances from the blood in extracorporeal apheresis constitutes an established therapeutic measure in the clinical routine of numerous diseases.

The CRP adsorber system (PentraSorb® CRP, Pentracor GmbH, Hennigsdorf, Germany) features an agarose-based resin, which contains a phosphocholine-derivative as ligand for CRP and is thereby capable of selectively depleting CRP from blood plasma with an efficiency of up to 94% (under laboratory conditions) [54]. The adsorber is regenerable and can be used up to a maximum cumulative treatment time of 24 h (contact with human plasma ≤24 h, according to CE license). In between treatments the adsorber has to be stored in sodium azide at 2–8 °C. CRP apheresis is executed in cycles, alternating between loading of the adsorber with plasma and regeneration of the column, that follows a fixed sequence of washing solutions. Loading and washing are controlled by a software module for automatic plasma flow management (ADAsorb, medicap clinic GmbH, Ulrichstein, Germany; Figure 2). Blood can be drawn via central or peripheral venous access (cubital veins). Plasma separation is performed by a blood centrifuge and blood is anti-coagulated 1:15 with citrate buffer (ACD-A; 3% citrate) or heparin. The usual plasma flow through the adsorber is between 25 to 35 mL/min. Blood flow ranges between 40 and 65 mL/min.

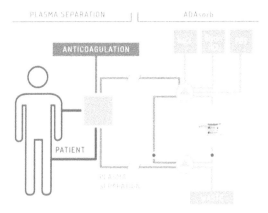

Figure 2. Schematic illustration of CRP apheresis. The procedure is described in detail by Ries et al. 2019 [45].

During one treatment, 6000 mL of plasma are usually processed in 12 cycles. A continuous monitoring of vital parameters, blood pressure and heart rate has to be carried out. Processing of 6000 mL blood plasma takes 4–5 h, depending on the blood flow. Patients can be treated an infinite amount of times with CRP apheresis, as the blood loss is only minimal. Depending on CRP level and indication, two to ten treatments on consecutive days are performed. So far, no side-effects have been reported [45,55–57].

The main advantages of CRP apheresis are the selective removal of the agent by the highly specific ligand and the good controllability of the process, since unlimited plasma volumes can be processed to achieve the desired CRP reduction. Drugs are not removed by CRP apheresis.

4. CRP Apheresis after Ischemic Tissue Damage

The extent of tissue damage during and after an acute traumatic incident defines outcome and follow-up health. Ischemic lesions, predominantly acute myocardial infarction (AMI) and ischemic stroke, generate initial organ damage in the acute zone by cell death due to oxygen deprivation and its magnitude is primarily determined by its duration [58]. Further, neighboring cells which are deprived of oxygen for a shorter duration or to a lesser extent are damaged but salvageable and constitute the area at risk (AMI) or penumbra (stroke) [58,59]. The first line of therapy constitutes the restoration of blood flow to limit the initial ischemic injury. This reperfusion, even though essential to decrease mortality and morbidity, is attended by an intense and maladaptive immune response, which augments and accelerates the organ damage and includes the still viable but damaged tissue [60,61]. The elimination of salvageable cells by CRP through this mechanism mediates reperfusion injury and critically contributes to the already existing deterioration [62,63]. CRP apheresis aims to remove circulating CRP after AMI and ischemic stroke in order to reduce acute tissue injury and ischemic reperfusion injury.

4.1. Myocardial Infarction

Patients who recover from AMI often suffer from reduced quality of life and very high risk of severe complications later on (e.g., second infarct), which implies a huge burden for the health system. This risk correlates significantly with the extent of myocardial injury and scarring [64,65].

It has long been established that inflammation especially mediated by the innate immune system extends myocardial injury, however, anti-inflammatory strategies to minimize myocardial necrosis have failed so far, maybe because these processes are also needed for healing and cardiac repair [3,4,52,66]. While baseline CRP levels in the healthy state are established as predictor of the incidence of cardiovascular disease [67–69], serum CRP concentration during and after AMI correlates with clinical outcome [16,17,70–74]. It is well known that high peak CRP levels during the acute phase response after AMI correlate with larger infarct size and higher mortality as well as incidence of major adverse events [17,74,75]. This has been described for more than two decades now and is in line with the described pathological function of CRP, eliminating cells in the area at risk [8,23,76]. This area contains cells, which could partially recover after revascularization and reperfusion, but are finally destroyed by immune-mediated mechanisms, as explained above and shown in detail in numerous experimental approaches focusing specifically on AMI [39,40,63,70,77,78]. Targeting CRP in AMI has therefore been proposed previously, but was never achieved due to non-functioning therapeutic approaches [43,79–81].

Preclinical studies on the efficacy of specific extracorporeal depletion of CRP have been successfully performed in a porcine animal model of AMI [41,42]. In this study, a mean reduction of CRP levels by about 50%, a significant reduction of the infarct size and a stabilization of the ejection fraction was observed. Interestingly, a completely different scar morphology was detected in animals after CRP apheresis compared to controls [41]. A smaller scar tissue and more vital heart muscle reflected the efficacy of this treatment strategy (Figure 3, previously published and taken from [41]). AMI was therefore selected as indication for the first clinical trial of CRP apheresis. CRP apheresis was applied in patients with ST-elevation myocardial infarction (STEMI) (CAMI-1 trial: "Selective depletion of C-reactive protein by therapeutic apheresis (CRP apheresis) in acute myocardial infarction", DRKS ID: DRKS00008988). Just recently, this multi-center clinical trial has been finished and first data were shown in Case reports and a publication describing 13 patients as a preliminary report [44,45,55,56].

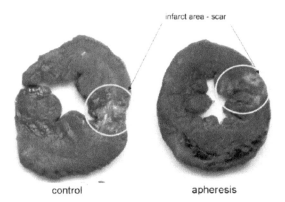

infarct area - scar

control   apheresis

Figure 3. Porcine Heart Slices after AMI with and without CRP apheresis. Slices of the left ventricle 14 days after AMI. Slices were generated after an Evans Blue staining of the heart. Circles localize a characteristic transmural scar of a control animals (left) versus spotted scar morphology after CRP apheresis (right). Figure previously published and taken from [41].

The CAMI-1 trial tested the hypothesis whether specific depletion of CRP by CRP apheresis can reduce myocardial infarct size in humans. Endpoints were safety, myocardial infarct size and function as well as CRP concentration in patients with acute STEMI. A total of 83 patients were recruited at 8 study centers. Plasma CRP levels were reduced by approximately 60% over all performed apheresis procedures in the CAMI-1 trial. Treatments were safe and well tolerated. There were no serious adverse effects associated with the treatment [45]. The magnitude of increase of CRP concentration during the acute phase response after STEMI correlated significantly with the infarct size in control patients. Patients with similar initial CRP increase, who subsequently underwent CRP apheresis, showed smaller infarct sizes as well as improved left ventricular function and wall motion (strains) compared to control patients (*unpublished data-submitted*). Currently, a CAMI-1 registry is on-going, collecting more data (DRKS00017481) [44].

4.2. Ischemic Stroke

Stroke is the third most frequent cause of death and the leading cause of serious, long-term disability worldwide. This disease has a tremendous personal, familiar and socioeconomic impact. More than 80% of patients suffer from ischemic stroke [82]. To date, restoring rapid reperfusion of the brain constitutes the only established therapeutic strategy to reduce the size of the infarct and the consequences of the disease [83]. However, similar mechanisms to AMI take place and inflammation plays an important role in various stages of ischemic stroke, because several humoral and cellular mechanisms are set in motion by the occlusion and subsequent therapeutic reperfusion [84,85]. These mechanisms may explain why some patients with ischemic stroke suffer from severe neurological symptoms despite early and successful recanalization. Several findings substantiate the hypothesis that CRP plays a similar pathological role as shown in AMI, facilitating the elimination of energetically challenged and compromised cells in the penumbra.

First, various publications have shown an association between the early inflammatory response after ischemic stroke and the clinical outcome. The early inflammatory response after stroke has been identified as a key prognostic factor [86,87]. Patients with favorable clinical outcome feature significantly lower levels of inflammatory parameters, especially CRP, compared to patients with poor outcome. Previous studies have described an association between high CRP values after acute stroke and negative prognosis [88–91]. Muir et al. have shown that CRP levels measured within 72 h after stroke predict mortality over an observation period of up to 4 years [92]. According to Winbek et al., CRP levels 24 and 48 h after onset of symptoms affect prognosis, but not their concentration at admission [87]. In another stroke study, patients who died during the study period had significantly higher CRP levels at admission compared to survivors and CRP levels correlated with the clinical outcome after 3 months follow-up [86]. Further, studies in a rat animal model have shown that infusion of human CRP enlarges cerebral infarct areas after acute occlusion via a complement-dependent mechanism [37].

Based on this background, a clinical trial investigating selective CRP apheresis after ischemic stroke was initiated (CASTRO1 trial: "Selective Depletion of C-reactive Protein by Therapeutic Apheresis (CRP-apheresis) in Ischemic Stroke", ID: NCT0441723). The CASTRO trial is designed as a randomized, controlled, multicentric interventional pilot trial. The aim of the CASTRO trial is to evaluate if CRP apheresis can be applied safely in patients with ischemic stroke and efficiently lower the CRP level. Therefore, the primary endpoint is the type and frequency of adverse events and serious adverse events after apheresis. In addition, potential effects of CRP apheresis on clinical outcome parameters (cognitive measures, infarct volume, laboratory parameters) will be investigated.

Participants for this trial need to have an ischemic stroke with or without intravenous lysis and recanalization therapy. The National Institutes of Health Stroke Scale (NIHSS) has to be between 1–24 in order to exclude patients with severe, potentially complicated disease courses. CRP needs to increase ≥5 mg/L within 72 h after the incident and/or serum CRP concentration needs to be larger than 10 mg/L. We aim to include 20 patients which are 1:1 randomly assigned to either the control group (standard guideline therapy) or CRP apheresis in addition to the standard guideline therapy. The standard therapy of acute ischemic stroke is carried out according to the guidelines of the European Academy of Neurology [93].

Exclusion criteria are severe dysphagia (risk of aspiration pneumonia), clinical or laboratory evidence of systemic infection, contraindications against apheresis, Modified Rankin Scale (mRS) before index event ≥ 3, intracranial hemorrhage, epileptic seizure in the context of the acute event, pregnancy, and lactation. Treatment and study regime will be implemented into the clinical standard diagnostic and therapeutic regime after stroke. Since CRP levels begin to rise approximately 8 h after the ischemic incident and reach their peak after 24 h, the first CRP apheresis will be carried out within 72 h after onset of symptoms. Therefore, CRP apheresis will not delay acute guideline therapies of stroke, such as intravenous lysis and intraarterial thrombectomy. The complete study flow is illustrated in Figure 4.

To investigate whether CRP apheresis improves clinical outcome parameters after ischemic stroke, patients will undergo assessments according to standardized clinical scales, namely National Institute of Health Stroke Scale (NIHSS) score, Barthel ADL index (BI), modified Rankin scale (mRS) and measurements of infarct volume (via magnetic resonance imaging; MRI). In addition, immunological and neurodegenerative biomarkers (interleukin-6, serum amyloid A) will be evaluated to objectify a potential beneficial effect of CRP apheresis on inflammatory pathways. Measurements of primary and secondary outcome parameters will be performed at baseline (before first apheresis), daily during apheresis, and 90 days after stroke.

Immunoadsorption with the PentraSorb® CRP is performed with the ADAsorb apheresis device as described in detail in 3. CRP apheresis is performed for a maximum amount of three times (three days) or until CRP concentration is below 10 mg/L.

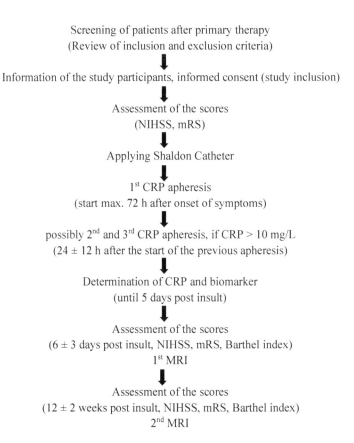

Figure 4. Study flow of the CASTRO1 trial. MRI magnetic resonance imaging; NIHSS National Institute of Health Stroke Scale; mRs modified Rankin scale.

5. CRP Apheresis in Other Indications

Both AMI and ischemic stroke feature a common underlying pathophysiology and the therapeutic application and benefit after AMI has been already shown. However, reduction of dramatically high CRP concentrations in other indications which are not defined by an ischemic pathophysiology could also be beneficial. The overcompensating immune reaction which often triggers SIRS after surgery, causes detrimental deterioration during acute pancreatitis, or mediates a cytokine storm after infection, could be dampened with CRP apheresis. Therefore, clinical trials investigating the safety and efficacy of CRP apheresis during pancreatitis and after coronary bypass surgery are ongoing (CAPRI1-study DRKS00014265; CABY1-study DRKS00013012). Further, first patients suffering from Covid-19 have been treated with CRP apheresis in order to inhibit the CRP-mediated autoimmune response leading to respiratory failure and multi-organ failure [57,94].

6. Conclusions and Outlook

CRP has been established as a general biomarker of inflammation and infection in clinical practice. Recently, its role as a stable and highly useful prognostic factor for cardiovascular and cerebral disease in healthy individuals has been widely acknowledged and utilized [95,96]. However, the characterization of CRP as not only a biomarker but also a mediator or even trigger of immunological destruction of tissue is widely ignored [8,37,39].

J. Clin. Med. **2020**, *9*, 2947

Therapeutic CRP removal by immunoadsorption might present a logical and promising therapy for pathologies in which the extent of tissue damage is aggravated by inflammation and correlated with a worse clinical outcome, including ischemic events.

CRP apheresis has been applied successfully in a controlled multi-center trial in patients with myocardial infarction (CAMI-1 trial). It showed very few and only moderate side effects and managed to significantly reduce CRP levels, thereby positively affecting infarct size and left ventricular ejection fraction [44,45,55,56]. Applying CRP apheresis in ischemic stroke is the next plausible step. However, the immunological situation in the brain is different. Neurons have a low tolerance to oxidative stress, and the physiologically important blood-brain-barrier may impair the effectiveness of this method [97–99].

The CASTRO study will show whether CRP apheresis can be safely performed in patients with ischemic stroke and also provide preliminary results whether reducing the concentration of serum CRP levels facilitates reduction of tissue damage of the brain, consequently improving clinical outcome measures compared to the control group.

Other anti-inflammatory therapies have been investigated in AMI and ischemic stroke, such as colchicine [100], anti-CD18 agents [101] and agents targeting IL-1 or IL-6 [102–104]. CRP removal intends to stop the destruction of tissue already during the acute event. Furthermore, targeting specifically and selectively CRP may constitute a superior choice because it does not cause a pleiotropic effect. The maximum removal of CRP in patients was 79% by now. This leaves enough CRP for potential repair processes. Importantly, cardiac or neural repair is not impaired by the intervention as opposed to former pharmacological interventions like the methylprednisolone trial in myocardial infarction which resulted in a catastrophic outcome [105].

Preliminary evidence suggests that CRP apheresis induces very few side effects and features a low risk profile [45]. One drawback is that the procedure takes relatively long. Nevertheless, CRP apheresis fits well into the management of stroke patients because it does not collide with acute measures and may therefore complement methods aiming at reperfusion.

The acute inflammatory response has two facets. For one thing it plays a key role in initial host defense against infections. But on the downside, it can cause collateral damage of tissues. Especially in situations with an inciting sterile stimulus, the cost-benefit ratio is unfavorable.

CRP as an ancient protein of the innate immune system physiologically disposes cells and reacts to almost every disturbance of tissue homeostasis. Therefore, the span of potential indications for CRP apheresis is broad, and the ongoing clinical trials will illuminate whether this therapy is beneficial in these specific indications.

Author Contributions: Conceptualization, S.K., P.B. and A.S.; writing—original draft preparation, S.K., A.S. and P.B.; writing—review and editing, K.A., J.D. and A.S.; All authors have read and agreed to the published version of the manuscript.

Funding: This research received no external funding.

Acknowledgments: We thank the CAMI1-study group for the realization of the CAMI-1 trial.

Conflicts of Interest: S.K. is an employee of Pentracor GmbH. J.D. received speaker honoraria and research fund from Fresenius Medical Care GmbH and Fresenius Medical Care Deutschland GmbH. A.S. is a founder, shareholder and managing director of Pentracor GmbH. P.B. and K.A. do not have any conflict of interest.

References

1. Netea, M.G.; Balkwill, F.; Chonchol, M.; Cominelli, F.; Donath, M.Y.; Giamarellos-Bourboulis, E.J.; Golenbock, U.; Gresnigt, M.S.; Heneka, M.T.; Hoffman, H.M.; et al. A guiding map for inflammation. *Nat. Immunol.* **2017**, *18*, 826–831. [CrossRef]
2. Eming, S.A.; Krieg, T.; Davidson, J.M. Inflammation in Wound Repair: Molecular and Cellular Mechanisms. *J. Investig. Dermatol.* **2007**, *127*, 514–525. [CrossRef] [PubMed]
3. Ong, S.-B.; Hernández-Reséndiz, S.; Crespo-Avilan, G.E.; Mukhametshina, R.T.; Kwek, X.-Y.; Cabrera-Fuentes, H.A.; Hausenloy, D.J. Inflammation following acute myocardial infarction: Multiple

players, dynamic roles, and novel therapeutic opportunities. *Pharmacol. Ther.* **2018**, *186*, 73–87. [CrossRef] [PubMed]

4. Anzai, T. Inflammatory Mechanisms of Cardiovascular Remodeling. *Circ. J.* **2018**, *82*, 629–635. [CrossRef]

5. Neher, M.D.; Weckbach, S.; Flierl, M.A.; Huber-Lang, M.; Stahel, P.F. Molecular mechanisms of inflammation and tissue injury after major trauma-is complement the "bad guy"? *J. Biomed. Sci.* **2011**, *18*, 90. [CrossRef]

6. Day, J.; Taylor, K. The systemic inflammatory response syndrome and cardiopulmonary bypass. *Int. J. Surg.* **2005**, *3*, 129–140. [CrossRef] [PubMed]

7. Tillett, W.S.; Francis, T. Serological Reactions in Pneumonia with a Non-Protein Somatic Fraction of Pneumococcus. *J. Exp. Med.* **1930**, *52*, 561–571. [CrossRef]

8. Kunze, R. C-Reactive Protein: From Biomarker to Trigger of Cell Death? *Ther. Apher. Dial.* **2019**, *23*, 494–496. [CrossRef]

9. Mortensen, R.F. C-Reactive Protein, Inflammation, and Innate Immunity. *Immunol. Res.* **2001**, *24*, 163–176. [CrossRef]

10. Du Clos, T.W. Pentraxins: Structure, Function, and Role in Inflammation. *ISRN Inflamm.* **2013**, *2013*, 1–22. [CrossRef]

11. Toniatti, C.; Arcone, R.; Majello, B.; Ganter, U.; Arpaia, G.; Ciliberto, G. Regulation of the human C-reactive protein gene, a major marker of inflammation and cancer. *Mol. Biol. Med.* **1990**, *7*, 199–212. [PubMed]

12. Zhang, D.; Sun, M.; Samols, D.; Kushner, I. STAT3 Participates in Transcriptional Activation of the C-reactive Protein Gene by Interleukin-6. *J. Biol. Chem.* **1996**, *271*, 9503–9509. [CrossRef] [PubMed]

13. Kramer, F.; Torzewski, J.; Kamenz, J.; Veit, K.; Hombach, V.; Dedio, J.; Ivashchenko, Y. Interleukin-1β stimulates acute phase response and C-reactive protein synthesis by inducing an NFκB- and C/EBPβ-dependent autocrine interleukin-6 loop. *Mol. Immunol.* **2008**, *45*, 2678–2689. [CrossRef] [PubMed]

14. Weinhold, B.; Bader, A.; Poli, V.; Rüther, U. Interleukin-6 is necessary, but not sufficient, for induction of the humanC-reactive protein gene in vivo. *Biochem. J.* **1997**, *325*, 617–621. [CrossRef] [PubMed]

15. Kushner, I.; Broder, M.L.; Karp, D. Control of the Acute Phase Response. *J. Clin. Investig.* **1978**, *61*, 235–242. [CrossRef] [PubMed]

16. Pietilä, K.; Harmoinen, A.; Hermens, W.; Simoons, M.L.; Van De Werf, F.; Verstraete, M. Serum C-reactive protein and infarct size in myocardial infarct patients with a closed versus an open infarct-related coronary artery after thrombolytic therapy. *Eur. Hear. J.* **1993**, *14*, 915–919. [CrossRef] [PubMed]

17. Dimitrijević, O.; Stojcevski, B.D.; Ignjatović, S.; Singh, N.M. Serial Measurements of C-Reactive Protein After Acute Myocardial Infarction in Predicting One-Year Outcome. *Int. Hear. J.* **2006**, *47*, 833–842. [CrossRef]

18. Gabriel, A.S.; Martinsson, A.; Wretlind, B.; Ahnve, S. IL-6 levels in acute and post myocardial infarction: Their relation to CRP levels, infarction size, left ventricular systolic function, and heart failure. *Eur. J. Intern. Med.* **2004**, *15*, 523–528. [CrossRef]

19. Szalai, A.J.; Briles, D.E.; Volanakis, J.E. Role of complement in C-reactive-protein-mediated protection of mice from Streptococcus pneumoniae. *Infect. Immun.* **1996**, *64*, 4850–4853. [CrossRef]

20. Mold, C.; Rodic-Polic, B.; Du Clos, T.W. Protection from Streptococcus pneumoniae Infection by C-Reactive Protein and Natural Antibody Requires Complement But Not Fcγ Receptors. *J. Immunol.* **2002**, *168*, 6375–6381. [CrossRef]

21. Chang, M.-K.; Binder, C.J.; Torzewski, M.; Witztum, J.L. C-reactive protein binds to both oxidized LDL and apoptotic cells through recognition of a common ligand: Phosphorylcholine of oxidized phospholipids. *Proc. Natl. Acad. Sci. USA* **2002**, *99*, 13043–13048. [CrossRef] [PubMed]

22. Li, Y.P.; Mold, C.; Du Clos, T.W. Sublytic complement attack exposes C-reactive protein binding sites on cell membranes. *J. Immunol.* **1994**, *152*, 2995–3005. [PubMed]

23. Sparkes, B.L.; Woods, K.; Roth, M.; Welti, R.; Fleming, S.D. Phospholipase A2 alters membrane lipid composition during ischemia/reperfusion (39.55). *J. Immunol.* **2009**, *182*, 39.55.

24. Yagami, T.; Yamamoto, Y.; Koma, H. The Role of Secretory Phospholipase A2 in the Central Nervous System and Neurological Diseases. *Mol. Neurobiol.* **2013**, *49*, 863–876. [CrossRef]

25. Murakami, M.; Taketomi, Y.; Sato, H.; Yamamoto, K. Secreted phospholipase A2 revisited. *J. Biochem.* **2011**, *150*, 233–255. [CrossRef] [PubMed]

26. Fujioka, D.; Kawabata, K.-I.; Ishimoto, Y.; Suzuki, N.; Hanasaki, K.; Sato, R.; Hasebe, H.; Kobayashi, T.; Saito, Y.; Kanazawa, M.; et al. Abstract 1435: Reduction in Myocardial Ischemia-reperfusion Injury in Group X Secretory Phospholipase A$_2$-deficient Mice. *Circulation* **2006**, *114*, II_275. [CrossRef]

27. Yano, T.; Fujioka, D.; Saito, Y.; Kobayashi, T.; Nakamura, T.; Obata, J.-E.; Kawabata, K.; Watanabe, K.; Watanabe, Y.; Mishina, H.; et al. Group V secretory phospholipase A2 plays a pathogenic role in myocardial ischaemia–reperfusion injury. *Cardiovasc. Res.* **2010**, *90*, 335–343. [CrossRef]
28. Nijmeijer, R.; Lagrand, W.K.; Baidoshvili, A.; Lubbers, Y.T.P.; Hermens, W.T.; Meijer, C.J.L.M.; Visser, C.A.; Hack, C.E.; Niessen, H.W.M. Secretory type II phospholipase A(2) binds to ischemic myocardium during myocardial infarction in humans. *Cardiovasc. Res.* **2002**, *53*, 138–146. [CrossRef]
29. Nijmeijer, R.; Willemsen, M.; Meijer, C.J.L.M.; Visser, C.A.; Verheijen, R.H.; Gottlieb, R.A.; Hack, C.E.; Niessen, H.W.M. Type II secretory phospholipase A2 binds to ischemic flip-flopped cardiomyocytes and subsequently induces cell death. *Am. J. Physiol. Circ. Physiol.* **2003**, *285*, H2218–H2224. [CrossRef]
30. Sproston, N.R.; Ashworth, J.J. Role of C-Reactive Protein at Sites of Inflammation and Infection. *Front. Immunol.* **2018**, *9*, 754. [CrossRef]
31. Goda, T.; Miyahara, Y. Calcium-independent binding of human C-reactive protein to lysophosphatidylcholine in supported planar phospholipid monolayers. *Acta Biomater.* **2017**, *48*, 206–214. [CrossRef] [PubMed]
32. Kushner, I.; Kaplan, M.H. Studies of acute phase protein: I. An Immunohistochemical method for the localization of cx-reactive protein in rabbits. Association with necrosis in local inflammatory lesions. *J. Exp. Med.* **1961**, *114*, 961–974. [CrossRef] [PubMed]
33. Narkates, A.J.; Volanakis, J.E. C-reactive protein binding specificities: Artificial and natural phospholipid bilayers. *Ann. N. Y. Acad. Sci.* **1982**, *389*, 172–182. [CrossRef] [PubMed]
34. Kushner, I.; Rakita, L.; Kaplan, M.H. Studies of acute-phase protein. II. Localization of Cx-reactive protein in heart in induced myocardial infarction in rabbits. *J. Clin. Investig.* **1963**, *42*, 286–292. [CrossRef] [PubMed]
35. Vogt, B.; Führnrohr, B.; Müller, R.; Sheriff, A. CRP and the disposal of dying cells: Consequences for systemic lupus erythematosus and rheumatoid arthritis. *Autoimmunity* **2007**, *40*, 295–298. [CrossRef]
36. Gaboriaud, C.; Juanhuix, J.; Gruez, A.; Lacroix, M.; Darnault, C.; Pignol, D.; Verger, D.; Fontecilla-Camps, J.C.; Arlaud, G.J. The Crystal Structure of the Globular Head of Complement Protein C1q Provides a Basis for Its Versatile Recognition Properties. *J. Biol. Chem.* **2003**, *278*, 46974–46982. [CrossRef] [PubMed]
37. Gill, R.; Kemp, J.A.; Sabin, C.; Pepys, M.B. Human C-Reactive Protein Increases Cerebral Infarct Size after Middle Cerebral Artery Occlusion in Adult Rats. *Br. J. Pharmacol.* **2004**, *24*, 1214–1218. [CrossRef]
38. Hack, C.; Wolbink, G.-J.; Schalkwijk, C.; Speijer, H.; Hermens, W.T.; Bosch, H.V.D. A role for secretory phospholipase A2 and C-reactive protein in the removal of injured cells. *Immunol. Today* **1997**, *18*, 111–115. [CrossRef]
39. Griselli, M.; Herbert, J.; Hutchinson, W.; Taylor, K.; Sohail, M.; Krausz, T.; Pepys, M.B. C-Reactive Protein and Complement Are Important Mediators of Tissue Damage in Acute Myocardial Infarction. *J. Exp. Med.* **1999**, *190*, 1733–1740. [CrossRef]
40. Nijmeijer, R.; Lagrand, W.K.; Lubbers, Y.T.P.; Visser, C.A.; Meijer, C.J.L.M.; Niessen, H.W.M.; Hack, C.E. C-Reactive Protein Activates Complement in Infarcted Human Myocardium. *Am. J. Pathol.* **2003**, *163*, 269–275. [CrossRef]
41. Sheriff, A.; Schindler, R.; Vogt, B.; Abdel-Aty, H.; Unger, J.K.; Bock, C.; Gebauer, F.; Slagman, A.; Jerichow, T.; Mans, D.; et al. Selective apheresis of C-reactive protein: A new therapeutic option in myocardial infarction? *J. Clin. Apher.* **2014**, *30*, 15–21. [CrossRef] [PubMed]
42. Slagman, A.; Bock, C.; Abdel-Aty, H.; Vogt, B.; Gebauer, F.; Janelt, G.; Wohlgemuth, F.; Morgenstern, R.; Yapici, G.; Puppe, A.; et al. Specific Removal of C-Reactive Protein by Apheresis in a Porcine Cardiac Infarction Model. *Blood Purif.* **2011**, *31*, 9–17. [CrossRef] [PubMed]
43. Pepys, M.B.; Hirschfield, G.M.; Tennent, G.A.; Gallimore, J.R.; Kahan, M.C.; Bellotti, V.; Hawkins, P.N.; Myers, R.M.; Smith, M.D.; Polara, A.; et al. Targeting C-reactive protein for the treatment of cardiovascular disease. *Nature* **2006**, *440*, 1217–1221. [CrossRef] [PubMed]
44. Ries, W.; Heigl, F.; Garlichs, C.; Sheriff, A.; Torzewski, J. *Die CRP-Apherese: Eine neue Therapiemöglichkeit bei Inflammation*; Nephro-News, Medicom VerlagsgmbH Bruck: Mur, Austria, 2019; pp. 23–27.
45. Ries, W.; Heigl, F.; Garlichs, C.; Sheriff, A.; Torzewski, J. Selective C-Reactive Protein-Apheresis in Patients. *Ther. Apher. Dial.* **2019**, *23*, 570–574. [CrossRef]
46. Braig, D.; Nero, T.L.; Koch, H.-G.; Kaiser, B.; Wang, X.; Thiele, J.R.; Morton, C.J.; Zeller, J.; Kiefer, J.; Potempa, L.A.; et al. Transitional changes in the CRP structure lead to the exposure of proinflammatory binding sites. *Nat. Commun.* **2017**, *8*, 14188. [CrossRef]

47. Thiele, J.R.; Habersberger, J.; Braig, D.; Schmidt, Y.; Goerendt, K.; Maurer, V.; Bannasch, H.; Scheichl, A.; Woollard, K.J.; Von Dobschütz, E.; et al. Dissociation of Pentameric to Monomeric C-Reactive Protein Localizes and Aggravates Inflammation. *Circulation* **2014**, *130*, 35–50. [CrossRef]
48. McFadyen, J.D.; Kiefer, J.; Braig, D.; Loseff-Silver, J.; Potempa, L.A.; Eisenhardt, S.U.; Peter, K. Dissociation of C-Reactive Protein Localizes and Amplifies Inflammation: Evidence for a Direct Biological Role of C-Reactive Protein and Its Conformational Changes. *Front. Immunol.* **2018**, *9*. [CrossRef]
49. Zhang, L.; Li, H.-Y.; Li, W.; Shen, Z.-Y.; Wang, Y.-D.; Ji, S.-R.; Wu, Y. An ELISA Assay for Quantifying Monomeric C-Reactive Protein in Plasma. *Front. Immunol.* **2018**, *9*, 9. [CrossRef]
50. Thiele, J.R.; Zeller, J.; Bannasch, H.; Stark, G.B.; Peter, K.; Eisenhardt, S.U. Targeting C-Reactive Protein in Inflammatory Disease by Preventing Conformational Changes. *Mediat. Inflamm.* **2015**, *2015*, 1–9. [CrossRef]
51. Caprio, V.; Badimon, L.; Di Napoli, M.; Fang, W.-H.; Ferris, G.R.; Guo, B.; Iemma, R.S.; Liu, D.; Zeinolabediny, Y.; Slevin, M. pCRP-mCRP Dissociation Mechanisms as Potential Targets for the Development of Small-Molecule Anti-Inflammatory Chemotherapeutics. *Front. Immunol.* **2018**, *9*. [CrossRef]
52. Frangogiannis, N.G.; Smith, C.W.; Entman, M.L. The inflammatory response in myocardial infarction. *Cardiovasc. Res.* **2002**, *53*, 31–47. [CrossRef]
53. Prasad, K. C-Reactive Protein (CRP)-Lowering Agents. *Cardiovasc. Drug Rev.* **2006**, *24*, 33–50. [CrossRef] [PubMed]
54. Mattecka, S.; Brunner, P.; Hähnel, B.; Kunze, R.; Vogt, B.; Sheriff, A. PentraSorb C-Reactive Protein: Characterization of the Selective C-Reactive Protein Adsorber Resin. *Ther. Apher. Dial.* **2019**, *23*, 474–481. [CrossRef] [PubMed]
55. Boljevic, D.; Nikolic, A.; Rusovic, S.; Lakcevic, J.; Bojic, M.; Balint, B. A Promising Innovative Treatment for ST-Elevation Myocardial Infarction: The Use of C-Reactive Protein Selective Apheresis: Case Report. *Blood Purif.* **2020**, 1–5. [CrossRef] [PubMed]
56. Ries, W.; Sheriff, A.; Heigl, F.; Zimmermann, O.; Garlichs, C.D.; Torzewski, J. "First in Man": Case Report of Selective C-Reactive Protein Apheresis in a Patient with Acute ST Segment Elevation Myocardial Infarction. *Case Rep. Cardiol.* **2018**, *2018*, 1–4. [CrossRef]
57. Torzewski, J.; Heigl, F.; Zimmermann, O.; Wagner, F.; Schumann, C.; Hettich, R.; Bock, C.; Kayser, S.; Sheriff, A. First-in-Man: Case Report of Selective C-Reactive Protein Apheresis in a Patient with SARS-CoV-2 Infection. *Am. J. Case Rep.* **2020**, *21*, e925020.
58. Xing, C.; Arai, K.; Lo, E.H.; Hommel, M. Pathophysiologic cascades in ischemic stroke. *Int. J. Stroke* **2012**, *7*, 378–385. [CrossRef]
59. Heusch, G.; Gersh, B.J. The pathophysiology of acute myocardial infarction and strategies of protection beyond reperfusion: A continual challenge. *Eur. Hear. J.* **2016**, *38*, 774–784. [CrossRef]
60. Kalogeris, T.; Baines, C.P.; Krenz, M.; Korthuis, R.J. Cell biology of ischemia/reperfusion injury. *Int. Rev. Cell Mol. Boil.* **2012**, *298*, 229–317. [CrossRef]
61. Yellon, D.M.; Hausenloy, D.J. Myocardial Reperfusion Injury. *N. Engl. J. Med.* **2007**, *357*, 1121–1135. [CrossRef]
62. Pegues, M.A.; McCrory, M.A.; Zarjou, A.; Szalai, A.J. C-reactive protein exacerbates renal ischemia-reperfusion injury. *Am. J. Physiol. Ren. Physiol.* **2013**, *304*, F1358–F1365. [CrossRef] [PubMed]
63. Valtchanova-Matchouganska, A.; Gondwe, M.; Nadar, A. The role of C-reactive protein in ischemia/reperfusion injury and preconditioning in a rat model of myocardial infarction. *Life Sci.* **2004**, *75*, 901–910. [CrossRef] [PubMed]
64. Stone, G.W.; Selker, H.P.; Thiele, H.; Patel, M.R.; Udelson, J.E.; Ohman, E.; Maehara, A.; Eitel, I.; Granger, C.B.; Jenkins, P.L.; et al. Relationship between Infarct Size and Outcomes Following Primary PCI. *J. Am. Coll. Cardiol.* **2016**, *67*, 1674–1683. [CrossRef]
65. De Waha, S.; Patel, M.R.; Granger, C.B.; Ohman, E.M.; Maehara, A.; Eitel, I.; Ben-Yehuda, O.; Jenkins, P.; Thiele, H.; Stone, G.W. Relationship between microvascular obstruction and adverse events following primary percutaneous coronary intervention for ST-segment elevation myocardial infarction: An individual patient data pooled analysis from seven randomized trials. *Eur. Hear. J.* **2017**, *38*, 3502–3510. [CrossRef]
66. Frangogiannis, N.G. Regulation of the Inflammatory Response in Cardiac Repair. *Circ. Res.* **2012**, *110*, 159–173. [CrossRef] [PubMed]
67. Danesh, J.; Wheeler, J.G.; Hirschfield, G.M.; Eda, S.; Eiriksdottir, G.; Rumley, A.; Lowe, G.D.O.; Pepys, M.B.; Gudnason, V. C-Reactive Protein and Other Circulating Markers of Inflammation in the Prediction of Coronary Heart Disease. *N. Engl. J. Med.* **2004**, *350*, 1387–1397. [CrossRef] [PubMed]

68. Koenig, W.; Sund, M.; Fröhlich, M.; Fischer, H.G.; Löwel, H.; Döring, A.; Hutchinson, W.L.; Pepys, M.B. C-Reactive protein, a sensitive marker of inflammation, predicts future risk of coronary heart disease in initially healthy middle-aged men: Results from the MONICA (Monitoring Trends and Determinants in Cardiovascular Disease) Augsburg Cohort Study, 1984 to 1992. *Circulation* **1999**, *99*, 237–242. [PubMed]
69. Verma, S.; Szmitko, P.E.; Ridker, P.M. C-reactive protein comes of age. *Nat. Clin. Pract. Neurol.* **2005**, *2*, 29–36. [CrossRef]
70. Beranek, J.T. C-reactive protein and complement in myocardial infarction and postinfarction heart failure. *Eur. Hear. J.* **1997**, *18*, 1834–1835. [CrossRef]
71. Liu, D.; Qi, X.; Li, Q.; Jia, W.; Wei, L.; Huang, A.; Liu, K.; Li, Z. Increased complements and high-sensitivity C-reactive protein predict heart failure in acute myocardial infarction. *Biomed. Rep.* **2016**, *5*, 761–765. [CrossRef]
72. Mani, P.; Puri, R.; Schwartz, G.G.; Nissen, S.E.; Shao, M.; Kastelein, J.J.P.; Menon, V.; Lincoff, A.M.; Nicholls, S.J. Association of Initial and Serial C-Reactive Protein Levels With Adverse Cardiovascular Events and Death After Acute Coronary Syndrome. *JAMA Cardiol.* **2019**, *4*, 314. [CrossRef] [PubMed]
73. Suleiman, M.; Khatib, R.; Agmon, Y.; Mahamid, R.; Boulos, M.; Kapeliovich, M.; Levy, Y.; Beyar, R.; Markiewicz, W.; Hammerman, H.; et al. Early Inflammation and Risk of Long-Term Development of Heart Failure and Mortality in Survivors of Acute Myocardial Infarction. *J. Am. Coll. Cardiol.* **2006**, *47*, 962–968. [CrossRef] [PubMed]
74. Stumpf, C.; Sheriff, A.; Zimmermann, S.; Schaefauer, L.; Schlundt, C.; Raaz, D.; Garlichs, C.D.; Achenbach, S. C-reactive protein levels predict systolic heart failure and outcome in patients with first ST-elevation myocardial infarction treated with coronary angioplasty. *Arch. Med. Sci.* **2017**, *5*, 1086–1093. [CrossRef]
75. Reindl, M.; Reinstadler, S.J.; Feistritzer, H.-J.; Klug, G.; Tiller, C.; Mair, J.; Mayr, A.; Jaschke, W.; Metzler, B. Relation of inflammatory markers with myocardial and microvascular injury in patients with reperfused ST-elevation myocardial infarction. *Eur. Hear. J. Acute Cardiovasc. Care* **2016**, *6*, 640–649. [CrossRef]
76. Mevorach, D.; Mascarenhas, J.O.; Gershov, D.; Elkon, K.B. Complement-dependent Clearance of Apoptotic Cells by Human Macrophages. *J. Exp. Med.* **1998**, *188*, 2313–2320. [CrossRef]
77. Lagrand, W.K.; Niessen, H.W.M.; Wolbink, G.-J.; Jaspars, L.H.; Visser, C.A.; Verheugt, F.W.; Meijer, C.J.; Hack, C.E. C-Reactive Protein Colocalizes With Complement in Human Hearts During Acute Myocardial Infarction. *Circulation* **1997**, *95*, 97–103. [CrossRef] [PubMed]
78. Barrett, T.D.; Hennan, J.K.; Marks, R.M.; Lucchesi, B.R. C-Reactive-Protein-Associated Increase in Myocardial Infarct Size after Ischemia/Reperfusion. *J. Pharmacol. Exp. Ther.* **2002**, *303*, 1007–1013. [CrossRef] [PubMed]
79. Krijnen, P.A.; Meischl, C.; Nijmeijer, R.; Visser, C.A.; Hack, C.E.; Niessen, H.W. Inhibition of sPLA2-IIA, C-reactive protein or complement: New therapy for patients with acute myocardial infarction? *Cardiovasc. Hematol. Disord. Drug Targets* **2006**, *6*, 113–123. [CrossRef]
80. Heinecke, J.W. Chemical knockout of C-reactive protein in cardiovascular disease. *Nat. Methods* **2006**, *2*, 300–301. [CrossRef]
81. Kitsis, R.N.; Jialal, I. Limiting Myocardial Damage during Acute Myocardial Infarction by Inhibiting C-Reactive Protein. *N. Engl. J. Med.* **2006**, *355*, 513–515. [CrossRef]
82. Virani, S.S.; Alonso, A.; Benjamin, E.J.; Bittencourt, M.S.; Callaway, C.W.; Carson, A.P.; Chamberlain, A.M.; Chang, A.R.; Cheng, S.; Delling, F.N.; et al. Heart Disease and Stroke Statistics—2020 Update: A Report From the American Heart Association. *Circulation* **2020**, *141*, e139–e596. [CrossRef]
83. Catanese, L.; Tarsia, J.; Fisher, M. Acute Ischemic Stroke Therapy Overview. *Circ. Res.* **2017**, *120*, 541–558. [CrossRef] [PubMed]
84. Anrather, J.; Iadecola, C. Inflammation and Stroke: An Overview. *Neurotherapeutics* **2016**, *13*, 661–670. [CrossRef] [PubMed]
85. Muir, K.W.; Tyrrell, P.; Sattar, N.; Warburton, E. Inflammation and ischaemic stroke. *Curr. Opin. Neurol.* **2007**, *20*, 334–342. [CrossRef] [PubMed]
86. Montaner, J.; Fernández-Cadenas, I.; Molina, C.A.; Ribo, M.; Huertas, R.; Rosell, A.; Penalba, A.; Ortega, L.; Chacoón, P.; Álvarez-Sabín, J. Poststroke C-Reactive Protein Is a Powerful Prognostic Tool Among Candidates for Thrombolysis. *Stroke* **2006**, *37*, 1205–1210. [CrossRef]
87. Winbeck, K.; Poppert, H.; Etgen, T.; Conrad, B.; Sander, D. Prognostic relevance of early serial C-reactive protein measurements after first ischemic stroke. *Stroke* **2002**, *33*, 2459–2464. [CrossRef]

88. Arenillas, J.F.; Álvarez-Sabín, J.; Molina, C.A.; Chacoón, P.; Montaner, J.; Rovira, A.; Ibarra, B.; Quintana, M. C-Reactive Protein Predicts Further Ischemic Events in First-Ever Transient Ischemic Attack or Stroke Patients with Intracranial Large-Artery Occlusive Disease. *Stroke* **2003**, *34*, 2463–2468. [CrossRef]

89. Di Napoli, M.; Papa, F.; Bocola, V. Prognostic Influence of Increased C-Reactive Protein and Fibrinogen Levels in Ischemic Stroke. *Stroke* **2001**, *32*, 133–138. [CrossRef]

90. Elkind, M.S.V.; Tai, W.; Coates, K.; Paik, M.C.; Sacco, R.L. High-Sensitivity C-Reactive Protein, Lipoprotein-Associated Phospholipase A2, and Outcome After Ischemic Stroke. *Arch. Intern. Med.* **2006**, *166*, 2073–2080. [CrossRef]

91. Woodward, M.; Lowe, G.D.; Campbell, D.J.; Colman, S.; Rumley, A.; Chalmers, J.P.; Neal, B.C.; Patel, A.; Jenkins, A.J.; E Kemp, B.; et al. Associations of Inflammatory and Hemostatic Variables with the Risk of Recurrent Stroke. *Stroke* **2005**, *36*, 2143–2147. [CrossRef]

92. Muir, K.W.; Weir, C.J.; Alwan, W.; Squire, I.B.; Lees, K.R. C-reactive protein and outcome after ischemic stroke. *Stroke* **1999**, *30*, 981–985. [CrossRef] [PubMed]

93. Ringleb, P.A.; Bousser, M.-G.; Ford, G.; Bath, P.; Brainin, M.; Caso, V.; Cervera, Á.; Chamorro, A.; Cordonnier, C.; Csiba, L.; et al. Ischaemic Stroke and Transient Ischaemic Attack. In *European Handbook of Neurological Management*; Wiley: Hoboken, NJ, USA, 2010; pp. 101–158.

94. Kayser, S.; Kunze, R.; Sheriff, A. Selective C-reactive protein apheresis for Covid-19 patients suffering from organ damage. *Ther. Apher. Dial.* **2020**. [CrossRef] [PubMed]

95. Di Napoli, M.; Schwaninger, M.; Cappelli, R.; Ceccarelli, E.; Di Gianfilippo, G.; Donati, C.; Emsley, H.; Forconi, S.; Hopkins, S.J.; Masotti, L.; et al. Evaluation of C-Reactive Protein Measurement for Assessing the Risk and Prognosis in Ischemic Stroke. *Stroke* **2005**, *36*, 1316–1329. [CrossRef] [PubMed]

96. Peters, S.A.E.; Visseren, F.L.; Grobbee, D.E. Screening for C-reactive protein in CVD prediction. *Nat. Rev. Cardiol.* **2012**, *10*, 12–14. [CrossRef] [PubMed]

97. Kuhlmann, C.R.; Librizzi, L.; Closhen, D.; Pflanzner, T.; Lessmann, V.; Pietrzik, C.U.; De Curtis, M.; Luhmann, H.J. Mechanisms of C-Reactive Protein-Induced Blood–Brain Barrier Disruption. *Stroke* **2009**, *40*, 1458–1466. [CrossRef]

98. Elwood, E.; Lim, Z.; Naveed, H.; Galea, I. The effect of systemic inflammation on human brain barrier function. *Brain Behav. Immun.* **2017**, *62*, 35–40. [CrossRef]

99. Lasek-Bal, A.; Jedrzejowska-Szypulka, H.; Student, S.; Warsz-Wianecka, A.; Zareba, K.; Puz, P.; Bal, W.; Pawletko, K.; Lewin-Kowalik, J. The importance of selected markers of inflammation and blood-brain barrier damage for short-term ischemic stroke prognosis. *J. Psysiol. Pharmacol.* **2019**, *70*, 209–217.

100. Khandkar, C.; Vaidya, K.; Patel, S. Colchicine for Stroke Prevention: A Systematic Review and Meta-analysis. *Clin. Ther.* **2019**, *41*, 582–590.e3. [CrossRef]

101. Dove, A. CD18 trials disappoint again. *Nat. Biotechnol.* **2000**, *18*, 817–818. [CrossRef]

102. Pawluk, H.; Woźniak, A.; Grześk, G.; Kołodziejska, R.; Kozakiewicz, M.; Kopkowska, E.; Grzechowiak, E.; Kozera, G. The Role of Selected Pro-Inflammatory Cytokines in Pathogenesis of Ischemic Stroke. *Clin. Interv. Aging* **2020**, *15*, 469–484. [CrossRef]

103. Mizuma, A.; Yenari, M.A. Anti-Inflammatory Targets for the Treatment of Reperfusion Injury in Stroke. *Front. Neurol.* **2017**, *8*, 467. [CrossRef] [PubMed]

104. Drieu, A.; Levard, D.; Vivien, D.; Rubio, M. Anti-inflammatory treatments for stroke: From bench to bedside. *Ther. Adv. Neurol. Disord.* **2018**, *11*, 1756286418789854. [CrossRef] [PubMed]

105. Roberts, R.; Demello, V.; Sobel, B.E. Deleterious effects of methylprednisolone in patients with myocardial infarction. *Circulation* **1976**, *53*, 204–206.

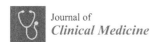

Journal of
Clinical Medicine

Review

Apheresis in Autoimmune Encephalitis and Autoimmune Dementia

Rosa Rössling [1,2] **and Harald Prüss** [1,2,*]

1   Department of Neurology and Experimental Neurology, Charité–Universitätsmedizin Berlin, Charitéplatz 1, 10117 Berlin, Germany; rosa.roessling@charite.de
2   German Center for Neurodegenerative Diseases (DZNE) Berlin, 10117 Berlin, Germany
*   Correspondence: harald.pruess@charite.de; Tel.: +49-(0)30-450-560399; Fax: +49-(0)30-450-539916

Received: 27 July 2020; Accepted: 10 August 2020; Published: 19 August 2020

Abstract: Autoimmune encephalitis (AE) is a rapidly progressive inflammatory neurological disease. Underlying autoantibodies can bind to neuronal surfaces and synaptic proteins resulting in psychiatric symptoms, focal neurological signs, autonomic dysfunction and cognitive decline. Early and effective treatment is mandatory to reduce clinical symptoms and to achieve remission. Therapeutic apheresis, involving both plasma exchange (PE) and immunoadsorption (IA), can rapidly remove pathogenic antibodies from the circulation, thus representing an important first-line treatment in AE patients. We here review the most relevant studies regarding therapeutic apheresis in AE, summarizing the outcome for patients and the expanding clinical spectrum of treatment-responsive clinical conditions. For example, patients with slowly progressing cognitive impairment suggesting a neurodegenerative dementia can have underlying autoantibodies and improve with therapeutic apheresis. Findings are encouraging and have led to the first ongoing clinical studies assessing the therapeutic effect of IA in patients with anti-neuronal autoantibodies and the clinical presentation of dementia. Therapeutic apheresis is an established and well tolerated option for first-line therapy in AE and, potentially, other antibody-mediated central nervous system diseases.

Keywords: autoimmune encephalitis; limbic encephalitis; NMDAR (N-Methyl-D-Aspartat); antibody; paraneoplastic; apheresis; plasma exchange; immunoadsorption

---

1. Introduction

Autoimmune encephalitis (AE) is a rapidly progressive inflammatory neurological disease with subacute onset. Patients may present with behavioral changes and altered mental status as well as reduced levels of consciousness and new focal neurological signs or epileptic seizures [1]. Furthermore, deficits in working or short-term memory frequently occur.

AE comprises both, antibody-mediated and paraneoplastic, i.e., cytotoxic T-cell-mediated, encephalitides. Clinical presentation is diverse and depends on the specific underlying antibody (Table 1). As more and more novel antibodies and new clinical phenotypes are being identified, the incidence is rising and currently estimated at 5–10 per 100,000 inhabitants per year [1]. Age and gender preferences are often specific for a given antibody. In some cases, the exact target of novel antibodies is not known yet. In other cases, even if the underlying antigen is known, the pathogenic relevance still awaits scientific clarification.

1.1. Antibody-Mediated AE

The most common and best-known form of antibody-mediated AE is NMDA (N-Methyl-D-Aspartat) receptor (NMDAR) encephalitis, defined by cerebrospinal fluid (CSF) IgG antibodies targeting the NMDA type glutamate receptor. Patients present with subacute onset of psychiatric symptoms, autonomic instability, focal neurological signs and behavioral changes as well as new-onset epileptic seizures and reduced levels of consciousness. Other AE-defining autoantibodies bind directly to excitatory transmitter receptors besides NMDAR (such as AMPA (α-amino-3-hydroxy-5-methyl-4-isoxazolepropionic acid) receptors), inhibitory transmitter receptors (GABAB (gamma-aminobutyric acid B), GABAA (gamma-aminobutyric acid A), glycine receptors), ion channel subunits and cell adhesion molecules (Caspr2 (contactin-associated protein 2), IgLON5) or soluble synaptic proteins (LGI1 (leucine-rich, glioma inactivated protein 1).

Autoimmune dementia might be considered a sub-form of AE with predominant cognitive deficits. Cognitive impairment is a common feature in AE. For instance, patients with encephalitis caused by LGI1 antibodies showed markedly impaired verbal and visuo-spatial memory as well as a significantly reduced hippocampal volume. A severe clinical course correlated with more pronounced structural damage of the hippocampus and correspondingly a worse overall memory performance [2]. As patients show good response to immunotherapy, especially in the early stage of disease, prompt and sufficiently "aggressive" treatment including apheresis is highly important. Interestingly, the cognitive deficits in LGI1 encephalitis can come in isolation and lead to the working diagnosis of a primary neurodegenerative disease such as Alzheimer's. Increasing awareness and the search for autoantibodies such as LGI1 are needed and can result in the early identification of dementia patients with an immunotherapy-responsive phenotype [3,4].

1.2. Paraneoplastic AE

In contrast to the neuronal surface antibodies, antibodies in classical paraneoplastic neurological syndromes (PNS) bind to intracellular antigens (such as Hu, Ri, Yo or Ma2 antibodies) and therefore do not cause the neurotoxicity directly; they rather serve as valuable biomarkers for an underlying tumor, often small cell lung cancer and gynecological tumors. The neuronal damage in these cases is, rather, caused by cytotoxic T-cells with oligoclonal T-cell receptor expansion and autoreactivity against neuronal structures. Among the antibodies targeting intracellular antigens, GAD (glutamic acid decarboxylase) and amphiphysin antibodies are an exception as they are not necessarily associated with a tumor and seem to be pathogenically relevant despite their intracellular antigen location [5].

Table 1. Most important antibodies and clinical syndromes.

Antigen	Clinical Presentation	Age/Gender	Tumor Type
	Antibodies against neurotransmitter receptors [6]		
NMDAR [7]	Schizophreniform psychosis, perioral dyskinesia, epileptic seizures, coma, dystonia, hypoventilation	All ages, peak in childhood and youth, 75% women	Ovarian teratoma
GABAaR	Epileptic seizures, schizophreniform syndrome, refractory status epilepticus and epilepsia partialis continua	Younger adults; m > f (1.5:1)	Hodgkin lymphoma
GABAbR	LE with frequent epileptic seizures	Older adults f = m	50% lung cancer (SCLC)
AMPAR	LE, Epileptic seizures, memory deficits, psychosis	Older Adults f > m (2.3:1)	In 70% lung/breast cancer
mGluR5	LE, Ophelia syndrome (depression, agitation, hallucination, memory deficits, personality changes)	Young adults, m > f (1.5:1)	Hodgkin lymphoma
GlycinR	PERM (progressive encephalomyelitis with rigidity and myoclonus), SPS, cognitive deficits	Older adults f = m	Thymoma (<10%)
DPPX	LE with tremor, myoclonus, hallucinations, therapy refractory diarrhea	Older adults f < m (1:2.3)	Not known

Table 1. *Cont.*

Antigen	Clinical Presentation	Age/Gender	Tumor Type
	Antibodies against ion channel subunits or cell adhesion molecules [8,9]		
LGI1	Facio-brachial dystonic seizures (FBDS), amnesia, psychosis, LE, hyponatremia	Adults > 40 years, m > f (2:1)	Rare
Caspr2	LE, neuro-myotonia, Morvan syndrome, can slowly progress over up to 1 year;similar to LGI1, but no hyponatremia	Elderly m > f (9:1)	Thymoma possible
IgLON5	REM- and non-REM sleep disorders, sleep apnea, stridor, dysarthria, dysphagia, dysautonomia, movement disorders, dementia	Older adults, f = m	Not known
	Antibodies against intracellular (onconeural) antigens [10,11]		
Hu (ANNA-1)	Encephalomyelitis, brainstem encephalitis, LE, Denny-Brown syndrome	Large variability, depending on tumor type	>90%, SCLC
Ri (ANNA-2)	OMS, CS, encephalomyelitis		>90%, Ovary, breast cancer
Yo (PCA-1)	CS		>90%, Ovary cancer
Ma2	LE, CS, diencephalic/hypothalamic involvement		>90%, Testicular, lung cancer
CV2 (CRMP5)	Encephalomyelitis, LE, CS		>90%, SCLC, thymoma
Amphiphysin	SPS		>90%, Breast, SCLC
GAD	SPS, LE, ataxia	Middle aged, f > m (4:1)	Tumor association rare

LE: limbic encephalitis, SPS: Stiff-person syndrome, OMS: Opsoclonus-myoclonus syndrome, CS: cerebellar syndrome, SCLC: small cell lung cancer, PCD: paraneoplastic cerebellar degeneration.

1.3. Therapy for AE

At this point, there is no clear evidence-based treatment standard for AE. Established treatment strategies for first-line therapy of AE include high-dose corticosteroids (three to five days course of 1000 mg intravenous methylprednisolone), intravenous immunoglobulins (IVIG) (2 g/kg body weight over three to five days), as well as therapeutic apheresis. Cyclophosphamide and the CD20-antibody rituximab (1000 mg, with the first two administrations at day 1 and day 15 followed by six months intervals) might be added in case of persisting or relapsing symptoms and as a long term maintenance therapy. Most centers favor a low threshold for rituximab initiation given its good safety profile and potential effect in preventing relapses. Many other treatments have been used with variable success, including mycophenolate mofetil, methotrexate or azathioprine. It is broadly agreed that immunotherapy needs to be started as early as possible after symptom onset to be most effective. Nevertheless, marked recovery can be seen in some patients with antibody-mediated AE in whom therapy is only started months after disease onset. The choice of adequate therapy depends on the clinical syndrome and the underlying antibody. However, comparative treatment studies in patients with AE are sparse and focus on the most common forms of AE, such as NMDAR encephalitis.

In paraneoplastic AE with antibodies targeting intracellular proteins, rituximab, intravenous immunoglobulins and therapeutic apheresis often have only little effect as the antibodies are not directly pathogenic. Here, neuronal damage is caused by cytotoxic T-cells. Evidence of a tumor requires prompt and complete removal in order to withdraw the auto-antigen expressed by the tumor that triggers the production of autoantibodies. Nevertheless, despite advanced immunotherapy and tumor removal, in many cases neuronal damage in paraneoplastic AE progresses.

Therapeutic apheresis and the removal of autoantibodies is a major therapeutic option in AE. The pathophysiological binding of antibodies to their antigens can thereby be reduced.

2. Search Strategy

To conduct the review, we followed the PRISMA (Preferred Reporting Items for Systematic Reviews and Meta-Analyses) guidelines and screened the articles independently for their respective eligibility [12].

2.1. Inclusion Criteria

We included all articles about patients with autoimmune encephalitis—antibody-mediated as well as paraneoplastic—treated with plasma exchange or immunoadsorption. Treatment regimen, such as concomitant immunotherapy, as well as details about the apheresis itself (plasma exchange (PE) or immunoadsorption (IA), number of courses) had to be specified in the article. Further, outcome measures, such as the modified Rankin Scale (mRS) or structured neuropsychological assessment had to be provided. The mRS ranges from zero (no symptoms) to six (death from the disease), and a change of ±1 mRS point is considered as clinically significant improvement or deterioration. Cut-off for independent living is at ≤2 mRS points.

2.2. Search Strategy

The following strategy was used to find previous literature and trials (Figure 1): MEDLINE (medical literature analysis and retrieval system online) was searched for articles published up until 30 June 2020 in English or German. The Medical Subject Headings (MeSH) terms used were "autoimmune encephalitis" and "apheresis" (37 hits), "plasma exchange" (104 hits) or "immunoadsorption" (12 hits). Furthermore, the references of the included articles were screened for potential additional articles.

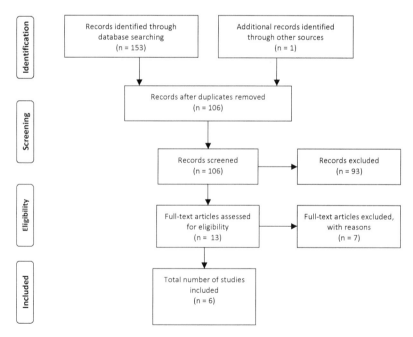

Figure 1. Preferred Reporting Items for Systematic Reviews and Meta-Analyses (PRISMA) flow diagram of the reviewed literature.

3. Results

3.1. Therapeutic Apheresis in Autoimmune Encephalitides

Therapeutic apheresis is an important treatment option in a range of inflammatory central nervous system diseases [13]. It has been proven to be beneficial in primary demyelinating disease as well as in encephalitis caused by antibodies targeting neuronal proteins [14] (Table 2).

Therapeutic apheresis has been shown to be safe and effective leading to measurable laboratory and clinical improvement in several inflammatory diseases of the central and peripheral nervous system, including myasthenia gravis, Guillain-Barré syndrome and multiple sclerosis. Apheresis is recommended by the German Society of Neurology as escalation treatment of severe courses of AE. Patients should be treated with apheresis at least five times every other day. In cases with predominant CSF antibodies seven to ten treatment courses are usually needed for relevant reduction of CSF antibody titers. Before receiving therapeutic apheresis, patients mostly show either severe clinical symptoms on hospital admission or an insufficient response to therapy with high-dose cortisone or IVIG.

Much has been learned from acquired myasthenia gravis, which represents a "model disease" for the much later discovered forms of autoantibody-mediated AE. It could first be demonstrated that removal of the disease-defining acetylcholine receptor antibodies using plasma-exchange led to marked symptom improvement [15]. Antibodies in antibody-mediated AE are mostly directed against neuronal surface antigens. Emerging studies have demonstrated that clinical symptoms relate directly to pathogenic autoantibodies. For example, isolated human monoclonal autoantibodies from patients with NMDAR encephalitis targeted the NR1 subunit of the NMDAR and were alone sufficient to induce morphological and electrophysiological changes in the neurons, and to lead to synaptic dysfunction by downregulation of NMDAR [16]. Thus, the pathogenic effect is caused by the antibodies themselves, indicating that removal of these antibodies can disrupt the disease-causing mechanisms.

Therapeutic apheresis has been shown to improve clinical symptoms in different antibody-mediated diseases. According to the American Society for apheresis (ASFA) guidelines PE and IA are strongly recommended for different antibody-mediated encephalitis forms ranging from low to moderate evidence. In contrast, the therapeutic role of apheresis is not yet established for paraneoplastic neurological syndromes and individual decision-making is necessary [23]. In NMDAR encephalitis, recovery and symptom remission often correlate with a reduction of antibodies, in particular with a decline in CSF titers. In this way, antibody titers can serve as intra-individual disease biomarkers and support treatment decisions [24]. Efficacy of therapeutic apheresis relates to the extracorporeal elimination of circulating serum antibodies, redistribution of antibodies from the extracellular space and a number of secondary immunomodulatory changes. The inflammatory processes during AE are likely to involve a leakier blood-brain barrier, which might support further redistribution of autoantibodies from the central nervous system into the blood [25].

Table 2. Overview of studies on therapeutic apheresis in autoimmune encephalitis (AE).

Author	Year	Journal	Study Type	AE Type	Sample Size	Procedure	Outcome Measurement	Results	Ref.
DeSena AD	2015	J Clin Aph	Retrospective	NMDAR	10	PE	Modified Rankin scale (mRS)	Steroids alone not as effective as steroids followed by PE	[17]
Ehrlich S	2012	Nervenarzt	Retrospective	Antibody-mediated, paraneoplastic	30	PE, IA	mRS	Improvement of mRS after PE or IA	[18]
Heine J	2016	J Neurol	Prospective	NMDAR, LGI1, Caspr2, GAD, mGluR5, Hu	21	PE, IA	mRS	Improvement of mRS in 60% of patients	[19]
Hempel P	2016	Ther Apher Dial	Prospective	agAAB	8	IA	Neuropsychological test	Stabilized cognitive performance after 4-day treatment	[20]
Köhler W	2014	Eur J Neurol	Retrospective	NMDAR, GABA, LGI1, GAD	13	IA	mRS	Improvement of mRS in 11/13 patients	[21]
Onugoren MD	2016	Neurol Neuroimmunol Neuroinflamm	Retrospective	LGI1, Caspr2, NMDAR, GAD	19	IA	mRS	Improvement of mRS in patients with LGI1, Caspr2, NMDAR, no improvement in patients with GAD	[22]

3.2. Therapeutic Procedure for Apheresis

Therapeutic apheresis offers two different procedures. On the one hand is plasma exchange (PE), where a defined plasma volume is removed and replaced by human albumin or fresh frozen plasma. On the other hand is immunoadsorption (IA), a procedure that more specifically removes immunoglobulins and immune complexes by passing the plasma over an adsorber column, allowing reinfusion of the patients' own plasma. Two different IA procedures were used in the reviewed articles: either a regenerative double column system or a disposable tryptophan column. Tolerability and therapeutic effects do not show relevant differences between PE and IA in recent studies [14,19,26]. Related to the procedure is a rare risk of pathogen transmission in PE due to substitution with donor-derived blood components, which is not existent in IA [19]. However, angiotensin-converting enzyme inhibitors need to be paused for a minimum of 48 h prior to IA, otherwise there exists a risk of IA-associated bradykinin-release syndrome. Main side effects are not caused by the apheresis directly, but are rather related to the necessary central venous catheter. They include bleedings, hematoma, infections, thrombosis or damage caused by the puncture [22].

Usually a minimum of five sessions of apheresis is performed. When patients show a CSF predominant antibody, more sessions are generally needed in order to eliminate the antibody in the central nervous system. Most studies included in this review describe a central venous catheter in an internal jugular vein as vascular access. Only Hempel et al. use a peripheral vein to perform IA and in order to treat patients as outpatients. However, they report significant patient drop-out due to a failure of repeatedly accessing the vein [20].

The treated plasma volumes can be calculated using Sprenger's formula [27]. Depending on the protocol, a total of 1.5–2.2 plasma volume is processed in PE, whereas in IA 2000–2500 mL plasma per session are treated [19,22]. Patients treated with PE receive a replacement solution, such as 4% human albumin or fresh frozen plasma. Treatments take place every other day, although the first two to three sessions can be conducted on consecutive days in selected cases. Due to the central venous catheter, anticoagulation is necessary to minimize the risk of thrombosis.

3.3. Initiation of Therapy with Apheresis and Prior Treatment

The specific mechanism of antibody removal has been shown to be a more beneficial treatment of NMDAR encephalitis than intravenous methylprednisolone alone. In a retrospective study 2/14 patients showed significant clinical improvement following steroids, whereas 9/14 patients who received additional PE improved in the mRS during the third and fifth cycle of apheresis [17]. This is likely to be related to the high therapeutic specificity and therefore efficacy of therapeutic apheresis compared to intravenous immunoglobulins (IVIG) or high-dose corticosteroids. Early diagnosis and prompt start of a sufficiently "aggressive" therapy are mandatory for symptom reduction and long-term remission. Interestingly, a study by Heine et al. showed that treatment delay was not associated with a significantly worsened outcome [19], whereas Onugoren et al. found that, in patients with irreversible damage of brain structures, such as fixed hippocampal sclerosis, no clinical improvement could be achieved by IA [22].

Many patients with AE treated with apheresis receive prior treatment with high-dose steroids or IVIG. The decision for treatment with apheresis is often only made after unsuccessful or incomplete recovery after these other therapies. It has been shown that both patients who did and patients who did not receive prior treatment benefitted from apheresis [19]. In all studies analysed, a substantial part of the patients (up to more than half) received apheresis as initial treatment.

In the study by Onugoren et al. all patients except one out of 19 were treated with high-dose prednisolone (median dose 4.9 g) in parallel to IA [22]. It is reported that in some patients immunosuppressive therapy with steroids is continued on a maintenance dose [18]. Especially, patients with antibodies to LGI1 respond well to continued treatment with steroids [8,9].

Apheresis in patients with AE is most established in the acute phase of the disease. However, repeated apheresis might also be applied in refractory disease with clinical signs of AE and constant detection of high antibody titers. Yet in one study, repeated IA after 4.5 months (median) in six patients with antibodies against NMDAR, LGI1, Caspr2 and GAD that responded insufficiently to a first series of IA, did not show any further clinical improvement measured by mRS [22].

In case of an underlying malignancy, tumor removal is essential for improving further disease course.

3.4. Effects of Treatment with Apheresis in Patients with AE

A better outcome in patients with NMDAR encephalitis was strongly associated with an early start of immunotherapy (less than 40 days after symptom onset) [28]. Response rate in general is considerably higher when therapy initiation is started early [29] and includes improvement in state-of-the-art imaging and neuropsychological assessments [30].

According to a prospective study, symptoms that responded best to apheresis include apathy, aphasia, stupor, sleep disorders, agitation, myoclonus and dystonia, sensory neuropathy, apraxia and seizures [19]. In another study, in the majority of patients the modified Rankin Scale (mRS) improved by ≥1 point. It is of note that no patient worsened during apheresis in these studies.

Treatment efficacy is more pronounced in patients with antibodies against cell surface antibodies (NMDAR, LGI1, Caspr2, mGluR5) or in patients with intracellular synaptic antibodies (GAD), whereas no positive treatment effect was observed in patients with paraneoplastic intracellular antigens (anti-Hu) [19,22]. Marked reduction of serum antibodies occurred during the first five sessions of IA, but titers dropped further when apheresis was continued. Five days after IA a median decrease in titers of 97% and 64% was noted for serum and CSF, respectively. Interestingly, the decrease further continued until the next follow-up (median time after IA 3.9 months) [22]. In a retrospective study, all cerebral magnetic resonance imaging (MRI) changes in 17 patients with NMDAR encephalitis decreased [18].

Marked and rapid effects of apheresis can be seen in patients with epileptic seizures concerning seizure frequency. This was seen for patients with LGI1 and Caspr2 antibodies, where five out of seven patients became seizure free immediately after initiation of therapy with IA [22]. This treatment effect results in reduction or even complete removal of antiepileptic drugs.

Several case reports point to the efficacy of PE in drug-resistant status epilepticus caused by AE in children and adults. Both convulsive and non-convulsive status have been described as being responsive to apheresis. In patients with abnormal electroencephalogram (EEG) prior to apheresis, EEG normalization was observed after 5 cycles of PE. EEG improvement correlated with decrease in antibody titers [31,32].

Treatment of severe AE complicated by status epilepticus or autonomic instability might need to take place on an intensive care unit. On the ICU, benefit from immunotherapy, including apheresis, strongly depends on medical complications associated with a prolonged ICU stay [33].

In patients with predominantly psychiatric symptoms related to treatable autoimmunity, corticosteroids are often hesitantly used given the potential side effect of steroid-induced psychosis. Overall, notable neuropsychiatric side effects can occur in up to 6% of patients who receive steroids [34]; however, in antibody-mediated AE the clinical improvement with immunotherapy quickly outrivals any steroid-related effects on psychiatric symptoms according to our experience.

In paraneoplastic AE with antibodies targeting intracellular proteins, therapeutic effects of rituximab, IVIG and therapeutic apheresis are usually limited as the antibodies are not directly pathogenic, but neuronal damage is caused by cytotoxic T-cells [19,26]. Furthermore, diagnosis in paraneoplastic disease is often delayed and substantial irreversible neuronal cell damage has already occurred at the time of therapy initiation. Discontinuation of therapy should be considered in patients in whom brain damage has progressed to an advanced stage in MRI after three to six months despite intensified immunotherapy.

After therapeutic apheresis with both PE and IA, a transient spurious intrathecal immunoglobulin synthesis of all three subclasses (IgG, IgA, IgM) can be observed. The transient intrathecal Ig fractions and increased IgG index are due to dropped serum IgG levels following apheresis. This "intrathecal pseudo-synthesis" regularly occurs in the first two days after apheresis in a majority of patients [35]. Thus, one needs to consider these abnormalities for interpretation of CSF results from lumbar puncture shortly after apheresis in order to prevent false diagnostic assumptions.

3.5. Future Treatment Options for Apheresis

Clinical indications for therapeutic apheresis in AE might expand to less recognized antibody-mediated conditions in the near future. We could recently demonstrate that asymptomatic mothers of a child requiring psychiatric in-patient diagnostics carried low-level pathogenic human NR1 antibodies more frequently than control mothers having a healthy child [36]. To better understand this possible connection, we developed a murine model of pregnancy-related materno-fetal antibody transfer. Here, human monoclonal NR1 antibodies diaplacentally transferred to the offspring, enriched in the fetal circulation and brain, caused neurotoxic effects during neonatal development, inducing brain network changes, and led to neuropathological disorders in the offspring persisting into adulthood [36]. Given the relatively high frequency of NR1 autoantibodies in the healthy human population, the findings indicate a novel disease principle with high clinical relevance for lifelong neuropsychiatric morbidity in the affected children [37]. Most importantly, these pathologies are potentially treatable with apheresis in asymptomatic mothers, but further studies are needed to better understand the frequency of autoantibodies, the susceptible window during pregnancy and the contribution of genetic and further risk factors. Further, this seems not to be limited to the NMDAR, as other maternal anti-neuronal autoantibodies may similarly cause neurodevelopmental disorders in the offspring, such as with antibodies against Caspr2 [38].

The use of therapeutic apheresis has been shown to be safe in pregnant women, both for mother and fetus. A recent Italian study evaluated the use of apheresis during pregnancy. Among 48 pregnant women receiving apheresis one had suspected autoimmune encephalitis. Adverse events occurred in 2.1% of all patients analysed, which is reported to be lower than the Italian average. Peripheral veins are preferred as a vascular access during pregnancy to avoid the risks associated with a central venous catheter [39].

3.6. Apheresis in Children with AE

Children with autoimmune disorders such as antibody-mediated AE can also be treated with therapeutic apheresis. PE was retrospectively evaluated in 22 children. All children had been treated with IVIG and/or steroids before PE. Each patient received a median number of six PE sessions. No PE-related mortality was observed and adverse events occurred in 2.2%, which is the expected average. Adverse events consisted of hypotension and urticaria. In total, three pediatric patients with antibody-mediated encephalitis were treated with PE, two patients improved and one patient showed partial recovery with persistent neurological deficits after three-year follow-up. One patient with paraneoplastic encephalitis did not benefit from PE and was lost to follow-up [40]. Another prospective observational study evaluated 535 children with acquired demyelinating syndrome or encephalitis treated with steroids, IVIG or PE. Here, pediatric patients with autoimmune encephalitis other than acute disseminated encephalomyelitis (ADEM) had the highest frequency of poor outcome. However, the individual treatment decisions were not specified [41].

3.7. Autoimmune Dementia and Treatment with Apheresis

Compared to 'classic' AE with subacute onset of neuropsychiatric as well as behavioral symptoms, antibody-associated dementias are a more slowly progressing group of diseases where decline in working and short-term memory as well as visuo-spatial deficits are the most prominent features. Detection of high-level autoantibodies in patients with dementia is rare, but autoimmune dementias represent a form of cognitive decline that is potentially treatable. A Mayo clinic study reported improvement of cognition in 64% of patients with suspected autoimmune dementia after immunomodulatory treatment [29]. An underlying autoimmune mechanism and response to immunotherapy is more likely when patients do not fulfill routine criteria for established neurodegenerative dementia forms, but rather present with subacute onset, psychiatric symptoms, fluctuating disease course, shorter delay to treatment, seropositivity for a specific autoantibody and inflammatory CSF [29].

In a retrospective study analyzing 286 CSF and serum samples of patients with different dementia forms, 16% of the serum samples had NMDAR IgA, IgM or IgG antibodies compared to 4.3% in a healthy control group [42]. Besides the spectrum of known and established pathogenic antibodies, there might be an even broader range of autoantibodies for which pathogenicity has not yet been confirmed. It is unclear from these studies whether anti-neuronal autoantibodies develop secondarily to neurodegeneration or whether they primarily contribute to and drive the disease. It is highly possible that neurodegeneration leads to the presentation of autoantigens from dying neurons with consecutive establishment of a specific autoimmune response. In this way, formed autoantibodies may contribute to synaptic dysfunction, further accelerate cognitive decline or contribute to clinical symptoms such as behavioral abnormalities commonly present in dementia patients.

Another recent target in dementia patients are autoantibodies against G protein-coupled receptors. In a small trial analyzing the effect of IA in patients with mild to moderate dementia and agonistic autoantibodies (agAAB) against α-adrenergic receptors, treatment with four cycles of IA not only caused disappearance of autoantibodies, but resulted in stabilization of the cognitive and mental condition during the follow-up period of 12–18 months [20]. Another study that is currently recruiting (ClinicalTrials.gov Identifier: NCT03132272) investigates the effects of IA in patients with Alzheimer's disease positive for agAAB. The group aims to demonstrate discontinuation of the vascular remodeling and slowing of cognitive decline following IA treatment.

Apheresis not only has an acute effect on disease activity but can be used for longer lasting immunomodulation. In case of uncertainty of the immunological findings, first-line therapy including steroids or apheresis may serve as a diagnostic test to support the autoimmune etiology [43]. In our experience, however, short-term treatment (such as intravenous high-dose steroids for three to five days) cannot demonstrate clinical improvement in autoimmune dementia in most cases, thus requiring longer administration for four to six weeks (e.g., daily 0.5 mg/kg prednisone).

Based on the new developments in this field, the ongoing identification of dementia-associated autoantibodies and the concern about overlooking treatable etiologies, we now offer diagnostic antibody testing in serum and CSF to every patient with suspected dementia in our memory clinic at the department of neurology at Charité. In this way we increasingly identify patients with a working diagnosis of Alzheimer's, frontotemporal dementia or atypical dementia who have new or established autoantibodies against neuronal and glial proteins, as exemplarily shown in the case vignette of an 81-year-old gentleman (Box 1).

Detection of antibodies against neurochondrin (Figure 2) in this patient led to immunotherapy with IA. The observed clinical improvement prompted B-cell depleting therapy with rituximab that led to long-term stabilization.

The patient participates in an ongoing clinical trial (DRKS00016017) analyzing the role of anti-neuronal and anti-glial surface antibodies in cognitive disorders and potential improvement following IA. The study aims to identify dementia patients who harbor autoantibodies against structures of the central nervous system using cell-based assays for detection of established autoantibodies as well as screening assays using indirect immunofluorescence on unfixed murine brain sections. Autoantibody-positive patients with cognitive decline can enroll in the study and receive therapeutic apheresis (Figure 3). Treatment includes five to six IA sessions over a 12-day course. Cognitive performance is evaluated prospectively and compared to historic controls. Patients further undergo structural und functional MRI before and after IA. CSF analysis evaluates the reduction of autoantibody levels over the course of IA and the potential utility of further biomarkers of neurodegeneration, such as micro-RNAs.

Box 1. Clinical case of autoimmune dementia.

An 81-year-old dementia patient presented to our outpatient memory clinic at the department of Neurology at Charité—Universitätsmedizin Berlin with deficits in working and short term memory as well as difficulties in concentration. Symptoms began nine months prior to presentation with increasing loss of orientation for place and time, confusion and reported visual hallucinations. Brain MRI at symptom onset was unremarkable apart from microangiopathic lesions in the left temporoparietal lobe (Figure 2A). Basic CSF analysis showed markedly increased protein. Symptoms improved after several weeks without specific therapy, but anterograde memory deficit persisted. During the following months, two episodes with re-appearance of confusion occurred, but lasted only for days.

In our center, the patient showed a persisting dysexecutive syndrome with amnestic and visuo-constructive deficits and apraxia. No other neurological deficits were observed. Montreal cognitive assessment showed mild cognitive impairment with a score of 21 out of 30. A second CSF analysis revealed normal cell count, but still increased protein of 1288 mg/L (normal <450 mg/L). No infectious cause was found. Extensive search for anti-neuronal autoantibodies in serum and CSF including indirect immunofluorescence staining on rodent brain sections detected neurochondrin IgG antibodies in the CSF (Figure 2B).

The diagnosis of AE with oligosymptomatic memory deficits was established. A three-day course of intravenous methylprednisolone with 1 g/day led to improved gait, but no impact on cognition was observed. Because of the persisting memory deficits, two months later five sessions of IA were administered every other day and resulted in reduction of CSF neurochondrin antibody titers (Figure 2C). The patient reported vertigo during IA, but vital signs were unremarkable at all times. After IA, the patient described improved concentration; his wife reported better organization of daily life and his ability to care for himself again. In the Bristol Activities of Daily Living Scale the patient improved from 20 points to 9 points.

The patient's autoantibodies targeted neurochondrin, a leucine-rich protein expressed not only in the brain, but also in bones and cartilage. As neurochondrin is located intracellularly, the pathogenicity of neurochondrin antibodies is unclear and they might only be a biomarker of autoimmunity including T-cell-mediated neurotoxicity [44]. Neurochondrin expression is highest in cerebellar Purkinje cells, brainstem, lateral parts of the central amygdala nuclei and the hippocampal pyramidal cells. Antibodies against neurochondrin bind robustly to the hippocampus, cerebellum and amygdala, while binding to the striatum, thalamus and cerebral cortex is less pronounced [45]. Patients described so far presented with rapidly progressing cerebellar ataxia, brainstem signs and neuropsychiatric symptoms.

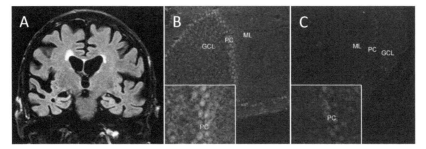

Figure 2. Autoantibodies against neurochondrin. (**A**) MRI T2/FLAIR (fluid-attenuated inversion recovery) of the 81-year-old dementia patient was largely unremarkable apart from few microangiopathic lesions in the left temporoparietal lobe. (**B**) Indirect immunofluorescence of murine cerebellum sections demonstrated CSF IgG antibodies against neurochondrin (GCL, granule cell layer; PC, Purkinje cells; ML, molecular layer). (**C**) Following immunotherapy with five sessions of IA, antibody titers in CSF were markedly reduced.

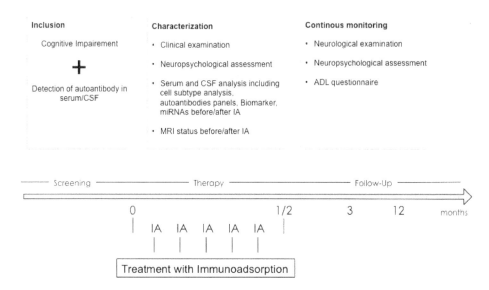

Figure 3. Immunoadsorption in autoantibody-positive patients with cognitive impairment—trial protocol. Patients with confirmed autoantibodies against central nervous system antigens and progressing cognitive impairment receive immunotherapy with five sessions of IA together with detailed neuropsychological, MRI and CSF biomarker assessment. Follow-up monitoring includes two visits after three and 12 months.

3.8. Closing Remarks and Outlook

Predictors for beneficial outcome after treatment with apheresis in patients with AE include start of the treatment early in the disease before substantial irreversible brain damage has occurred. Nevertheless, after longer periods from symptom onset to therapy initiation, apheresis can also result in symptom improvement. Immunotherapy with steroids or IVIG prior to apheresis does not seem to have an effect on the overall outcome. Especially in patients with severe disease courses apheresis is a major treatment option and should be initiated early, possibly together with other immune therapies.

For selected patient groups such as children and pregnant women as well as patients requiring ICU treatment, the safety and efficacy of apheresis could also be shown.

According to all studies reviewed, the ASFA guidelines and the recommendations given by the German Society of Neurology, no benefit of apheresis in patients with onco-neuronal antibodies could be shown. Here, results are inconsistent, with most patients showing no therapeutic effect after apheresis, or even further deterioration, but in single patients clinical improvement could sometimes be seen. A clear treatment response to apheresis, both, PE and IA, is established in patients with antibodies against surface antigens or synaptic antigens. In the articles screened for this review, there was no difference in outcome of patients treated with PE or IA. Therapeutic apheresis is a valuable option within the complex multimodal immune therapy of AE. The benefit of treating patients with antibody-mediated AE with apheresis by far outweighs the possible side effects that were not severe and were mainly associated with the central venous catheter. Furthermore treatment with apheresis may be complicated by the necessity of an ICU setting and poor patient cooperation.

Although predominant humoral autoimmunity seems to be rare in dementia patients and requires further study, the search for autoantibodies in these patients allows the detection of potentially treatable dementia forms and holds the potential to prevent further cognitive decline in selected patients. Thus, therapeutic apheresis is not only an important first-line therapy in patients with AE but may be increasingly considered in further patients who are positive for autoantibodies against neuronal structures. This already includes patients with cognitive decline but may in the future expand to novel clinical indications ranging from antibody-associated psychosis to autoantibody-positive pregnant women.

Author Contributions: Conceptualization, R.R. and H.P.; methodology, R.R. and H.P.; validation, R.R. and H.P.; formal analysis, R.R. and H.P.; investigation, R.R.; resources, H.P.; data curation, R.R.; writing—original draft preparation, R.R.; writing—review and editing, H.P.; visualization, R.R. and H.P.; supervision, H.P.; project administration, H.P.; funding acquisition, H.P. All authors have read and agreed to the published version of the manuscript.

Funding: This research was funded by grants from the German Research Foundation (DFG) to H.P. (PR1274/2-1, 3-1, 4-1 and 5-1).

Conflicts of Interest: HP received research funding from Diamed. The funders had no role in the design of the study; in the collection, analyses, or interpretation of data; in the writing of the manuscript, or in the decision to publish the results.

Ethics Approval : Vote of the Ethics committee is available (EA1/052/18).

Consent for Publication: Patient gave written informed consent for participation in the study and publication.

References

1. Graus, F.; Titulaer, M.J.; Balu, R.; Benseler, S.; Bien, C.G.; Cellucci, T.; Cortese, I.; Dale, R.C.; Gelfand, J.M.; Geschwind, M.; et al. A clinical approach to diagnosis of autoimmune encephalitis. *Lancet Neurol.* **2016**, *15*, 391–404. [CrossRef]
2. Finke, C.; Prüss, H.; Heine, J.; Reuter, S.; Kopp, U.A.; Wegner, F.; Bergh, F.T.; Koch, S.; Jansen, O.; Münte, T.; et al. Evaluation of cognitive deficits and structural hippocampal damage in encephalitis with leucine-rich, glioma-inactivated 1 antibodies. *JAMA Neurol.* **2017**, *74*, 50. [CrossRef] [PubMed]
3. Reintjes, W.; Romijn, M.D.; Hollander, D.; Ter Bruggen, J.P.; Van Marum, R.J. Reversible dementia: Two nursing home patients with voltage-gated potassium channel antibody-associated limbic encephalitis. *J. Am. Med. Dir. Assoc.* **2015**, *16*, 790–794. [CrossRef] [PubMed]
4. Marquetand, J.; Lessen, M.; Bender, B.; Reimold, M.; Elsen, G.; Stoecker, W.; Synofzik, M. Slowly progressive LGI1 encephalitis with isolated late-onset cognitive dysfunction: A treatable mimic of Alzheimer's disease. *Eur. J. Neurol.* **2016**, *23*, 28–29. [CrossRef]
5. Saiz, A.; Blanco, Y.; Sabater, L.; González, F.; Bataller, L.; Casamitjana, R.; Ramió-Torrentà, L.; Graus, F. Spectrum of neurological syndromes associated with glutamic acid decarboxylase antibodies: Diagnostic clues for this association. *Brain* **2008**, *131*, 2553–2563. [CrossRef]
6. Dalmau, J.; Graus, F. Antibody-mediated encephalitis. *N. Engl. J. Med.* **2018**, *378*, 840–851. [CrossRef]
7. Dalmau, J.; Armangué, T.; Planagumà, J.; Radosevic, M.; Mannara, F.; Leypoldt, F.; Geis, C.; Lancaster, E.; Titulaer, M.J.; Rosenfeld, M.R.; et al. An update on anti-NMDA receptor encephalitis for neurologists and psychiatrists: Mechanisms and models. *Lancet Neurol.* **2019**, *18*, 1045–1057. [CrossRef]
8. Gaig, C.; Graus, F.; Compta, Y.; Högl, B.; Bataller, L.; Brüggemann, N.; Giordana, C.; Heidbreder, A.; Kotschet, K.; Lewerenz, J.; et al. Clinical manifestations of the anti-IgLON5 disease. *Neurology* **2017**, *88*, 1736–1743. [CrossRef]
9. Irani, S.R.; Alexander, S.; Waters, P.; Kleopa, K.A.; Pettingill, P.; Zuliani, L.; Peles, E.; Buckley, C.; Lang, B.; Vincent, A. Antibodies to Kv1 potassium channel-complex proteins leucine-rich, glioma inactivated 1 protein and contactin-associated protein-2 in limbic encephalitis, Morvan's syndrome and acquired neuromyotonia. *Brain* **2010**, *133*, 2734–2748. [CrossRef]
10. Graus, F.; Delattre, J.Y.; Antoine, J.C.; Dalmau, J.; Giometto, B.; Grisold, W.; Honnorat, J.; Smitt, P.S.; Vedeler, C.; Verschuuren, J.; et al. Recommended diagnostic criteria for paraneoplastic neurological syndromes. *J. Neurol. Neurosurg. Psychiatry* **2004**, *75*, 1135–1140. [CrossRef]
11. Gultekin, S.H.; Rosenfeld, M.R.; Voltz, R.; Eichen, J.; Posner, J.B.; Dalmau, J. Paraneoplastic limbic encephalitis: Neurological symptoms, immunological findings and tumour association in 50 patients. *Brain* **2000**, *123*, 1481–1494. [CrossRef] [PubMed]
12. Moher, D.; Liberati, A.; Tetzlaff, J.; Altman, U.G. Preferred reporting items for systematic reviews and meta-analyses: The PRISMA statement. *PLoS Med.* **2009**, *6*, e1000097. [CrossRef] [PubMed]

13. Sorgun, M.H.; Erdogan, S.; Bay, M.; Ayyıldız, E.; Yücemen, N.; Iihan, O.; Yücesan, C.; Ayyildiz, E. Therapeutic plasma exchange in treatment of neuroimmunologic disorders: Review of 92 cases. *Transfus. Apher. Sci.* **2013**, *49*, 174–180. [CrossRef] [PubMed]

14. Weinshenker, B.G.; O'Brien, P.C.; Petterson, T.M.; Noseworthy, J.H.; Lucchinetti, C.F.; Dodick, D.W.; Pineda, A.A.; Stevens, L.N.; Rodriguez, M. A randomized trial of plasma exchange in acute central nervous system inflammatory demyelinating disease. *Ann. Neurol.* **1999**, *46*, 878–886. [CrossRef]

15. Pinching, A.J.; Peters, D.K. Remission of myasthenia gravis following plasma-exchange. *Lancet* **1976**, *308*, 1373–1376. [CrossRef]

16. Kreye, J.; Wenke, N.K.; Chayka, M.; Leubner, J.; Murugan, R.; Maier, N.; Jurek, B.; Ly, L.-T.; Brandl, D.; Rost, B.R.; et al. Human cerebrospinal fluid monoclonal N-methyl-D-aspartate receptor autoantibodies are sufficient for encephalitis pathogenesis. *Brain* **2016**, *139*, 2641–2652. [CrossRef]

17. DeSena, A.D.; Noland, D.K.; Matevosyan, K.; King, K.; Phillips, L.; Qureshi, S.S.; Greenberg, B.M.; Graves, D. Intravenous methylprednisolone versus therapeutic plasma exchange for treatment of anti-n-methyl-d-aspartate receptor antibody encephalitis: A retrospective review. *J. Clin. Apher.* **2015**, *30*, 212–216. [CrossRef]

18. Ehrlich, S.; Fassbender, C.; Blaes, C.; Finke, C.; Günther, A.; Harms, L.; Hoffmann, F.; Jahner, K.; Klingel, R.; Kraft, A.; et al. Therapeutische Apherese bei autoimmuner Enzephalitis. *Der Nervenarzt* **2013**, *84*, 498–507. [CrossRef]

19. Heine, J.; Ly, L.-T.; Lieker, I.; Slowinski, T.; Finke, C.; Prüss, H.; Harms, L. Immunoadsorption or plasma exchange in the treatment of autoimmune encephalitis: A pilot study. *J. Neurol.* **2016**, *263*, 2395–2402. [CrossRef]

20. Hempel, P.; Heinig, B.; Jerosch, C.; Decius, I.; Karczewski, P.; Kassner, U.; Kunze, R.; Steinhagen-Thiessen, E.; Bimmler, M. Immunoadsorption of agonistic autoantibodies against α1-adrenergic receptors in patients with mild to moderate dementia. *Ther. Apher. Dial.* **2016**, *20*, 523–529. [CrossRef]

21. Kohler, W.; Ehrlich, S.; Dohmen, C.; Haubitz, M.; Hoffmann, F.; Schmidt, S.; Klingel, R.; Kraft, A.; Neumann-Haefelin, T.; Topka, H.; et al. Tryptophan immunoadsorption for the treatment of autoimmune encephalitis. *Eur. J. Neurol.* **2014**, *22*, 203–206. [CrossRef] [PubMed]

22. Onugoren, M.D.; Golombeck, K.S.; Bien, C.; Abu-Tair, M.; Brand, M.; Bulla-Hellwig, M.; Lohmann, H.; Münstermann, D.; Pavenstädt, H.; Thölking, G.; et al. Immunoadsorption therapy in autoimmune encephalitides. *Neurol. Neuroimmunol. Neuroinflamm.* **2016**, *3*, e207. [CrossRef] [PubMed]

23. Padmanabhan, A.; Connelly-Smith, L.; Aqui, N.; Balogun, R.A.; Klingel, R.; Meyer, E.; Pham, H.P.; Schneiderman, J.; Witt, V.; Wu, Y.; et al. Guidelines on the use of therapeutic apheresis in clinical practice—evidence-based approach from the writing committee of the american society for apheresis: The eighth special issue. *J. Clin. Apher.* **2019**, *34*, 171–354. [CrossRef] [PubMed]

24. Gresa-Arribas, N.; Titulaer, M.J.; Torrents, A.; Aguilar, E.; McCracken, L.; Leypoldt, F.; Gleichman, A.J.; Balice-Gordon, R.; Rosenfeld, M.R.; Lynch, D.; et al. Antibody titres at diagnosis and during follow-up of anti-NMDA receptor encephalitis: A retrospective study. *Lancet Neurol.* **2013**, *13*, 167–177. [CrossRef]

25. Dalmau, J.; Gleichman, A.J.; Hughes, E.G.; Rossi, J.E.; Peng, X.; Lai, M.; Dessain, S.K.; Rosenfeld, M.R.; Balice-Gordon, R.; Lynch, D.R. Anti-NMDA-receptor encephalitis: Case series and analysis of the effects of antibodies. *Lancet Neurol.* **2008**, *7*, 1091–1098. [CrossRef]

26. Fassbender, C.; Klingel, R.; Köhler, W. Immunoadsorption for autoimmune encephalitis. *Atheroscler. Suppl.* **2017**, *30*, 257–263. [CrossRef]

27. Sprenger, K.B.G.; Huber, K.; Kratz, W.; Henze, E. Nomograms for the prediction of patient's plasma volume in plasma exchange therapy from height, weight and hematocrit. *J. Clin. Apher.* **1987**, *3*, 185–190. [CrossRef]

28. Irani, S.R.; Vincent, A. NMDA receptor antibody encephalitis. *Curr. Neurol. Neurosci. Rep.* **2011**, *11*, 298–304. [CrossRef]

29. Flanagan, E.P.; McKeon, A.; Lennon, V.A.; Boeve, B.F.; Trenerry, M.R.; Tan, K.M.; Drubach, D.A.; Josephs, K.A.; Britton, J.W.; Mandrekar, J.N.; et al. Autoimmune dementia: Clinical course and predictors of immunotherapy response. *Mayo Clin. Proc.* **2010**, *85*, 881–897. [CrossRef]

30. Finke, C.; Kopp, U.A.; Pajkert, A.; Behrens, J.R.; Leypoldt, F.; Wuerfel, J.T.; Ploner, C.J.; Prüss, H.; Paul, F. Information, P.E.K.F.C. structural hippocampal damage following anti-n-methyl-d-aspartate receptor encephalitis. *Biol. Psychiatry* **2016**, *79*, 727–734. [CrossRef]

31. Bektaş, Ö.; Yılmaz, A.; Kendirli, T.; Şıklar, Z.; Deda, G.; Yilmaz, A.; Kendirli, T. Hashimoto encephalopathy causing drug-resistant status epilepticus treated with plasmapheresis. *Pediatr. Neurol.* **2012**, *46*, 132–135. [CrossRef] [PubMed]

32. Pari, E.; Rinaldi, F.; Premi, E.; Codella, M.; Rao, R.; Paghera, B.; Panarotto, M.B.; De Maria, G.; Padovani, A. A follow-up 18F-FDG brain PET study in a case of Hashimoto's encephalopathy causing drug-resistant status epilepticus treated with plasmapheresis. *J. Neurol.* **2014**, *261*, 663–667. [CrossRef] [PubMed]

33. Mittal, M.K.; Rabinstein, A.A.; Hocker, S.E.; Pittock, S.J.; Wijdicks, E.F.M.; McKeon, A. Autoimmune encephalitis in the ICU: Analysis of phenotypes, serologic findings, and outcomes. *Neurocritical Care* **2015**, *24*, 240–250. [CrossRef] [PubMed]

34. Dubovsky, A.N.; Arvikar, S.; Stern, T.A.; Axelrod, L. The neuropsychiatric complications of glucocorticoid use: Steroid psychosis revisited. *Psychosomatics* **2012**, *53*, 103–115. [CrossRef]

35. Berger, B.; Hottenrott, T.; Leubner, J.; Dersch, R.; Rauer, S.; Stich, O.; Prüss, H. Transient spurious intrathecal immunoglobulin synthesis in neurological patients after therapeutic apheresis. *BMC Neurol.* **2015**, *15*, 1–6. [CrossRef]

36. Jurek, B.; Chayka, M.; Kreye, J.; Lang, K.; Kraus, L.; Fidzinski, P.; Kornau, H.; Dao, L.; Wenke, N.K.; Long, M.; et al. Human gestational N -methyl- d -aspartate receptor autoantibodies impair neonatal murine brain function. *Ann. Neurol.* **2019**, *86*, 656–670. [CrossRef]

37. Dahm, L.; Ott, C.; Steiner, J.; Stepniak, B.; Teegen, B.; Saschenbrecker, S.; Hammer, C.; Borowski, K.; Begemann, M.; Lemke, S.; et al. Seroprevalence of autoantibodies against brain antigens in health and disease. *Ann. Neurol.* **2014**, *76*, 82–94. [CrossRef]

38. Coutinho, E.; Jacobson, L.; Pedersen, M.G.; Benros, M.E.; Nørgaard-Pedersen, B.; Mortensen, P.B.; Harrison, P.J.; Vincent, A. CASPR2 autoantibodies are raised during pregnancy in mothers of children with mental retardation and disorders of psychological development but not autism. *J. Neurol. Neurosurg. Psychiatry* **2017**, *88*, 718–721. [CrossRef]

39. Colpo, A.; Marson, P.; Pavanello, F.; Tison, T.; Gervasi, M.T.; Zambon, A.; Ruffatti, A.; De Silvestro, G.; Hoxha, A. Therapeutic apheresis during pregnancy: A single center experience. *Transfus. Apher. Sci.* **2019**, *58*, 652–658. [CrossRef]

40. Özkale, M.; Erol, I.; Özkale, Y.; Kozanoğlu, I. Overview of therapeutic plasma exchange in pediatric neurology: A single-center experience. *Acta Neurol. Belg.* **2018**, *118*, 451–458. [CrossRef]

41. Armangue, T.; Olivé-Cirera, G.; Martínez-Hernandez, E.; Sepulveda, M.; Ruiz-Garcia, R.; Muñoz-Batista, M.; Ariño, H.; González-Álvarez, V.; Felipe-Rucián, A.; Martínez-González, M.J.; et al. Associations of paediatric demyelinating and encephalitic syndromes with myelin oligodendrocyte glycoprotein antibodies: A multicentre observational study. *Lancet Neurol.* **2020**, *19*, 234–246. [CrossRef]

42. Doss, S.; Wandinger, K.-P.; Hyman, B.T.; Panzer, J.A.; Synofzik, M.; Dickerson, B.; Mollenhauer, B.; Scherzer, C.R.; Ivinson, A.J.; Finke, C.; et al. High prevalence of NMDA receptor IgA/IgM antibodies in different dementia types. *Ann. Clin. Transl. Neurol.* **2014**, *1*, 822–832. [CrossRef] [PubMed]

43. Flanagan, E.P.; Drubach, D.A.; Boeve, B.F. Autoimmune dementia and encephalopathy. *Handb. Clin. Neurol.* **2016**, *133*, 247–267. [CrossRef] [PubMed]

44. Miske, R.; Gross, C.C.; Scharf, M.; Golombeck, K.S.; Hartwig, M.; Bhatia, U.; Schulte-Mecklenbeck, A.; Bönte, K.; Strippel, C.; Schöls, L.; et al. Neurochondrin is a neuronal target antigen in autoimmune cerebellar degeneration. *Neurol. Neuroimmunol. Neuroinflamm.* **2016**, *4*, e307. [CrossRef]

45. Weisenhorn, D.M.V.; Floss, T.; Wurst, W.; Istvánffy, R. Expression of neurochondrin in the developing and adult mouse brain. *Dev. Genes Evol.* **2004**, *214*, 206–209. [CrossRef]

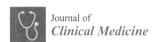

Journal of
Clinical Medicine

Review

Therapeutic Apheresis in Acute Relapsing Multiple Sclerosis: Current Evidence and Unmet Needs—A Systematic Review

Leoni Rolfes [1,*,†], Steffen Pfeuffer [1,†], Tobias Ruck [1], Nico Melzer [1], Marc Pawlitzki [1], Michael Heming [1], Marcus Brand [2], Heinz Wiendl [1] and Sven G. Meuth [1]

[1] Department of Neurology with Institute of Translational Neurology, University Hospital Muenster, Albert-Schweitzer-Campus 1, 48149 Muenster, Germany; steffen.pfeuffer@ukmuenster.de (S.P.); tobias.ruck@ukmuenster.de (T.R.); nico.melzer@ukmuenster.de (N.M.); marc.pawlitzki@ukmuenster.de (M.P.); michaeloleg.heming@ukmuenster.de (M.H.); heinz.wiendl@ukmuenster.de (H.W.); sven.meuth@ukmuenster.de (S.G.M.)
[2] Department of Internal Medicine D, University Hospital Münster, Albert-Schweitzer-Campus 1, 48149 Muenster, Germany; marcus.brand@ukmuenster.de
*   Correspondence: leoni.rolfes@ukmuenster.de; Tel.: +49-(0)251-83-44463; Fax: +49-(0)251-83-46812
†   Both authors contributed equally.

Received: 16 September 2019; Accepted: 2 October 2019; Published: 4 October 2019

Abstract: Multiple sclerosis (MS) is the most abundant inflammatory demyelinating disorder of the central nervous system. Despite recent advances in its long-term immunomodulatory treatment, MS patients still suffer from relapses, significantly contributing to disability accrual. In recent years, apheresis procedures such as therapeutic plasma exchange (TPE) and immunoadsorption (IA) have been recognized as two options for treating MS relapses, that do not respond to standard treatment with corticosteroids. TPE is already incorporated in most international guidelines, although evidence for its use resulted mostly from either case series or small unblinded and/or non-randomized trials. Data on IA are still sparse, but several studies indicate comparable efficacy between both apheresis procedures. This article gives an overview of the published evidence on TPE and IA in the treatment of acute relapses in MS. Further, we outline current evidence regarding individual outcome predictors, describe technical details of apheresis procedures, and discuss apheresis treatment in children and during pregnancy.

Keywords: immunoadsorption; acute relapsing multiple sclerosis; plasma exchange; therapeutic apheresis

1. Introduction

In multiple sclerosis (MS), the complex interplay between environmental factors and susceptibility genes leads to the development of inflammatory brain lesions defined by oligodendrocyte death and axonal damage, recovery of function and structural repair, post-inflammatory gliosis, and neurodegeneration. Besides, disruption of the blood–brain barrier (BBB) and enhanced transendothelial migration of immune cells early in the course of MS likely contribute to the disturbance of neuronal integrity [1]. Numerous reports describe MS as a primarily T cell-mediated disorder [2,3]. However, findings such as immunoglobulin and complement deposits in demyelinating brain lesions, the presence of intrathecal immunoglobulin synthesis, and results from clinical trials on B cell depletion therapies suggest a pivotal role for B cells as well [4–6]. Several well-accepted roles for B cells in MS include the secretion of the central nervous system (CNS)-directed autoantibodies, B cell-dependent maturation of autoreactive CD4[+] T cells, and dysregulation of cytokine responses [7–9].

Despite great advances in disease-modifying treatment, treatment for acute MS relapses has remained largely unaltered for the past 20 years, namely treatment with intravenous or oral corticosteroids [10]. The administration of high-dose intravenous methylprednisolone (IVMPS; up to 1000 mg daily) over a period of three to five days usually represents the first step in acute MS relapse treatment and has been endorsed by national and international guidelines, ever since a first prospective, randomized trial showed superiority of IVMPS compared to placebo [9,11]. The rationale here is primarily attributed to a non-genomic response, including a direct effect on cellular membranes, leading to a suppression of cell-mediated processes (suppression of immune-cell-migration, restitution of BBB integrity), as well as dose-dependent induction of T- cell apoptosis [12,13]. Although there is evidence for faster recovery of relapses by IVMPS treatment, there have been notable proponents for no effect of IVMPS treatment on long-term disability [14]. Furthermore, approximately one-quarter of the patient's clinical improvement is not sufficient after the first course of IVMPS [15]. In this context, apart from extending steroid treatment to a higher dose (up to 2000 mg daily for five additional days), apheresis procedures, such as therapeutic plasma exchange (TPE) and immunoadsorption (IA) are considered as an alternative after their proven success in other neurological diseases [16–18]. Here, the lead (immuno)-pathogenetic principle for both apheresis modalities (TPE and IA) is based on the removal of circulating, pathogenic humoral factors such as autoantibodies, immune complexes and inflammatory cytokines, and the modification of pro-inflammatory mediators and co-stimulatory signals linked to T and B cell-mediated autoimmunity [19–21].

However, guidelines have no uniform recommendations on using TPE or IA in acute steroid-refractory MS relapses. Both procedures are recommended by the German Society of Neurology for escalation treatment of acute relapsing-remitting MS (RRMS) exacerbations not responding to the first IVMPS course [22]. The American Academy of Neurology also advises the use of TPE for adjunctive treatment of relapsing forms of MS (Level B), while IA is not addressed [23]. In 2016, the American Society for Apheresis published evidence-based guidelines for the clinical use of therapeutic apheresis, considering 16 neurological disorders. The modality recommended for most of these disorders was TPE. The clinical indication category assigns TPE for treatment of MS to category II ("apheresis accepted as second-line therapy") and IA for treatment of RRMS to category III ("optimum role of apheresis therapy is not established") [23].

Since several studies demonstrated that residual deficits persist after MS relapses and contribute to a stepwise progression of disability, fast and adequate therapy of relapses is indispensable, and the optimal treatment sequence has to be well defined [24,25]. Thus, we here aimed to conduct a review of the published literature that provides a general overview of available evidence using apheresis treatment in inflammatory demyelinating relapses, and in more detail outlines specific treatment-determining aspects.

2. Search Strategy

To conduct this review, we followed PRISMA (Preferred Reporting Items for Systematic Reviews and Meta-Analyses) guidelines [26]. The articles were independently screened for eligibility.

2.1. Inclusion Criteria

Studies had to meet the following inclusion criteria:

a. Cohort: Reporting response rates of at least one patient with an established diagnosis of clinically-isolated syndrome (CIS) or RRMS (according to the McDonald or Poser criteria) or optic neuritis (ON) in absence of any other infectious or inflammatory disease of the CNS after treatment due to an acute relapse that is unresponsive to steroids [27–30].

b. Treatment regimens: Apheresis was preceded by relapse therapy with high-dose steroids. No concomitant immunomodulatory relapse treatment was carried out simultaneously while using the apheresis procedures. Technical details of apheresis procedures adhered to current guidelines described in the 2016 consensus paper (number of TPE/IA courses: 4–7 (mean);

patient's estimated plasma volume (EPV) per session: 0.6–2.5; for TPE: Fluid replacement with albumin) [31].

c. Outcome measure: Reporting at least one clinical outcome measure of apheresis; such as the expanded disability status scale (EDSS), its functional systems scores (FSS), or visual acuity (VA) [32].

Application of inclusion criteria: a. was mandatory for inclusion. If criteria b. and/or c. were not met, authors were contacted for additional data. Only in the case of insufficient information were the studies ultimately excluded.

2.2. Search Strategy

To identify studies, MEDLINE was searched for relevant articles published between 1 January 1980 and 30 April 2019 (in the English or German language). Additionally, we decided to evaluate abstracts from international conferences, namely Annual Meeting - American Academy of Neurology (AAN) and European/ Americas committee for treatment and research in multiple sclerosis (ECTRIMS/ ACTRIMS). Medical Subject Headings (MeSH) terms used were 'multiple sclerosis', and 'plasma exchange' or 'immunoadsorption'. Furthermore, reference lists of published articles and abstracts were screened for additional studies (Figure 1).

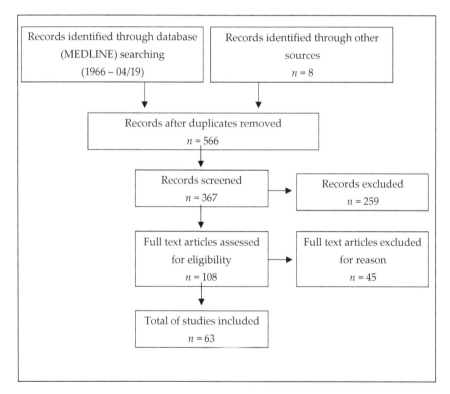

Figure 1. PRISMA flow diagram of the reviewed literature.

3. Results

3.1. General Efficacy of Apheresis Procedures

3.1.1. Therapeutic Plasma Exchange in Acute MS Relapse

TPE is an extracorporeal blood purification technique separating plasma from blood and involves the removal of patient plasma and the replacement with another fluid. TPE treatment of isolated ON, acute RRMS, and CIS, refractory to conventional pulsed IVMPS, has been evaluated in several studies [19,33–42]. Unfortunately, studies assessing functional outcomes of apheresis treatment used different outcome measures, usually referring to either the EDSS or its FSS. Reasoning that the most sensitive outcome was likely to be the one that addressed relapse-related disability, several studies primarily assessed changes in the 'target neurologic deficit' (TND), defined as the predominant symptom matching the FSS [19,34,35,38,42]. To simplify the statistical analysis, the majority of the reviewed studies classified recovery according to the response categories 'no, mild, moderate, and marked' (Table 1) [19,34–36,38,41,43–45]. Satisfying treatment success was mainly defined as 'marked to moderate' response. However, some studies also contained different classifications and/or other outcome parameters such as visual evoked potentials or gait/power scales from Weinshenker [33,39,42,46,47].

Table 1. Classification of treatment response in the reviewed literature.

Level of Improvement	Definition
'no response'	the same or even worse compared to baseline
'mild response'	clinically detectable improvement but not relevant to function score
'moderate response'	changes in function score
'marked response'	major improvement or restitution of function

Here we outline both the response rates defined by the individual studies, as well as a uniform transformation of the data according to the 'FSS-based relapse recovery model' implemented by Conway and colleagues (Figure 2) [48]. The outcome model was based on the changes between the peak deficit and maximum recovery in FSS related to relapse (ΔFSS = FSS relapse peak – FSS maximum recovery). Relapse specific changes in FSS were defined as a 'good', 'average', or 'worse' response to apheresis. Although patients' individual EDSS or FSS were not outlined consistently throughout the different trials, we extracted the indicated FSS of ON, RRMS, and CIS patients where possible, taking all limitations of comparability into account. Table 2 gives an overview of published TPE data.

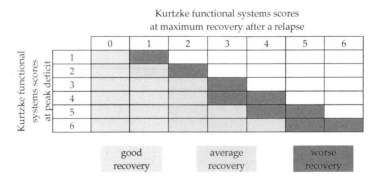

Figure 2. Functional systems score (FSS) based relapse recovery model. Good, average, and worse recovery is assigned based on the peak FSS, and the amount of final stabilized recovery FSS reached. Modified from Conway et al. [48].

J. Clin. Med. **2019**, *8*, 1623

Table 2. Overview of publications on therapeutic plasma exchange in acute MS relapses.

Author	Publ. Year	Journal	Study Design	Disease Entity (no)	Sample Size	Outcome Parameter	Results in Regard to RRMS/CIS Patients	Results according to the Conway Matrix	Reference
Weinshenker BG.	1999	Ann Neurol	Prospective randomized, sham-controlled	RRMS (13), other IIDD (9)	22	EDSS (TND), gait/power scale	Relevant improvement in 8/19 patients (42%) after TPE vs. 1/17 (6%) after sham	N/A	[33]
Trebst C.	2009	Blood Purification	Prospective	RRMS (15), CIS (3), NMO (2)	20	EDSS (TND), VA, VEP	Marked to moderate improvement in 18/20 patients (90%)	Good response: 1/20 (5%) average response: 11/20 (55%), worse response: 8/20 (40%)	[34]
Schilling S.	2006	Nervenarzt	Retrospective	RRMS (6), CIS (5), NMO (2)	13	FSS, VA	Marked to moderate improvement in 8/11 patients (73%)	Good response: 1/11 (9%) average response: 4/11 (36%), worse response: 6/11 (55%)	[35]
Schroeder A.	2009	Aktuelle Neurologie	Retrospective	RRMS (22), CIS (9), SPMS (2), NMO (2)	35	EDSS (TND), VA	Improvement in 28/35 patients (80%)	Good response: 7/35 (20%) average response: 19/35 (54%), worse response: 9/35 (26%)	[19]
Habek M.	2010	Ther Apher Dial.	Retrospective	RRMS	4	EDSS	Marked to moderate improvement in 3/4 patients (75%)	Good response: 1/4 (25%) average response: 2/4 (50%), worse response: 1/4 (25%)	[36]
Ehler J.	2014	Ther Apher Dial.	Retrospective	CIS	11	EDSS (TND)	Marked improvement in 2/11 patients (18%), mild improvement in 8/11 patients (73%)	Good response: 1/11 (9%) average response: 7/11 (64%), worse response: 3/11 (27%)	[38]
Llufriu S.	2009	Neurology	Retrospective, multicentre	RRMS (22), CIS (5), other IIDD (17)	41	EDSS	Improvement in 11/24 patients (46%)	N/A	[39]
Magana SM.	2012	Arch Neurol.	Retrospective	RRMS (55), CIS (5) NMO 26), other IIDD (67)	153	EDSS (TND)	Marked to moderate improvement in 38/60 patients (63%)	N/A	[41]
Pfeuffer S.	2018	Multiple Sclerosis Journal	Retrospective	CIS, RRMS	99	EDSS (TND), FSS	N/A	Good response: 33/99 (33%) average response: 45/99 (46%), worse response: 21/99 (21%)	[42]

Abbreviations: CIS (clinically isolated syndrome), EDSS (Expanded Disability Status Scale), FSS (functional systems score), IIDD (idiopathic inflammatory demyelinating disorder), TND (target neurologic deficit), N/A (not applicable), NMO (neuromyelitis optica), RRMS (relapsing-remitting multiple sclerosis), SPMS (secondary-progressive multiple sclerosis), VA (visual acuity), VEP (visual evoked potentials).

Studies

Up to now, only two prospective studies have been carried out [33,34]. In 1999, Weinshenker and colleagues conducted a randomized, sham-controlled and double-blind crossover trial, including 22 patients with acute, steroid-refractory relapses. While 13 patients were diagnosed with RRMS according to the Poser criteria, the other nine patients suffered from more or less specifically defined demyelinating disorders [30,33]. Half of the patients received TPE, while the others underwent a sham procedure in which the blood was separated within the apheresis system but recombined again prior to re-infusion. Patients that did not achieve a marked or moderate improvement crossed over to the other treatment arm. At discharge, 8 out of 19 patients (42%) had improved relevantly during the two-week course of active treatment, compared to 1 out of 17 patients (6%) in the sham group.

The second perspective but not the placebo-controlled study, published in 2009 by Trebst and colleagues, evaluated 20 patients with acute MS relapses and found a marked to moderate improvement in 18 out of the 20 patients (90%) following apheresis therapy [34].

Findings in the two prospective studies were underscored by several retrospective trials [19,35,36,38–41]. Two groups demonstrated comparable TPE response rates, revealing a marked to moderate response in 8 out of 11 patients (73%) and in 28 out of 35 patients (80%) at discharge [19,35]. Corroborating results from a small case series recorded a marked to moderate response in 3 out of 4 (71%) one month after TPE [36]. Contrastingly, Ehler and colleagues considered the response rate to be much lower: Following apheresis therapy, they detected a marked to moderate response in only 2 out of 11 patients (18%), while a mild response was observed in 8 out of 11 patients (73%) [38]. However, the remaining demographic characteristics and technical details of apheresis, including cycles and processed plasma volumes (PPV) did not differ substantially compared to other reviewed studies (Table 3). A slightly lower response rate was also demonstrated in a multicentre study conducted by Llufriu and colleagues with an improvement (not otherwise specified) in 11 out of 24 patients (46%) only [39]. As this study evaluated outcomes after six months, and thus later than the other trials, the sustainability of effects observed after TPE was questionable. Of note, Magana and colleagues also assessed the clinical course of 60 RRMS and CIS patients six months following TPE and revealed a rate of moderate or even marked response of 68% [41]. Several other studies with long-term data on apheresis-treated patients revealed sustained or even increased functionality during follow-up (1 to 14 months) with no new relapses occurring in between [19,34,35].

Table 3. Overview of technical details on therapeutic plasma exchange (TPE) and immunoadsorption (IA)in acute MS relapse.

Author	IVMPS Refractory	Number of Cycles (range)	Possessed Plasma Volume	Replacement Fluid	Vascular Access	Reference
			Therapeutic plasma exchange			
Weinshenker BG.	yes	7–14	1.1 EVP	5% albumin	CVA	[33]
Trebst C.	yes	3–7	3.0–4.2 L	5% albumin	CVA	[34]
Schilling S.	yes	4–6	3.0 L	4% albumin	CVA	[35]
Schroeder A.	yes	4–6	50 mL/KgBW	5% albumin	CVA	[19]
Habek M.	yes	5–10	1.5 L	5% albumin	N/A	[36]
Ehler J.	yes	3–8	2.2–3.5 L	5% albumin	PV, CVA	[38]
Llufriu S.	yes	5–15	125–166 EPV	5% albumin	N/A	[39]
Magana SM.	yes	2–20	1.1–1.4 EPV	5% albumin, FFP	N/A	[41]
Lammerding L.	yes	5	15 EPV	5% albumin	CVA	[42]
			Immunoadsorption (tryptophan-based)			
Koziolek M.	yes	5	2.5 L	None	CVA	[40]
Mauch E.	yes	5–6	2.0 L	None	PV, CVA	[47]
Schimrigk S.	yes	3–6	2.0–2.5 L	None	CVA	[44]
Schimrigk S.	yes	3–6	2.0–2.5 L	None	CVA	[45]
Trebst C.	yes	5–7	2.5 L	None	CVA	[44]
Heigl F.	yes	6	2.0 L	None	PV, CVA	[49]

Abbreviations: CVA (central venous access), EPV (estimated plasma volume), FFP (fresh-frozen plasma), IVMPS (intravenous methylprednisolone), kgBW (kilogram per body weight), liter (L), PV (peripheral vein).

For a uniform transformation of data, according to the Conway model (Figure 2), six studies were accessible, outlining the patient's FSS before apheresis and at discharge [19,34–36,38,42]. In total, 181 patients were included in this analysis. Forty-four patients (24%) experienced a good response, 89 patients (49%) an average response, and 48 patients (27%) a worse response.

3.1.2. Immunoadsorption in Acute MS Relapse

IA has entered the field of MS treatment as a new important method for selective extracorporeal adsorption. In contrast to standard TPE, the eluted plasma can be reinfused during IA, suggesting a better tolerability and safety profile [50]. Two technical options have been developed: Single-use tryptophan-based adsorbers and reusable IgG Protein A containing staphylococci-based adsorbers (PrA-adsorbers). Single-pass devices are used for only one session, while their capacity is limited to approximately 2.0 to 2.5 L (L) of plasma volume. A treatment with tryptophan adsorber and conventional plasma separator results in an elimination of 30% of immunoglobulin IgG and IgM, 15% of IgA, 10% of the patient's total protein and approximately 60%–70% of the fibrinogen during a single treatment, with a PPV of 2 L [51,52].

In contrast, a semi-selective (defined by the adsorption of mainly immunoglobulins (>95%), but not directed against a specific antibody) reusable PrA based devices can provide continuous IA to treat more than one EPV per session. Strong affinity for Fc fragments of immunoglobulins from any source is a remarkable characteristic of protein A. After one session with a PPV of 2,5 L a decrease in total serum IgG level of 87%, 55% of the IgA and 56% of the IgM level occur, without a clinically significant loss of fibrinogen (less than 15%) [53].

In the last two decades, six studies have been published on IA therapy for RRMS or CIS, including one prospective study [43–47,49]. All studies used tryptophan based adsorbers (Table 3). In order to compare these to the TPE studies, we separately reviewed the response rates for ON, RRMS, and CIS patients where possible and further assessed the patient's FSS according to the Conway outcome assessment tool [48]. Table 4 gives an overview of the published IA data.

Table 4. Overview of publications on immunoadsorption in acute MS relapse.

Author	Publication Year	Journal	Study Design	Disease Entity (no)	Sample Size	Outcome Parameter	Results in Regard to RRMS/CIS	Results according to the Conway Matrix	Reference
Koziolek M.	2012	J. Neuro- Inflamm.	Prospective	RRMS, CIS	11	VA, VEP	Significant improvement in 8/11 patients (73%)	N/A	[-]
Mauch E.	2011	Nervenarzt	Retrospective	RRMS (11), SPMS (2); NMO (1)	14	EDSS (TND), VA	Significant improvement in 12/14 patients (86%)	Good response: 2/14 (14%) average response: 7/14 (50%), worse response: 5/14 (36%)	[-]
Schimrigk S.	2012	Aktuelle Neurologie	Retrospective, multicentr	RRMS (15), SPMS (9)	24	EDSS, VA	Marked to moderate improvement in 12/15 patients (80%)	Good response: 2/24 (8%) average response: 11/24 (46%), worse response: 11/24 (46%)	[-]
Schimrigk S.	2016	Eur Neurol.	Retrospective, multicentre	RRMS (111), SPMS (36)	147	EDSS	Marked to moderate improvement in 105/147 patients (71%)	N/A	[-]
Trebst C.	2012	Blood Purif	Retrospective	RRMS (8), CIS (2)	10	EDSS, VA, VEP	Marked to moderate improvement in 5/10 patients (50%)	Good response: 1/10 (10%) average response: 2/10 (20%), worse response: 7/10 (30%)	[-]
Heigl F.	2013	Athero-sclerosis supp.	Retrospective	RRMS	60	EDSS, VA	Marked to mild improvement in 53/60 patients (88%)	N/A	[-]

Abbreviations: CIS (clinically isolated syndrome), EDSS (Expanded Disability Status Scale), N/A (not applicable), NMO (neuromyelitis optica), ON (optic neuritis), RRMS (relapsing-remitting multiple sclerosis), SPMS (secondary-progressive multiple sclerosis), TND (target neurological deficit), VA (visual acuity), VEP (visual evoked potentials).

J. Clin. Med. **2019**, *8*, 1623

Studies

One prospective study has been conducted on IA in acute RRMS [46]. Koziolek and colleagues reported a significant improvement (defined as improved VA with 0.6 cc or more) in 8 out of 11 patients (73%) suffering from acute steroid-refractory ON (mean VA at baseline 0.12 ± 0.12 compared to 0.47 ± 0.32 at discharge). In four out of six patients (67%), visual evoked potentials could not be identified before treatment but were re-detectable after IA [46].

Various retrospective studies are in line with these data [43–45,47,49]. Mauch and colleagues reviewed the clinical course of 14 patients suffering from acute relapses of either RRMS (*n* = 12) or secondary-progressive multiple sclerosis (SPMS, *n* = 2). TND in 12 out of 14 patients (86%) significantly improved (assessed via EDSS, FSS not further specified) [47]. Corroborating results from Schimrigk and colleagues revealed 12 out of 15 patients (80%) with a marked to moderate response to IA [44]. In a subsequent retrospective multicenter study, Schimrigk and colleagues analyzed the largest cohort of MS patients treated with IA thus far, comprising six sites with 147 patients and 786 single IA treatments [45]. All patients suffered from an acute relapse of either RRMS (111 patients) or SPMS (36 patients). In 105 patients (71%), the affected TND improved functionally, including 88 patients (60%) with marked and 17 patients (11%) with moderate treatment response. Further studies indicated a marked to moderate response in 5 out of 10 patients (50%), and a marked to mild response (not precisely differentiated) in 53 out of 60 patients (88%) at discharge [43,49].

As the patient's individual EDSS and FSS was not outlined consistently throughout the IA trials, a uniform transformation of data was not possible (only the data of 48 patients out of 3 individual studies were accessible) [43,44,47].

Comment

Guidelines on apheresis therapies currently refer to TPE only, since data on IA are considered less substantial [54]. Nevertheless, existing studies with individual outcome assessments indicated IA as effective with similar response rates compared to TPE (42%–90% for TPE vs. 50%–86% for IA) [19,33–36,38,43–47,49]. The limitations regarding the comparability of studies must be considered though. Criteria for patient selection and diagnosis significantly changed over time, and, therefore, characteristics of RRMS trial populations are diverging, probably resulting in lead-time bias [28,29]. In this context, a significant number of novel pharmacological agents have not just entered the field but even defined the treatment of active MS to date.

Additionally, the time points for apheresis therapy and evaluation of outcome parameters selected differed considerably throughout the trials. While EDSS assessment is universally familiar to MS clinicians and accepted by regulators, it has shortcomings in its variability between examiners, heavy emphasis on walking, and especially nonlinearity [55]. Consequently, several relapses associated with upper limb involvement are not reflected in terms of pre-existing gait impairment. Moreover, trials do not reflect whether a particular patient does not reconstitute at discharge or goes on to develop a persistent disability. In this context, in addition to evaluating the overall response, future studies should also cover the time between discharge and recovery, since complete but delayed recovery may still mean loss of independence and a need for rehabilitation or intermediate care. The main recovery has been suggested to take place within the first three months following relapse [24]. Hence, if an outcome is measured at discharge only, it may not be a suitable marker for overall improvement. On the other hand, a longer observation period carries the risk of detecting disabilities resulting from new relapses; confirmed disability progression at six months should be included as an outcome parameter in future study designs.

3.1.3. Comparison of Apheresis Treatments (TPE vs. IA)

Despite the multitude of studies evaluating TPE or IA treatment of acute MS relapses separately, only a few studies compared both extracorporeal blood purification methods in terms of clinical efficacy, safety profile, and serological changes [21,54,56,57]. Assessing IA effectiveness is complicated even more by the co-existence of different IA systems (tryptophan based absorbers and PrA-based absorbers).

Studies

Two retrospective studies directly compared the efficacy of both apheresis treatments and described IA and TPE as equally effective for treating steroid-refractory relapses of MS [21,54]. Muhlhausen and colleagues included 140 patients with steroid-refractory exacerbation of MS and neuromyelitis optica (NMO), while Palm et al. compared the clinical efficacy of TPE and IA in acute relapses of RRMS as well as progressive forms, respectively [21,54].

In terms of treatment safety, IA is associated with fewer side effects and fewer contraindications [56,57]. Accordingly, the reviewed studies revealed a lower rate of adverse events (AE) during and following IA compared to TPE. Side effects and discomfort were apparent in 0.8%–15% of IA treatments [43–45,47,49]. In contrast, Koziolek and colleagues reported a higher side effect rate, with 22% mild and moderate AEs occurring during IA (12/55 IA treatments) [46]. Most AEs were classified according to the Common Terminology Criteria for Adverse Events (CTCAE) category I–II and were related to symptoms such as transient hypotension accompanied by dizziness and nausea, chest pain, palpitations, and headache. Side effects classified as CTCAE categories III–IV were mainly caused by vascular access and catheter-associated complications [45–47,49]. In this context, catheter dislocations (1/266 patients from all reviewed IA studies, specifying AEs in detail (Table 4)) and infections (3/266 IA patients), and catheter-associated thrombosis (6/266 patients) with one case of pulmonary embolism represent the most relevant risks after IA [45–47,49]. Moreover, one case of heparin-induced thrombocytopenia and one case of bradykinin-associated shock following a single administration of an ACE inhibitor have been described [49]. No study observed AEs classified as CTCAE category V following IA.

Notably, side effects reported for TPE were classified higher and were apparent in 24%–80% of all TPE treatments [19,33–36,38,39,42]. In particular, the risk of apheresis-related AEs with CTCAE categories I–III was higher for TPE than IA. Apart from the symptoms listed above, TPE AEs were also related to coagulopathy (including fibrinogen decrease), hypogammaglobulinamia, an allergic rash, paraesthesia, and anemia [33,35,38,39,42]. The rate of catheter-associated AEs were slightly higher compared to those of IA patients, with catheter dislocations (7/246 patients out of all reviewed TPE studies, specifying AEs in detail (Table 2), catheter-associated thrombosis (9/246 patients) and catheter-associated infections (11/246 patients), including one case of severe sepsis [19,33–36,38,39,42]. Additionally, one patient developed a catheter-associated phrenic nerve palsy, one patient a pneumothorax, and another patient experienced gastrointestinal bleeding, associated with hypofibrinogenemia [33,35,42]. Moreover, one patient died due to pulmonary embolism following TPE [33].

Comment

Based on the current literature, both treatments appear comparably effective. However, several studies described particular advantages in terms of safety for IA versus TPE [56,57]. IA avoids the removal of key plasma components with a milder impact on the cardiovascular system and a lower risk of allergic reactions and coagulopathy potentially underlying the more favorable safety outcomes.

According to American (ClinicalTrials.gov) and European (EudraCT) registries, further clinical comparative studies are in preparation. A prospective randomized trial, comparing both procedures in 60 RRMS and CIS patients with acute relapses, has been completed recently (NCT02671682); study results thus far unpublished.

In terms of technical options, all current IA studies employ single-use tryptophan-based absorber columns. Although PrA-based absorbers have been shown to be more effective in pure antibody depletion, the two techniques have not been compared in MS treatment thus far [58]. However, the responsiveness of steroid-refractory MS relapses to apheresis therapy is unlikely to depend on antibody clearance alone, since the clinical course of the disease is not correlated with autoantibody titers, and identification of crucial antibody targets remains elusive [59,60].

3.2. Individual Predictors of Apheresis Outcome

Comprehensive predictive models of individual treatment response to apheresis are lacking. This includes clinical, radiographic, and serological features to characterize individual differences in apheresis outcome. Several factors may exhibit a predictive value for apheresis response, including age, sex, monofocal or multifocal relapse manifestation, the affected functional system, previous success or failure to apheresis procedures in a preceding relapse, as well as technical aspects of TPE and IA [41,61]. However, the current literature is controversial, and whether predictors should be included in clinical decisions remains to be defined.

Using individual patient data from the respective studies, we performed an analysis of the literature using the Conway Matrix (Figure 2) to identify predictive factors for the TPE response. We included all studies that met the above inclusion criteria and outlined the complete sets of individual patient data, including all predictors we aimed to analyze. Overall, we included five studies with a total of 146 patients [34–36,42,62]. Statistical analysis was performed with R 3.6.1. The mean of the predictors was determined and categorized by the TPE response. Next, the data were scaled, centered, and depicted in a heatmap (Figure 3A). In order to determine the adjusted odds ratio of the predictors, a multivariate binomial logistic regression was performed (Figure 3B). Adjusted odds ratios with confidence intervals were displayed in a forest plot. Due to insufficient data in the IA arm, analysis in this cohort was not possible.

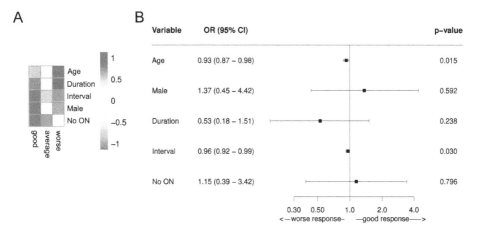

Figure 3. Predictive values of TPE response assessed by the functional systems score (FSS)-based relapse recovery model. (**A**) Predictive risk heatmap, applicable in individual patients, using three different outcome classifications (good, average, and worse) according to the Conway matrix (Figure 2) [48]. The heatmap depicts the scaled means of the variables. The red color indicates older patients (Age), with a higher prevalence of not suffering the first demyelinating event (Duration), a long interval between symptom onset and initiation of TPE (Interval), higher occurrence of male patients (Male), and a higher prevalence of relapse manifestations other than optic neuritis (no ON). (**B**) A forest plot of the predictive values of the TPE response in a multivariate logistic regression analysis. The x-axis represents the respective adjusted odd ratios for a worse versus good response. Odds ratios are outlined with a 95% confidence interval (CI; OR >1 no predictive value of treatment response, <1 statistic significant value associated with beneficial apheresis response). Data were generated in the RRMS and CIS patient cohort of five individual studies, including a total of 146 patients. All patients received TPE due to steroid unresponsive relapse [34–36,42,62].

3.2.1. Patient Dependent Variables (age, sex, neurological status, disease duration, and previous success or failure to apheresis)

Several studies have shown that the relapse recovery after IVMPS treatment linearly declines with age [48,63]. Correspondingly, our analysis of the literature revealed a positive association between poor TPE outcome and older age (Figure 3) [34–36,42,62]. This finding was statistically significant, as the adjusted OR for age was 0.93 (0.87–0.98, p <0.05).

Moreover, one observational study associated the male sex with a more favorable treatment response [61]. Of note, our analysis confirmed this observation, also indicating a trend towards a beneficial TPE response in male patients (Figure 3). However, this finding was not statistically significant.

Magana and colleagues further postulated a shorter disease course to be associated with a favorable TPE outcome [11]. We evaluated the impact of the disease course by implementing two groups: The first demyelinating event vs. not the first demyelinating event. Our analysis showed the superiority of the first demyelinating event compared to not, for treatment response to TPE and thus confirmed the above-mentioned observation (Figure 3) [34–36,42,62]. However, this finding was not statistically significant either.

Additionally, a retrospective study by Llufriu and colleagues revealed a positive correlation between the absence of disease modifying treatment (DMT) and more frequent response to TPE [39]. Since the respective demographic data of these patients are not mentioned in this study, it is not possible to specify whether this finding is based on a younger patient cohort or a shorter disease course. However, the predictive value of DMT has not been corroborated by other studies [41,62].

In addition, it can be assumed that a favorable response to apheresis in a preceding relapse provides a beneficial predictive value. In this context, rare individual case reports from the literature support this assumption [19,36]. However, the number of cases is small (n = 3) and not accessible for a systematic analysis.

Comment

To date, no patient-related response predictors have been confirmed for apheresis. However, regarding the discussed aspects above, our analysis revealed that older age, longer disease duration, and female sex were associated with poorer TPE outcomes (Figure 3) [34–36,42,62]. Although we performed uniform evaluation techniques and only included original studies that contained both the same patient cohort and a comparable TPE protocol according to current guidelines, we have to be aware of limitations concerning the validity of our findings, such as bias in the search strategy or methodological bias.

In the long-term, further clinical trials are needed to break new ground towards personalized MS relapse therapy. Apart from the factors mentioned, there are others of interest that have not been addressed in the studies thus far. These include the baseline annualized relapse rate, radiological, and immunological findings.

3.2.2. Impact of the Affected Functional System

It has been discussed whether both subsequent long-term disability and post-relapse recovery are linked to the site of relapse manifestation [41,63–65]. Magana and colleagues described the highest response rates after TPE for brainstem and cerebellar impairments [41]. However, a relapse manifesting as ON has also been described to be associated with more favorable treatment response [48,65]. This is worth mentioning, as the proportion of patients suffering from acute ON varies considerably throughout the reviewed trials (TPE: 0%–100% [19,34–36,42,62]; IA: 25%–100% [43–47,49].

To provide better comparability, we analyzed the study data and extracted the indicated VA, transforming the values into a standardized outcome assessment tool as described above (Figure 2) [48]. Of note, demographic features such as age and sex, the dose of received steroids, the duration between symptom onset and apheresis treatment, and the number of treatment cycles did not differ between the trials.

We were able to extract a total of 151 patients from the 10 studies, treated with either TPE (*n* = 92) or IA (*n* = 59) due to acute steroid-refractory ON [19,34,35,38,42–45,47,49]. Based on the described outcome definition, 30 out of 151 patients (20%) showed "good" recovery, 66 out of 151 patients (44%) showed "average" recovery, and 55 out of 151 patients (36%) showed "worse" recovery at discharge.

IA resulted in a slightly higher proportion of patients with "good" recovery (14/59 patients, 24%) compared to TPE (16/92 patients, 17%). However, regarding the rate of non-responders, the available data indicated the inferiority of IA (31/59 patients, 52%) compared to TPE (24/92 patients, 26%).

In contrast, nine studies outlined the data of patients with relapse other than ON, including in a total of 119 patients [19,34–36,38,42–44,47]. As the respective studies did not further specify the affected functional system consistently, we included all these patients in one comparison between ON and relapses other than ON. Compared to the findings above, 29 out of 119 patients (24%) showed a good recovery (27/90 patients (30%) in the TPE, 2/29 patients (7%) in the IA group), 55 out of 119 (46%) an average recovery (40/90 patients (44%) in the TPE, 15/29 patients (52%) in the IA group), and 35 out of 119 (30%) a worse recovery (23/90 patients (26%) in the TPE, 12/29 patients (41%) in the IA group), at discharge.

Data on the comparison of ON vs. relapses other than ON regarding the TPE modality are separately outlined in Figure 3 (ON vs. No ON).

Comment

Except for acute ON, individual FSS was not indicated in the majority of the reviewed studies. This prevented further analysis of whether a specific disorder or symptom would respond more favorably to apheresis than another. Transforming VA to the new outcome model allowed us to analyze the response rate of ON to apheresis throughout the respective trials and compare them to relapses other than ON. Response rates to apheresis were homogeneously distributed, except for the study from Trebst and colleagues [19,34,35,38,42–45,47,49]. In this study, all five patients with ON showed a "worse" response to IA, and also during follow-up, only one patient improved [43]. Since both the technical data of apheresis and the demographic features of the patients did not differ from other trials, the cause for non-improvement remains elusive.

As already mentioned, we generated a heat map from the TPE data to demonstrate predictive factors of the TPE response (Figure 3). Although the finding was not statistically significant, there is a trend towards a favorable TPE outcome for relapses other than ON (no_ON, Figure 3). Unfortunately, we were not able to perform a corresponding analysis in the IA group due to missing data points. Nevertheless, findings encourage further investigations. Randomized controlled trials, investigating the response rates to both apheresis techniques regarding the relapse manifestation, with the treatment of the same individual plasma volume by TPE and IA, respectively, are needed.

3.2.3. Time to Treatment Induction/Escalation

Time from symptom onset to apheresis initiation has been of interest in many studies [34,35,39, 42,43,61]. Llufriu and colleagues demonstrated that time from relapse onset to TPE initiation was significantly shorter in patients who improved after treatment compared with those who did not respond [39]. When the days from symptom onset to apheresis initiation were stratified as ≤5 days, 16–60 days, and ≥60 days, a corresponding decrease of response rate was found (67% vs. 43% vs. 8%, respectively). Other groups also confirmed this time dependency [46,61]. Nonetheless, several studies demonstrated that even with a late TPE start patients markedly improved or recovered fully [34,38,49]. In this context, Trebst and colleagues showed treatment success with IA following a mean interval of 47.2 days—with patients being successfully treated even after more than 100 days following relapse onset [43].

Our analysis of the literature using the Conway outcome assessment tool revealed a slight, but statistically significant better TPE outcome, when initiated shortly after symptom onset (adjusted OR for shorter interval = 0.96 (0.92–0.99, *p* <0.05)) (Figure 3).

Comment

A short time interval between relapse onset and apheresis initiation is considered as a strong predictor of a good outcome, assuming nerve conduction in the early stages is blocked but not irreversibly damaged [19,35,39]. Consequently, it is recommended to initiate apheresis within six weeks after relapse onset [35,61]. However, apheresis should also be considered at later stages in patients with persistent symptoms. Unfortunately, no data exist thus far to aid the identification of potential responders. Nevertheless, we assume time to apheresis is one important modifying factor related to treatment outcome.

3.2.4. Pre-Treatment with Steroids

Currently, there is no satisfying estimation of the contribution of steroid-treatment before apheresis to treatment success. The reviewed literature includes patients having received 2.0–15 g IVMPS prior to apheresis [19,33,34,36,38,43,45–47,49]. Steroids were administered after a median of 8–12 days (range: 1 to 68 days) after symptom onset and the time interval between the start of IVMPS and apheresis varied between 3 to 92 days. A limitation in all the studies is the absence of a placebo-treated control group. Thus, a spontaneous late improvement or a delayed effect of corticosteroids cannot be formally excluded. However, several aspects suggest the effects are directly associated with the apheresis procedure: No obvious correlation was apparent between the IVMPS dosage and treatment outcome, even when accounting for demographic and clinical features such as FSS, age, or sex [34,35,43]. Further, after a period of non-recovery prior to apheresis, symptoms began to improve soon after TPE or IA initiation [19,38,47,49]. In this context, several studies showed that most of the patients started to improve after the third cycle [19,38,47,49].

Further, we recently completed the first retrospective comparative study of double dose steroids and TPE in acute relapses of RRMS and CIS, including 145 patients [42]. All patients received 5g IVMPS before escalating treatment with either extended dose of IVMPS (2g/day over additionally five days), TPE (five cycles every other day, one EPV per session) or the combination of both (IVMPS, subsequently TPE). The treatment response was assessed according to the FSS-related outcome assessment tool described above (Figure 2). Good/average/worse recovery of relapse symptoms at discharge was observed in 60.9%/32.6%/6.5% of TPE patients vs. 15.2%/14.1%/70.7% of IVMPS patients. Of note, in patients who received TPE after escalated IVMPS treatment, the outcome was significantly inferior compared to those who received TPE as a first-line escalation treatment (multivariate odd's ratio for worse recovery = 39.01 (10.41–146.18; *p* <0.001)).

Comment

Thus far, there is no standard treatment approach for ongoing relapse regarding steroids and apheresis modalities. Consequently, guidelines recommend both therapies as possible options for relapse escalation treatment but give no recommendations towards a specific treatment sequence [66].

Our retrospective comparison of escalated IVMPS vs. TPE revealed significantly higher response rates at discharge in the TPE group and in patients who underwent only one course of IVMPS prior to TPE [42]. As a possible explanation, it can be hypothesized that restoring BBB permeability with IVMPS treatment may, in fact, hinder the elimination of inflammatory mediators within the CNS via apheresis. Another explanation could be the longer time to apheresis treatment when conducted as the second instead of first escalation treatment.

Based on both assumptions, it may be preferable to choose a more aggressive therapy (TPE or IA) in cases of severe relapse, rather than the escalated IVPMS treatment. However, we recommend that the rapid admission of steroid-refractory patients to apheresis treatment without escalated IVMPS treatment should be prospectively evaluated.

3.2.5. Number of Apheresis Courses and the Impact of the PPV

Guidelines currently recommend five to seven courses of apheresis treatment with a PPV according to 1.0 to 1.5 EPV [16]. An extension of further cycles can be considered on an individual basis in cases of non-response [22]. These recommendations are mostly derived from calculations of antibody concentrations. Antibody removal during a single TPE or IA treatment is limited, since (pathogenic) antibodies are often produced in abundance, with high tissue concentrations, and slowly equilibrated between their extravascular and intravascular distribution [67,68]. At least five separate treatments are required to eliminate 90% of the initial total antibody burden [69]. Further, especially for TPE, it is preferable to perform procedures every other day since exchange volumes per session are limited by the cumulative alteration of global hemostasis parameters and potentially increased bleeding risk [70,71]. Correspondingly, fibrinogen requires 48 h to recover to half of the pre-treatment level [70]. With regard to the studies discussed in this review, a comparable protocol was applied with regard to the technical aspects of therapeutic apheresis such as the volume of whole blood processed (number of cycles, number of plasma volumes exchanges per cycle), and replacement solution and vascular access, in line with recent national and international guidelines (Table 3) [31].

Comment

Current recommendations are based on calculations of antibody equilibration rates. However, there is plenty of evidence that apheresis treatment also eliminates additional soluble factors involved in acute inflammation [21]. Thus far, no studies exist examining the elimination kinetics of these additional factors. For clinical routine, the optimal number of cycles needs to be balanced in terms of achieving the best resolution of symptoms on the one hand, and keeping hospitalization times as short as possible on the other hand. In the reviewed studies, the first therapeutic effects typically occurred after a median of three apheresis cycles [19,38,47,49]. Consequently, based on kinetic considerations and clinical observations, a minimum of three to five cycles should be performed.

3.3. Apheresis Treatment in Special Situations

Although apheresis is an established therapy for adults, there is limited experience and literature on the application of apheresis in childhood or during pregnancy. The International Pediatric Multiple Sclerosis Study Group currently recommends TPE for children with severe relapses who do not improve after high-dose IVMPS or have contraindications; IA has not been implemented in the guideline [72]. However, established treatment standards for children are still lacking, and most apheresis protocols are derived from studies in adult patients [73].

Additionally, every fourth woman with MS experiences a relapse during pregnancy, and nearly every third suffers from a relapse in the first three months after birth [74]. Although the amounts of IVMPS in breastmilk are low, breastfeeding should be avoided for several hours after a high maternal dose and might occasionally cause temporary loss of milk supply [75]. Moreover, especially within the first trimester of pregnancy, high doses of IVMPS bear serious risks (preterm birth, a lower bodyweight of the child, and/or facial/palatal cleft) [76,77]. Thus, alternative treatment options are warranted. According to international guidelines, both apheresis procedures are recommended as an escalation or second-line therapy in pregnant patients with steroid unresponsive relapses [66,78].

Studies

In 2013, Koziolek and colleagues reported on the largest cohort of children undergoing apheresis treatment for severe attacks of demyelinating disorders (including RRMS; NMO-spectrum disorders and acute disseminated encephalomyelitis) refractory to IVMPS, demonstrating high and sustained recovery rates (88%) after five cycles of either TPE or IA [79]. These findings correspond to a retrospective study by Bigi and colleagues [80]. Five pediatric patients (median baseline EDSS 2.0; range: 0–3.5) were treated with TPE due to a severe attack of RRMS (median EDSS of relapse 6.5;

range 4 to 7). The mean reduction in EDSS at discharge was 3 points, sustained at follow-up after three months.

Concerning treatment safety, De Silvestro and colleagues outlined a 5.6% rate of AEs in pediatric apheresis [81]. Corroborating rates were observed by Koziolek and colleagues, indicating four relevant side effects (hypotension, acute dyspnoea, catheter dislocation, and decreased serum fibrinogen) in 50 treatment courses in 4 patients (8%) [79]. However, in a retrospective study by Michon and colleagues, a much higher AE rate was detected for pediatric patients treated with either TPE or IA (55% of all procedures, *n* = 137) compared to adult patients (16.2% of all procedures, *n* = 86) [82].

Further, one retrospective study and several case reports suggest TPE and IA treatment for acute RRMS relapse during pregnancy and breastfeeding, considering them as rather a safe option [75,83,84]. In 2018, Hoffmann and colleagues conducted the largest retrospective study on this special cohort thus far, analyzing the use of tryptophan IA during pregnancy and breastfeeding in 24 patients. Twenty patients were treated with IA during pregnancy, and four patients received IA postnatal during the breastfeeding period. In 83% of patients, a rapid and marked improvement of the TND was achieved, defined either as an EDSS decrease of ≥1.0 point or improvement in VA ≥20% at discharge. Moreover, no clinically relevant side effects were reported in connection with the 138 IA treatments [75].

Comment

Published experience of apheresis procedures in children is limited, and most of the indications for treatment and the technical and procedural aspects of the procedure are also extrapolated from adult data and experience [82].

Koziolek and colleagues showed that apheresis in children suffering from acute relapses of demyelinating disorders seems to be as effective compared to treating adult patients [79]. However, special risk factors need consideration, including citrate toxicity, extravascular volume shifts, and difficulty related to vascular access [82]. Therefore, apheresis therapy in children requires a multidisciplinary approach involving expertise in children, intensive care medicine, and nephrology. Prospective studies are clearly warranted to optimize treatment protocols and to avoid permanent disabilities in this sensitive age group.

During pregnancy, apheresis represents a therapeutic option both in first and second-line relapse treatment. In this context, IA can be considered superior to TPE for several reasons. Plasma levels of numerous hormones undergo pronounced shifts during pregnancy [85]. The protective effect of pregnancy on MS disease activity seems to be at least in part, mediated by the immunomodulatory effects of these hormones. This supports the use of IA to preserve protective plasma proteins, instead of discarding them as with TPE. A further advantage of avoiding plasma substitution is the reduced risk of allergic reactions and infections, as well as the reduced impact of coagulation factors [86]. In contrast to TPE, most coagulation factors remain unaffected by IA, except fibrinogen, especially in terms of tryptophan based IA [87]. However, no fibrinogen substitution was required in pregnancy IA studies [75]. Thus, reduced bleeding risk in the perinatal period and reduced thrombotic risk due to the reduction of antithrombin can be achieved with IA treatment compared to TPE [88]. Moreover, since IA has a milder impact on the cardiovascular system, including hypotension, it can be assumed that it is superior in terms of placenta perfusion.

3.4. Closing Remarks and Outlook

Relapses are a hallmark of MS and often associated with significant functional impairment and decreased quality of life. Consequently, MS relapses need to be recognized and treated quickly using valid therapeutic methods. Although evidence for apheresis treatment in MS relapse is mostly derived from either case series or unblinded or retrospective cohorts—especially IA has thus far not been considered in international guidelines—both procedures have become an alternative to escalated and repeated pulsed steroid therapy. In respect to our recent comparison of escalated IVMPS and TPE, apheresis procedures should even be considered as a first-line escalation treatment [42].

In regard to the preferred apheresis modality and according to the literature, IA should be regarded as a method of equivalent therapeutic efficacy compared to TPE, probably offering greater safety in its use. This is particularly relevant in special populations such as children and during pregnancy.

As the long-term goal is to enable personalized MS relapse therapy, the predictive value for apheresis response is of high interest. In this regard, our analysis and several studies highlighted time to treatment as an important and modifiable factor related to outcome (Figure 3) [39,46,61]. Consequently, apheresis should be applied as early as possible in the course of a relapse. However, since some cases describe full recovery for patients even late after symptom onset, a strict regimentation to the suggested six-week period is not recommendable. Further, our analysis considers younger age, male sex, shorter MS disease duration, and a relapse not manifesting as ON to be associated with beneficial apheresis response (Figure 3). However, these parameters (eventually apart from sex) are associated with beneficial relapse outcomes in general [89,90]. Of note, using binomial regression models, both predictive values—male sex and shorter interval between apheresis initiation and symptom onset—were statistically significant (adjusted Odd-Ratio (OR) for age: 0.93 (0.87–0.98, p <0.05); OR for shorter interval = 0.96 (0.92–0.99, p <0.05). However, as in all systematic reviews, we have to deal with several limitations, such as bias from selection and publication of studies, availability of data, choice of relevant outcome, methods of analysis, and interpretation of heterogeneity. Therefore, we should keep in mind that systematic analyses should neither be a replacement for well-designed randomized studies.

In this regard, intervention studies with a prospective, randomized, controlled design are required to compare:

(I)   TPE vs. IA (with the same plasma volume exchange (TPE) or adsorbed (IA)), and

(II)   Escalated IVMPS vs. apheresis.

With regard to the study protocol, at least five cycles should be performed every other day. Considering the diversity of MS presentation, multiple patient-related clinical outcomes should be combined with surrogate endpoints [91]. Both outcome analyses at discharge and in the long-term (follow-up period of at least three months) are recommendable. Since it remains largely unclear by which cellular and molecular pathways apheresis affect disease activity, an analysis of blood samples and IA columns would also be of high interest.

There are several hypotheses regarding the mechanism of action of the different apheresis techniques, but their discussion is beyond the scope of this review. In this regard, previous studies provided evidence that the response to apheresis treatment is associated with the immunopathological pattern, indicating that the pattern of the two patients who showed signs of a humoral immune response benefited the most [40]. Anyways, knowledge about the predominant lesion pathology is usually unavailable in clinical routine as MS patients do not undergo a brain biopsy. Given the strong effects in the overall population of both TPE and IA, the procedures should be offered to all patients with severe and/or refractory relapses. We assume that, currently, the selection of the definitive technique will be determined by side effect profile and availability. However, trials are ongoing and will be published in the nearer future.

Author Contributions: L.R.: Review concept and design, research of literature, analysis, and interpretation, writing the manuscript—original draft preparation. S.P.: Review concept and design, research of literature, analysis, and interpretation, writing the manuscript. T.R.: Critical revision of the manuscript for intellectual content—review and editing. N.M.: Critical revision of the manuscript for intellectual content—review and editing. M.P.: Critical revision of the manuscript for intellectual content—review and editing. M.H.: Statistical analysis, critical revision of the manuscript for intellectual content—review and editing. M.B.: Critical revision of the manuscript for intellectual content—review and editing. H.W.: Critical revision of the manuscript for intellectual content—review and editing. S.G.M.: Review concept and design, supervision, critical revision of manuscript for intellectual content.

Funding: This research received no external funding.

Conflicts of Interest: Leoni Rolfes: Received travel reimbursements from Merck Serono, Novartis, and Sanofi Genzyme. Steffen Pfeuffer: Received travel reimbursements from Sanofi-Genzyme and Merck Serono, honoraria

J. Clin. Med. **2019**, *8*, 1623

for lecturing from Sanofi Genzyme, Biogen, and Mylan Healthcare, and research support from Merck Serono, Diamed, and the German Multiple Sclerosis Society. Tobias Ruck: Received travel expenses and financial research support from Genzyme and Novartis, and received honoraria for lecturing from Roche, Merck, Genzyme, Biogen, and Teva. Nico Melzer: Received honoraria for lecturing and travel expenses for attending meetings from Biogen Idec, GlaxoSmith Kline, Teva, Novartis Pharma, Bayer Healthcare, Genzyme, Alexion Pharmaceuticals, Fresenius Medical Care, and Diamed, and has received financial research support from Euroimmun, Fresenius Medical Care, Diamed, Alexion Pharmaceuticals, and Novartis Pharma. Marcus Brand: Received honoraria for lecturing and travel expenses for attending meetings from Fresenius Medical Care, Alexion Pharmaceuticals, and Diamed. Marc Pawlitzki: Received speaker honoraria from Roche, Genzyme, and Novartis and travel/accommodation/meeting expenses from Novartis, Biogen Idec, Genzyme, and MERCK Serono Michael Heming: None. Heinz Wiendl: Received compensation for serving on the Scientific Advisory Boards/Steering Committees from Bayer, Biogen, Sanofi Genzyme, Merck Serono, and Novartis, honoraria for lecturing and travel reimbursements from Bayer, Biogen, CSL Behring, EMD Serono, Fresenius Medical Care, Sanofi Genzyme, Merck Serono, Omniamed, Novartis, and Sanofi Aventis. He received compensation as a consultant from Biogen Idec, Merck Serono, Novartis, Roche, and Sanofi Genzyme, and research support from Bayer, Biogen, Merck Serono, Novartis, Sanofi Genzyme, Sanofi US, Teva, and Novartis. Sven G. Meuth: Received honoraria for lecturing, and travel expenses for attending meetings from Almirall, Amicus Therapeutics Germany, Bayer Health Care, Biogen, Celgene, Diamed, Genzyme, MedDay Pharmaceuticals, Merck Serono, Novartis, Novo Nordisk, ONO Pharma, Roche, Sanofi-Aventis, Chugai Pharma, QuintilesIMS and Teva. His research was funded by the German Ministry for Education and Research (BMBF), Deutsche Forschungsgemeinschaft (DFG), Else Kröner Fresenius Foundation, German Academic Exchange Service, Hertie Foundation, Interdisciplinary Center for Clinical Studies (IZKF) Muenster, German Foundation Neurology and Almirall, Amicus Therapeutics Germany, Biogen, Diamed, Fresenius Medical Care, Genzyme, Merck Serono, Novartis, ONO Pharma, Roche, and Teva.

References

1. Kermode, A.G.; Thompson, A.J.; Tofts, P.; MacManus, D.G.; Kendall, B.E.; Kingsley, D.P.; Moseley, I.F.; Rudge, P.; McDonald, W.I. Breakdown of the blood-brain barrier precedes symptoms and other MRI signs of new lesions in multiple sclerosis. Pathogenetic and clinical implications. *Brain* **1990**, *113*, 1477–1489. [CrossRef] [PubMed]
2. Lucchinetti, C.; Bruck, W.; Parisi, J.; Scheithauer, B.; Rodriguez, M.; Lassmann, H. Heterogeneity of multiple sclerosis lesions: Implications for the pathogenesis of demyelination. *Ann. Neurol.* **2000**, *47*, 707–717. [CrossRef]
3. Weiner, H.L. Multiple sclerosis is an inflammatory T-cell-mediated autoimmune disease. *Arch. Neurol.* **2004**, *61*, 1613–1615. [CrossRef] [PubMed]
4. Esiri, M.M. Immunoglobulin-containing cells in multiple-sclerosis plaques. *Lancet* **1977**, *2*, 478. [CrossRef]
5. Monson, N.L.; Cravens, P.D.; Frohman, E.M.; Hawker, K.; Racke, M.K. Effect of rituximab on the peripheral blood and cerebrospinal fluid B cells in patients with primary progressive multiple sclerosis. *Arch. Neurol.* **2005**, *62*, 258–264. [CrossRef]
6. Baker, D.; Pryce, G.; Amor, S.; Giovannoni, G.; Schmierer, K. Learning from other autoimmunities to understand targeting of B cells to control multiple sclerosis. *Brain* **2018**, *141*, 2834–2847. [CrossRef]
7. Colombo, M.; Dono, M.; Gazzola, P.; Roncella, S.; Valetto, A.; Chiorazzi, N.; Mancardi, G.L.; Ferrarini, M. Accumulation of clonally related B lymphocytes in the cerebrospinal fluid of multiple sclerosis patients. *J. Immunol.* **2000**, *164*, 2782–2789. [CrossRef]
8. Constant, S.L. B lymphocytes as antigen-presenting cells for CD4+ T cell priming in vivo. *J. Immunol.* **1999**, *162*, 5695–5703.
9. Goodin, D.S.; Frohman, E.M.; Garmany, G.P.; Halper, J.; Likosky, W.H.; Lublin, F.D.; Silberberg, D.H.; Stuart, W.H.; van den Noort, S. Therapeutics and Technology Assessment Subcommittee of the American Academy of Neurology and the MS Council for Clinical Practice Guidelines. Disease modifying therapies in multiple sclerosis: Report of the Therapeutics and Technology Assessment Subcommittee of the American Academy of Neurology and the MS Council for Clinical Practice Guidelines. *Neurology* **2002**, *58*, 169–178.
10. Berkovich, R.R. Acute Multiple Sclerosis Relapse. *Continuum (Minneap. Minn.)* **2016**, *22*, 799–814. [CrossRef]
11. Beck, R.W. The Optic Neuritis Treatment Trial. *Arch. Ophthalmol.* **1988**, *106*, 1051–1053. [CrossRef] [PubMed]
12. Gold, R.; Buttgereit, F.; Toyka, K.V. Mechanism of action of glucocorticosteroid hormones: Possible implications for therapy of neuroimmunological disorders. *J. Neuroimmunol.* **2001**, *117*, 1–8. [CrossRef]
13. Schmidt, J.; Gold, R.; Schonrock, L.; Zettl, U.K.; Hartung, H.P.; Toyka, K.V. T-cell apoptosis in situ in experimental autoimmune encephalomyelitis following methylprednisolone pulse therapy. *Brain* **2000**, *123*, 1431–1441. [CrossRef] [PubMed]

14. Myhr, K.M.; Mellgren, S.I. Corticosteroids in the treatment of multiple sclerosis. *Acta Neurol. Scand.* **2009**, *120*, 73–80. [CrossRef]

15. Stoppe, M.; Busch, M.; Krizek, L.; Then Bergh, F. Outcome of MS relapses in the era of disease-modifying therapy. *BMC Neurol.* **2017**, *17*, 151. [CrossRef]

16. Szczepiorkowski, Z.M.; Winters, J.L.; Bandarenko, N.; Kim, H.C.; Linenberger, M.L.; Marques, M.B.; Sarode, R.; Schwartz, J.; Weinstein, R.; Shaz, B.H.; et al. Guidelines on the use of therapeutic apheresis in clinical practice—Evidence-based approach from the Apheresis Applications Committee of the American Society for Apheresis. *J. Clin. Apher.* **2010**, *25*, 83–177. [CrossRef]

17. Valbonesi, M.; Garelli, S.; Mosconi, L.; Zerbi, D.; Forlani, G. Plasma exchange in the management of patients with multiple sclerosis: Preliminary observations. *Vox Sang.* **1981**, *41*, 68–73. [CrossRef]

18. Oliveri, R.L.; Valentino, P.; Russo, C.; Sibilia, G.; Aguglia, U.; Bono, F.; Fera, F.; Gambardella, A.; Zappia, M.; Pardatscher, K.; et al. Randomized trial comparing two different high doses of methylprednisolone in MS: A clinical and MRI study. *Neurology* **1998**, *50*, 1833–1836. [CrossRef]

19. Schroder, A.; Linker, R.A.; Gold, R. Plasmapheresis for neurological disorders. *Expert Rev. Neurother.* **2009**, *9*, 1331–1339. [CrossRef]

20. Koziolek, M.J.; Kitze, B.; Muhlhausen, J.; Muller, G.A. Immunoadsorption in steroid-refractory multiple sclerosis. *Atheroscler. Suppl.* **2013**, *14*, 175–178. [CrossRef]

21. Palm, M.; Behm, E.; Schmitt, E.; Buddenhagen, F.; Hitzschke, B.; Kracht, M.; Kundt, G.; Meyer-Rienecker, H.; Klinkmann, H. Immunoadsorption and plasma exchange in multiple sclerosis: Complement and plasma protein behaviour. *Biomater. Artif. Cells Immobil. Biotechnol.* **1991**, *19*, 283–296. [CrossRef]

22. Gold, R.; Chan, A.; Flachenecker, P.; Haghikia, A.; Hellwig, K.; Kappos, L. *DGN/KKNMS Leitlinie zur Diagnose und Therapie der MS*; German Society of Neurology: Berlin, Germany, 2012.

23. Schwartz, J. Evidence-based guideline update: Plasmapheresis in neurologic disorders. *Neurology* **2011**, *77*, e105–e106. [PubMed]

24. Lublin, F.D.; Baier, M.; Cutter, G. Effect of relapses on development of residual deficit in multiple sclerosis. *Neurology* **2003**, *61*, 1528–1532. [CrossRef] [PubMed]

25. Koch-Henriksen, N.; Thygesen, L.C.; Sorensen, P.S.; Magyari, M. Worsening of disability caused by relapses in multiple sclerosis: A different approach. *Mult. Scler. Relat. Disord.* **2019**, *32*, 1–8. [CrossRef] [PubMed]

26. Moher, D.; Liberati, A.; Tetzlaff, J.; Altman, D.G.; Group, P. Preferred reporting items for systematic reviews and meta-analyses: The PRISMA statement. *PLoS Med.* **2009**, *6*, e1000097. [CrossRef]

27. McDonald, W.I.; Compston, A.; Edan, G.; Goodkin, D.; Hartung, H.P.; Lublin, F.D.; McFarland, H.F.; Paty, D.W.; Polman, C.H.; Reingold, S.C.; et al. Recommended diagnostic criteria for multiple sclerosis: Guidelines from the International Panel on the diagnosis of multiple sclerosis. *Ann. Neurol.* **2001**, *50*, 121–127. [CrossRef]

28. Thompson, A.J.; Banwell, B.L.; Barkhof, F.; Carroll, W.M.; Coetzee, T.; Comi, G.; Correale, J.; Fazekas, F.; Filippi, M.; Freedman, M.S.; et al. Diagnosis of multiple sclerosis: 2017 revisions of the McDonald criteria. *Lancet Neurol.* **2018**, *17*, 162–173. [CrossRef]

29. Polman, C.H.; Reingold, S.C.; Edan, G.; Filippi, M.; Hartung, H.P.; Kappos, L.; Lublin, F.D.; Metz, L.M.; McFarland, H.F.; O'Connor, P.W.; et al. Diagnostic criteria for multiple sclerosis: 2005 revisions to the "McDonald Criteria". *Ann. Neurol.* **2005**, *58*, 840–846. [CrossRef]

30. Poser, C.M.; Paty, D.W.; Scheinberg, L.; McDonald, W.I.; Davis, F.A.; Ebers, G.C.; Johnson, K.P.; Sibley, W.A.; Silberberg, D.H.; Tourtellotte, W.W. New diagnostic criteria for multiple sclerosis: Guidelines for research protocols. *Ann. Neurol.* **1983**, *13*, 227–231. [CrossRef]

31. Schwartz, J.; Padmanabhan, A.; Aqui, N.; Balogun, R.A.; Connelly-Smith, L.; Delaney, M.; Dunbar, N.M.; Witt, V.; Wu, Y.; Shaz, B.H. Guidelines on the Use of Therapeutic Apheresis in Clinical Practice-Evidence-Based Approach from the Writing Committee of the American Society for Apheresis: The Seventh Special Issue. *J. Clin. Apher.* **2016**, *31*, 149–162. [CrossRef]

32. Kurtzke, J.F. Rating neurologic impairment in multiple sclerosis: An expanded disability status scale (EDSS). *Neurology* **1983**, *33*, 1444–1452. [CrossRef] [PubMed]

33. Weinshenker, B.G.; O'Brien, P.C.; Petterson, T.M.; Noseworthy, J.H.; Lucchinetti, C.F.; Dodick, D.W.; Pineda, A.A.; Stevens, L.N.; Rodriguez, M. A randomized trial of plasma exchange in acute central nervous system inflammatory demyelinating disease. *Ann. Neurol.* **1999**, *46*, 878–886. [CrossRef]

34. Trebst, C.; Reising, A.; Kielstein, J.T.; Hafer, C.; Stangel, M. Plasma exchange therapy in steroid-unresponsive relapses in patients with multiple sclerosis. *Blood Purif.* **2009**, *28*, 108–115. [CrossRef] [PubMed]

35. Schilling, S.; Linker, R.A.; Konig, F.B.; Koziolek, M.; Bahr, M.; Muller, G.A.; Paulus, W.; Gartner, J.; Bruck, W.; Chan, A.; et al. Plasma exchange therapy for steroid-unresponsive multiple sclerosis relapses: Clinical experience with 16 patients. *Nervenarzt* **2006**, *77*, 430–438. [CrossRef] [PubMed]

36. Habek, M.; Barun, B.; Puretic, Z.; Brinar, V.V. Treatment of steroid unresponsive relapse with plasma exchange in aggressive multiple sclerosis. *Ther. Apher. Dial.* **2010**, *14*, 298–302. [CrossRef]

37. Brunot, S.; Vukusic, S.; Fromont, A.; Couvreur, G.; Mousson, C.; Giroud, M.; Confavreux, C.; Moreau, T. Plasma exchanges in severe and acute inflammatory demyelinating attacks of the central nervous system. *Press. Med.* **2011**, *40*, e271–e278. [CrossRef]

38. Ehler, J.; Koball, S.; Sauer, M.; Hickstein, H.; Mitzner, S.; Benecke, R.; Zettl, U.K. Therapeutic plasma exchange in glucocorticosteroid-unresponsive patients with Clinically Isolated Syndrome. *Ther. Apher. Dial.* **2014**, *18*, 489–496. [CrossRef]

39. Llufriu, S.; Castillo, J.; Blanco, Y.; Ramio-Torrenta, L.; Rio, J.; Valles, M.; Lozano, M.; Castella, M.D.; Calabia, J.; Horga, A.; et al. Plasma exchange for acute attacks of CNS demyelination: Predictors of improvement at 6 months. *Neurology* **2009**, *73*, 949–953. [CrossRef]

40. Keegan, M.; Konig, F.; McClelland, R.; Bruck, W.; Morales, Y.; Bitsch, A.; Panitch, H.; Lassmann, H.; Weinshenker, B.; Rodriguez, M.; et al. Relation between humoral pathological changes in multiple sclerosis and response to therapeutic plasma exchange. *Lancet* **2005**, *366*, 579–582. [CrossRef]

41. Magana, S.M.; Keegan, B.M.; Weinshenker, B.G.; Erickson, B.J.; Pittock, S.J.; Lennon, V.A.; Rodriguez, M.; Thomsen, K.; Weigand, S.; Mandrekar, J.; et al. Beneficial plasma exchange response in central nervous system inflammatory demyelination. *Arch. Neurol.* **2011**, *68*, 870–878. [CrossRef]

42. Lammerding, L.; Pfeuffer, S.; Bormann, E.; Sauerland, C.; Ruck, T.; Brand, M.; Schilling, M.; Kleinschnitz, C.; Wiendl, H.; Meuth, S.G. Comparison of high-dose intravenous corticosteroids and therapeutic plasma exchange in acute relapsing multiple sclerosis. *Mult. Scler. J.* **2018**, *24* (Suppl. S2), 121–327. [CrossRef]

43. Trebst, C.; Bronzlik, P.; Kielstein, J.T.; Schmidt, B.M.; Stangel, M. Immunoadsorption therapy for steroid-unresponsive relapses in patients with multiple sclerosis. *Blood Purif.* **2012**, *33*, 1–6. [CrossRef] [PubMed]

44. Schimrigk, S.; Adibi, I.; Eberl, A.; Selka, I.; Galle, J.; Schmidt, S.; Fritz, H.G.; Fassbender, C.; Klingel, R.; Füchtemann, D.; et al. Immunadsorption zur Eskalation der Schubtherapie bei Multipler Sklerose. *Akt. Neurol.* **2012**, *39*, 174–179. [CrossRef]

45. Schimrigk, S.; Faiss, J.; Kohler, W.; Gunther, A.; Harms, L.; Kraft, A.; Ehrlich, S.; Eberl, A.; Fassbender, C.; Klingel, R.; et al. Escalation Therapy of Steroid Refractory Multiple Sclerosis Relapse with Tryptophan Immunoadsorption—Observational Multicenter Study with 147 Patients. *Eur. Neurol.* **2016**, *75*, 300–306. [CrossRef]

46. Koziolek, M.J.; Tampe, D.; Bahr, M.; Dihazi, H.; Jung, K.; Fitzner, D.; Klingel, R.; Muller, G.A.; Kitze, B. Immunoadsorption therapy in patients with multiple sclerosis with steroid-refractory optical neuritis. *J. Neuroinflamm.* **2012**, *9*, 80. [CrossRef]

47. Mauch, E.; Zwanzger, J.; Hettich, R.; Fassbender, C.; Klingel, R.; Heigl, F. Immunoadsorption for steroid-unresponsive multiple sclerosis-relapses: Clinical data of 14 patients. *Nervenarzt* **2011**, *82*, 1590–1595. [CrossRef]

48. Conway, B.L.; Zeydan, B.; Uygunoglu, U.; Novotna, M.; Siva, A.; Pittock, S.J.; Atkinson, E.J.; Rodriguez, M.; Kantarci, O.H. Age is a critical determinant in recovery from multiple sclerosis relapses. *Mult. Scler.* **2018**, 1352458518800815. [CrossRef]

49. Heigl, F.; Hettich, R.; Arendt, R.; Durner, J.; Koehler, J.; Mauch, E. Immunoadsorption in steroid-refractory multiple sclerosis: Clinical experience in 60 patients. *Atheroscler. Suppl.* **2013**, *14*, 167–173. [CrossRef]

50. Sanchez, A.P.; Cunard, R.; Ward, D.M. The selective therapeutic apheresis procedures. *J. Clin. Apher.* **2013**, *28*, 20–29. [CrossRef]

51. Braun, N. *Fundamentals and Applications of Immunoadsorption*; Uni-Med Science: Bremen, Germany, 2009; Volume 2, p. 103.

52. Ohkubo, A.; Okado, T.; Sakurasawa, T.; Maeda, T.; Itagaki, A.; Yamamoto, H.; Miyamoto, S.; Seshima, H.; Kurashima, N.; Mori, T.; et al. Removal Characteristics of Immunoadsorption with the Tryptophan-Immobilized Column Using Conventional and Selective Plasma Separators in the Treatment of Myasthenia Gravis. *Ther. Apher. Dial.* **2019**, *23*, 271–278. [CrossRef]
53. Belak, M.; Borberg, H.; Jimenez, C.; Oette, K. Technical and clinical experience with protein A immunoadsorption columns. *Transfus. Sci.* **1994**, *15*, 419–422. [CrossRef]
54. Muhlhausen, J.; Kitze, B.; Huppke, P.; Muller, G.A.; Koziolek, M.J. Apheresis in treatment of acute inflammatory demyelinating disorders. *Atheroscler. Suppl.* **2015**, *18*, 251–256. [CrossRef] [PubMed]
55. Meyer-Moock, S.; Feng, Y.S.; Maeurer, M.; Dippel, F.W.; Kohlmann, T. Systematic literature review and validity evaluation of the Expanded Disability Status Scale (EDSS) and the Multiple Sclerosis Functional Composite (MSFC) in patients with multiple sclerosis. *BMC Neurol.* **2014**, *14*, 58. [CrossRef] [PubMed]
56. Loschiavo, C.; Greco, M.; Polo, A.; Del Colle, R. The use of therapeutic apheresis in neurological diseases and comparison between plasma exchange and immunoadsorption. *G. Ital. Nefrol.* **2015**, *32*.
57. Kohler, W.; Bucka, C.; Klingel, R. A randomized and controlled study comparing immunoadsorption and plasma exchange in myasthenic crisis. *J. Clin. Apher.* **2011**, *26*, 347–355. [CrossRef]
58. Somnier, F.E.; Langvad, E. Plasma exchange with selective immunoadsorption of anti-acetylcholine receptor antibodies. *J. Neuroimmunol.* **1989**, *22*, 123–127. [CrossRef]
59. Kuerten, S.; Pauly, R.; Blaschke, S.; Rottlaender, A.; Kaiser, C.C.; Schroeter, M.; Fink, G.R.; Addicks, K. The significance of a B cell-dependent immunopathology in multiple sclerosis. *Fortschr. Neurol. Psychiatr.* **2011**, *79*, 83–91. [CrossRef]
60. Wilson, H.L. B cells contribute to MS pathogenesis through antibody-dependent and antibody-independent mechanisms. *Biologics* **2012**, *6*, 117–123. [CrossRef]
61. Keegan, M.; Pineda, A.A.; McClelland, R.L.; Darby, C.H.; Rodriguez, M.; Weinshenker, B.G. Plasma exchange for severe attacks of CNS demyelination: Predictors of response. *Neurology* **2002**, *58*, 143–146. [CrossRef]
62. Ehler, J.; Koball, S.; Sauer, M.; Mitzner, S.; Hickstein, H.; Benecke, R.; Zettl, U.K. Response to Therapeutic Plasma Exchange as a Rescue Treatment in Clinically Isolated Syndromes and Acute Worsening of Multiple Sclerosis: A Retrospective Analysis of 90 Patients. *PLoS ONE* **2015**, *10*, e0134583. [CrossRef]
63. Leone, M.A.; Bonissoni, S.; Collimedaglia, L.; Tesser, F.; Calzoni, S.; Stecco, A.; Naldi, P.; Monaco, F. Factors predicting incomplete recovery from relapses in multiple sclerosis: A prospective study. *Mult. Scler.* **2008**, *14*, 485–493. [CrossRef] [PubMed]
64. Kalincik, T. Multiple Sclerosis Relapses: Epidemiology, Outcomes and Management. A Systematic Review. *Neuroepidemiology* **2015**, *44*, 199–214. [CrossRef] [PubMed]
65. Riise, T.; Gronning, M.; Fernandez, O.; Lauer, K.; Midgard, R.; Minderhoud, J.M.; Nyland, H.; Palffy, G.; Poser, S.; Aarli, J.A. Early prognostic factors for disability in multiple sclerosis, a European multicenter study. *Acta Neurol. Scand.* **1992**, *85*, 212–218. [CrossRef] [PubMed]
66. Cortese, I.; Chaudhry, V.; So, Y.T.; Cantor, F.; Cornblath, D.R.; Rae-Grant, A. Evidence-based guideline update: Plasmapheresis in neurologic disorders: Report of the Therapeutics and Technology Assessment Subcommittee of the American Academy of Neurology. *Neurology* **2011**, *76*, 294–300. [CrossRef]
67. Kaplan, A.A. Therapeutic plasma exchange: A technical and operational review. *J. Clin. Apher.* **2013**, *28*, 3–10. [CrossRef]
68. Hohenstein, B.; Passauer, J.; Ziemssen, T.; Julius, U. Immunoadsorption with regenerating systems in neurological disorders—A single center experience. *Atheroscler. Suppl.* **2015**, *18*, 119–123. [CrossRef]
69. Charlton, B.; Schindhelm, K.; Farrell, P.C. Effect of extracorporeal IgG removal on IgG kinetics. *Trans. Am. Soc. Artif. Intern. Organs* **1983**, *29*, 724–729.
70. Orlin, J.B.; Berkman, E.M. Partial plasma exchange using albumin replacement: Removal and recovery of normal plasma constituents. *Blood* **1980**, *56*, 1055–1059. [CrossRef]
71. Tholking, G.; Mesters, R.; Dittrich, R.; Pavenstadt, H.; Kumpers, P.; Reuter, S. Assessment of Hemostasis after Plasma Exchange Using Rotational Thrombelastometry (ROTEM). *PLoS ONE* **2015**, *10*, e0130402. [CrossRef]
72. Pohl, D.; Waubant, E.; Banwell, B.; Chabas, D.; Chitnis, T.; Weinstock-Guttman, B.; Tenembaum, S.; International Pediatric, M.S.S.G. Treatment of pediatric multiple sclerosis and variants. *Neurology* **2007**, *68*, S54–S65. [CrossRef]
73. Goldstein, S.L. Therapeutic apheresis in children: Special considerations. *Semin. Dial.* **2012**, *25*, 165–170. [CrossRef] [PubMed]

74. Hellwig, K.; Haghikia, A.; Rockhoff, M.; Gold, R. Multiple sclerosis and pregnancy: Experience from a nationwide database in Germany. *Ther. Adv. Neurol. Disord.* **2012**, *5*, 247–253. [CrossRef] [PubMed]

75. Hoffmann, F.; Kraft, A.; Heigl, F.; Mauch, E.; Koehler, J.; Harms, L.; Kumpfel, T.; Kohler, W.; Ehrlich, S.; Bayas, A.; et al. Tryptophan immunoadsorption during pregnancy and breastfeeding in patients with acute relapse of multiple sclerosis and neuromyelitis optica. *Ther. Adv. Neurol. Disord.* **2018**, *11*, 1756286418774973. [CrossRef] [PubMed]

76. Park-Wyllie, L.; Mazzotta, P.; Pastuszak, A.; Moretti, M.E.; Beique, L.; Hunnisett, L.; Friesen, M.H.; Jacobson, S.; Kasapinovic, S.; Chang, D.; et al. Birth defects after maternal exposure to corticosteroids: Prospective cohort study and meta-analysis of epidemiological studies. *Teratology* **2000**, *62*, 385–392. [CrossRef]

77. Gur, C.; Diav-Citrin, O.; Shechtman, S.; Arnon, J.; Ornoy, A. Pregnancy outcome after first trimester exposure to corticosteroids: A prospective controlled study. *Reprod. Toxicol.* **2004**, *18*, 93–101. [CrossRef]

78. Multiple Sclerosis Therapy Consensus, G.; Wiendl, H.; Toyka, K.V.; Rieckmann, P.; Gold, R.; Hartung, H.P.; Hohlfeld, R. Basic and escalating immunomodulatory treatments in multiple sclerosis: Current therapeutic recommendations. *J. Neurol.* **2008**, *255*, 1449–1463. [CrossRef]

79. Koziolek, M.; Muhlhausen, J.; Friede, T.; Ellenberger, D.; Sigler, M.; Huppke, B.; Gartner, J.; Muller, G.A.; Huppke, P. Therapeutic apheresis in pediatric patients with acute CNS inflammatory demyelinating disease. *Blood Purif.* **2013**, *36*, 92–97. [CrossRef]

80. Bigi, S.; Banwell, B.; Yeh, E.A. Outcomes after early administration of plasma exchange in pediatric central nervous system inflammatory demyelination. *J. Child. Neurol.* **2015**, *30*, 874–880. [CrossRef]

81. De Silvestro, G.; Tison, T.; Vicarioto, M.; Bagatella, P.; Stefanutti, C.; Marson, P. The Italian Registry of Pediatric Therapeutic Apheresis: A report on activity during 2005. *J. Clin. Apher.* **2009**, *24*, 1–5. [CrossRef]

82. Michon, B.; Moghrabi, A.; Winikoff, R.; Barrette, S.; Bernstein, M.L.; Champagne, J.; David, M.; Duval, M.; Hume, H.A.; Robitaille, N.; et al. Complications of apheresis in children. *Transfusion* **2007**, *47*, 1837–1842. [CrossRef]

83. Rubio Tabares, J.; Amaya Gonzalez, P.F. Plasma exchange therapy for a severe relapse of Devic's disease in a pregnant woman: A case report and concise review. *Clin. Neurol. Neurosurg.* **2016**, *148*, 88–90. [CrossRef] [PubMed]

84. Cox, J.L.; Koepsell, S.A.; Shunkwiler, S.M. Therapeutic plasma exchange and pregnancy: A case report and guidelines for performing plasma exchange in a pregnant patient. *J. Clin. Apher.* **2017**, *32*, 191–195. [CrossRef] [PubMed]

85. Gold, S.M.; Voskuhl, R.R. Pregnancy and multiple sclerosis: From molecular mechanisms to clinical application. *Semin. Immunopathol.* **2016**, *38*, 709–718. [CrossRef] [PubMed]

86. Hewitt, P.E.; Ijaz, S.; Brailsford, S.R.; Brett, R.; Dicks, S.; Haywood, B.; Kennedy, I.T.; Kitchen, A.; Patel, P.; Poh, J.; et al. Hepatitis E virus in blood components: A prevalence and transmission study in southeast England. *Lancet* **2014**, *384*, 1766–1773. [CrossRef]

87. Koessler, J.; Kobsar, A.; Kuhn, S.; Koessler, A.; Yilmaz, P.; Weinig, E.; Putz, E.; Boeck, M.; Klinker, E. The effect of immunoadsorption with the Immusorba TR-350 column on coagulation compared to plasma exchange. *Vox Sang.* **2015**, *108*, 46–51. [CrossRef]

88. Marson, P.; Gervasi, M.T.; Tison, T.; Colpo, A.; De Silvestro, G. Therapeutic apheresis in pregnancy: General considerations and current practice. *Transfus. Apher. Sci.* **2015**, *53*, 256–261. [CrossRef]

89. Scott, T.F.; Schramke, C.J. Poor recovery after the first two attacks of multiple sclerosis is associated with poor outcome five years later. *J. Neurol. Sci.* **2010**. [CrossRef]

90. Binquet, C.; Quantin, C.; Le Teuff, G.; Pagliano, J.F.; Abrahamowicz, M.; Moreau, T. The prognostic value of initial relapses on the evolution of disability in patients with relapsing-remitting multiple sclerosis. *Neuroepidemiology* **2006**, *27*, 45–54. [CrossRef]

91. Lavery, A.M.; Verhey, L.H.; Waldman, A.T. Outcome measures in relapsing-remitting multiple sclerosis: Capturing disability and disease progression in clinical trials. *Mult. Scler. Int.* **2014**, *2014*, 262350. [CrossRef]

MDPI

St. Alban-Anlage 66

4052 Basel

Switzerland

Tel. +41 61 683 77 34

Fax +41 61 302 89 18

www.mdpi.com

Journal of Clinical Medicine Editorial Office

E-mail: jcm@mdpi.com

www.mdpi.com/journal/jcm

Ingram Content Group UK Ltd.
Milton Keynes UK
UKHW050627060623
422904UK00004B/200